ANTIDEPRESSANTS, ANTIPSYCHOTICS, AND STIMULANTS

DANGEROUS DRUGS ON TRIAL

The Soaring Heights Series

By Dr. David W. Tanton, Ph.D.

DISCLAIMER:

Every effort has been made by the author to ensure that the information in this book is as complete and accurate as possible, although the author cannot, and does not render judgment or advice regarding a particular individual. As our bodies are each unique, we will not always experience the same results that another might from the very same therapy.

The author believes in both prevention and the superiority of a natural non-invasive approach over drugs and surgery.

The information herein is presented by an independent research scientist, whose sources of information include 45 years of his own personal experience, along with researching the world's medical and scientific literature, patient records, and other clinical and anecdotal reports for decades.

The leading cause of death and disability today appears to be the lack of awareness of natural therapies, by both doctors and their patients, known to prevent and treat many common degenerative diseases. This book is dedicated to making as many as possible aware that they no longer need to suffer and die needlessly from diseases that may already have cures. Unfortunately, the general public is seldom aware of many valuable resources available for preventing or effectively eliminating serious health conditions, as they are often suppressed due to their lack of profitability.

Those who read this book and make decisions regarding their health or medical care based on ideas contained in this book, do so as their constitutional right. Please do not use this book if you are unwilling to assume responsibility for results that arise from the use of any of the suggestions, preparations or procedures in the book. The author and publisher are not responsible for any adverse effects or consequences resulting from the use of any of the suggestions or information contained in the book, but offer this material as information that the public has a right to hear and utilize at their own discretion.

Published by *Soaring Heights Publishing* 2007

Library of Congress Control Number: 2007903866
ISBN: 978-0-9772703-2-3
SAN: 257-1641

Printed in the United States by Morris Publishing
3212 East Highway 30
Kearney, NE 68847
1-800-650-7888

Additional copies of this book can be ordered at http://www.drtanton.com.

For single book purchases, send check or money order for $24.95 to:
Soaring Heights Publishing
PO Box 2138
Jasper, OR 97438

For wholesale prices or quantity purchases:
Email: books@drtanton.com
Or Call: (541) 726-5959

TABLE OF CONTENTS

INTRODUCTION

Although I will be playing the part of the prosecutor throughout this book, I will also be defending every vulnerable person from what I consider to be, one of the most serious threats we are currently facing in the nation today - a very dangerous class of mind-altering drugs. Possibly the most immediate concern is the very aggressive, well-orchestrated campaign called TeenScreen, which was recently established in order to promote the placing of as many of our children as possible on several very profitable, although (as you will soon learn), extremely dangerous drugs. You, in turn, will be in a unique position as not only a member of the jury, but possibly even a defendant as well. It basically depends on whether either you or your children are currently one of those at risk. Just get out your pen and notepad, as you're about to encounter a ton of damaging evidence. From years of research, I have come well prepared, so we'll just let the undeniable evidence speak for itself.

What you are about to learn is likely obvious from the title: *Antidepressants, Antipsychotics, and Stimulants – Dangerous Drugs on Trial.* Our focus will basically be on these three classes of drugs that so many in the nation are unnecessarily taking. Although Prozac™ was the first Selective Serotonin Reuptake Inhibitor (SSRI) antidepressant produced, and thus the best known, there are now many others on the market, such as Paxil™, Zoloft™, and Celexa™, that can at times pose an even greater risk. For the sake of convenience, in some cases I may just refer to Prozac™. The same also applies to the stimulant drug Ritalin™, as there are also newer versions of that same basic drug as well. And we now have an additional class of drugs known as atypical antipsychotics, which are being aggressively promoted as well. It has become an extremely profitable business, and has absolutely nothing to do with mental health, but instead actually threatening our mental health.

You will soon discover that these drugs not only pose a "serious threat" to both you, and your children, but in some cases, the developing fetus as well! Possibly the very best news is, **you basically don't need them,** and there are "much better" drug-free solutions, proven more effective!

You will soon learn many important things that even most doctors are totally unaware of. For example, **you will learn exactly how Prozac™ contributes to diabetes, obesity, cancer, and even "brain damage", and in more than one way.** It's also a major thyroid suppressant, lowering the metabolism, which potentially contributes to as many as 47 different conditions (including depression). You will then find that just one 30 mg dose of Prozac™ actually increases the stress hormone cortisol by an amazing 200%! And of particular concern, is that elevated cortisol actually damages the area in the brain where hormones are regulated, and "long term memories are stored". Not only that, but it also causes elevated blood sugar and insulin, (and does so on a daily basis), which as we're aware is the primary cause of type II diabetes, (one of Prozac's side effects).

Possibly worst of all is, **every single molecule of Prozac™ actually contains three molecules of the highly toxic fluoride,** (a major concern). Fluoride is considered by scientists as an environmental toxin, and is known to damage the DNA, (it's a cancer risk). Study after study, dating as far back as 1854, has proven beyond a doubt, that fluoride is an iodine antagonist, which disrupts iodine receptors in both the body and brain, suppressing the thyroid and lowering the metabolism. In fact, in 1950, there was a broad study, which included "300 references" detailing the known biochemical findings associated with fluoride, which basically goes to show that there were many people concerned about the serious problems that fluoride posed. You will learn that even low doses of fluoride in the drinking water were found to lower children's IQs, and greatly increase the rate of children acquiring cancer.

Most importantly, you will learn exactly how these drugs can create tremendous damage to both the body and brain, in everyone from fetuses to seniors. And you will find that I always provide adequate scientific proof to substantiate my claims. Then as usual, I never identify a problem without, in turn, providing a solution. You will likely be quite amazed at how many different options are available for you to choose from, and how simple and inexpensive they can be. Absolutely no one needs these dangerous mind-altering drugs that contribute to major disease, and reduce your mental capacity!

As the drugs we will be addressing pose such a "serious threat" to anyone taking them, and the fact that they are now being "aggressively marketed" to our children, you will find that throughout this book, I deliberately provide multiple findings by credible sources to back up all my claims. Also, in order to better emphasize important issues pertinent to the subjects I will be discussing, the bold print or underlining in quotes throughout this book, may at times be mine, although the text will remain unchanged. Once you learn the facts, I believe that you will be as amazed as I am, that they are not only still legal, but even encouraged for pregnant mothers, and young children's use! You will soon discover that they are "far more dangerous" than some drugs already removed from the market, due to their known risks. I believe that anyone who takes the time to read this book, and seriously consider the well-documented facts presented, will be totally amazed that companies are allowed to continue marketing them.

Other than the companies producing these drugs, very few (including most doctors) are fully aware of the serious conditions (both physical and mental) that these drugs can contribute to. Most importantly, there are many drug-free solutions proven to be "more effective". There is, in my opinion, no valid excuse for a doctor to prescribe any of them. We find that the well-known and highly respected **Dr. Julian Whitaker, M.D. claims that, with the 40,000 patients treated in his clinic in Los Angeles, California, over the years, never once has he found it necessary to prescribe an antidepressant to anyone!** In my opinion, there is no valid reason whatsoever, for any doctor to prescribe antidepressants, (irrespective of his or her specialty).

We must keep in mind that we are all unique, often referred to as our bio-individuality. At least partly due to genetics, or possibly how we were raised, we all have different personalities, (something we can at least partially influence). Some of us are naturally extroverts, while others tend to be introverts. The problem is, even being timid is now considered a mental condition, which drugs can now be prescribed for! Some of the brightest children are often not adequately challenged, thus labeled as having ADHD, and drugged into submission just because they are more active. These drugs tend to remove emotions, change personalities, and in the case of children, attempt to force them into a "convenient" mold so they will be easier to manage. Unfortunately, they are also creating major diseases in our children in the process; diseases that were, until recently, considered as adult diseases.

Due to our bio-individuality and our dietary habits, as well as any foods or additives we might be allergic to, our solutions will not always be the same. The important issue is, there are "always" drug-free solutions, and in my opinion, absolutely no one needs to resort to the use of drugs for any physical or mental condition. In the majority of cases, just a simple diet modification, combined with appropriate nutritional supplements, is normally adequate to resolve depression and change behavior. In several studies, just a dietary change was found to be effective in improving both children's behavior and grades.

I have attempted to cover all the bases, so absolutely no one would be left out. Thus, we will also be addressing some less common conditions as well. If you prefer, you can just skip those that possibly don't apply to you, or a loved one. Although, if you're like me, and inclined to be curious, you can always read the book in its entirely.

Never forget that, although some drugs are legal, they are still potent, and can potentially create several serious physical and mental conditions. Also keep in mind that cocaine, heroin, and LSD, were once legal, and produced by the very same companies that are now producing the "legal drugs" currently being aggressively promoted, (even to pregnant mothers and very young children). Not only that, but they were also approved as safe by the FDA. And most importantly, they are seldom, (if ever), necessary! The importance of truly resolving the underlying condition, rather than just suppressing symptoms, is a major issue that can't be overemphasized. Otherwise, a lifetime of symptom-causing nutrient-depleting drugs is necessary. Then, the more drugs you are on, and the longer you remain on them, the worse your health will become.

The good news is that we have more than enough natural options to choose from. Although it is important to note that, as we are all unique (our bio-individuality), we won't all experience the same results on the very same regimen. The supplements and dosages that are the most effective can at times vary between individuals, although I will normally provide you with the typical recommended dosage. A prime example is regarding vitamin C. Following surgery, or when we have a virus such as a cold or the flu, we might need up to ten times as much vitamin C as we normally would. And we can't forget that our diet, the condition of our liver, our metabolism, and especially any medications we might be taking, all come into play as well.

Although some of the information in this book might possibly seem a little overwhelming to some, it's important for validation purposes, that I support my claims with sufficient well-substantiated facts that would hopefully convince any skeptics who might possibly be of the opinion that drugs are the only solution. Just keep in mind that my objective is to present the facts in as simple unscientific terms as possible. You would likely find it nearly impossible to decipher some of the scientific papers that I sometimes come across. In my opinion, that same information could be quite easily explained in much simpler terminology, that you could easily understand, and that will be my objective.

I would guess that if anything in my book might appear at all difficult to follow, it would likely not be due to the terminology, but instead the inherent complexity of some issues and the many variables sometimes involved. If so, I would suggest that you take your time, and just re-read parts of the text if necessary. For instance, as vitamins and minerals have so many different benefits, and are often co-dependent (do not work independently), both an adequate supply, as well as the proper balance of each, can at times be critical. You will learn that all drugs, be they legal or illegal, are basically inorganic chemicals (foreign to the body), and have been proven to deplete many critical nutrients. Thus, depending on them makes it nearly impossible to maintain adequate levels (or proper balance) of any nutrient. We cannot expect to force our body (against its will), with <u>in</u>organic chemicals, and somehow expect to experience positive results – it just won't happen! We must learn to trust in Our Creator, and our body's innate intelligence. All we have to do is provide the necessary nutrients, allowing our body to manage the details, (something it is very efficient at).

Your life-changing adventure is about to begin, and I guarantee you, your time will be well spent, so why don't we get started?

CHAPTER ONE

The Primary Reason For This Book:
The Aggressive Marketing Of Psychiatric Drugs That Are Contributing To Disease Backed By Our Government, Forced On Our Children!

Although it was the current, very aggressive, promotion of the potentially dangerous drugs to our children that prompted me to write this book, I soon realized that millions of adults have already been taking them for years. That especially applies to the SSRI antidepressants, although recently, many more adults have begun taking Ritalin™ as well. It's basically a legal stimulant, very similar to cocaine, just in a milder form. Unfortunately, it greatly increases the risk of eventually graduating to more serious drugs, such as cocaine. And not only do antidepressants contribute to the development of diabetes, cancer, and obesity in children, but adults also experience the very same problems, although with adults it's much easier to place the blame elsewhere.

The problem originates with the powerful and very profitable pharmaceutical companies, who are constantly looking for the most effective ways to market their drugs. Although in the past, children seldom had the many different conditions that adults are normally prescribed medications for, it appears that drug companies have now come up with a new plan to change all that, (and on a large scale). They have been very busy behind the scenes working with the American Psychiatric Association (APA), creating hundreds of different mental conditions that any doctor or psychiatrist, could now use to justify placing our children on one or more of their very profitable psychiatric drugs on.

At last count, it was 374 different mental conditions! I'd say that psychiatrists have to be "extremely creative" to come up with that many different mental conditions. Just about anyone who was having a bad day, or any child who possibly ate too much sugar for breakfast, would likely qualify for at least one label. Just one brief evaluation is normally all it takes to justify placing a child on Ritalin™ or an antidepressant such as Prozac™.

Getting legislation drafted and approved is surprisingly easy when you collectively, (via PhRMA), have more lobbyists than senators and congressmen combined. Some lobbyists are either prior legislators, or legislative aids, who already have connections in Washington, and can thus be very persuasive. You will soon learn about their tremendous clout, in order to get the recent legislation passed, mandating that all our school children should now receive a psychiatric exam, (beginning in preschool). It's hard to imagine getting legislation that ridiculous passed, especially if you consider the expense involved. Psychiatrists' time for the evaluation doesn't come cheap; nor does the cost of years of very expensive psychiatric drugs that would eventually follow. Unfortunately, as you will soon discover, that's just the beginning, as drugs such as Ritalin™ and Prozac™ can contribute to cancer, diabetes, or heart disease, and thus more drugs would soon follow.

Millions of children have already been placed on stimulating, mind-altering drugs such as Prozac™ and Ritalin™, (very similar in action to cocaine). Now, with the recently passed legislation, that number is rapidly escalating, and can be expected to skyrocket in the very near future, unless we intervene. We absolutely must put a stop to the madness before more children's lives are unnecessarily sacrificed! It's interesting that we continually hear on the news how many children are beginning to experience adult diseases such as diabetes and cancer, as well as obesity. Other than their diet, they can't seem to find a plausible explanation, (although I can), and you soon will discover that **"the primary contributor is surprisingly not their diet."** I'm not saying that their diet is not a contributing factor, as it obviously is; it's just not the basic culprit. Our children have been eating junk food for decades, and a lot of unhealthy and totally inappropriate foods are still being served in the school cafeterias, (which obviously should stop). Although this is definitely an area that must be addressed in the future, as strange as it might seem, it's not actually the primary concern.

And we can't forget that millions of adults have been, and are continuing to be, placed on these very same potentially dangerous antidepressants. And more often than not, they are left on them for years, (and even decades), as doctors seldom recommend their withdrawal. Few doctors are familiar enough with using nutrition to help prevent the potentially serious reactions patients can at times experience from withdrawal, (especially after years of use). Most doctors are unfamiliar with even the basics of nutrition, or disease prevention, which obviously should be every doctor's primary objective. They are rather like an army of soldiers, armed with ammunition that often misfires, and can at times be outright dangerous. Unfortunately, a lot of talent is being totally wasted, as most traditionally trained medical doctors have been hijacked in medical school by the pharmaceutical industry. It's amazing how many mental conditions the "experts" have recently concocted, and how they managed to turn doctors into their legal drug pushers, with their patients paying the ultimate price with their health, (and at times even their life)! Following is just one more example of yet another mental condition, that a well-connected psychiatrist apparently dreamt up, in which he suggested that an SSRI antidepressant (such as Prozac™) should, in his opinion, help resolve.

The Latest New Mental Disorder! Is It Really Science, or Just Science Fiction? – You Decide!

It seems like psychiatrists must stay awake nights, dreaming up new mental disorders. At last count, to the best of my knowledge, it was 374, although now it's likely 375! My guess is, with that many mental conditions, the majority of the population would likely qualify for at least one, even on a normal day. And we now have a new mental condition called **Intermittent Explosive Disorder (IED)** - what in the world will they come up with next?

The following was reported by the Associated Press in *The Washington Post* (June 6, 2006):

"Road Rage" Gets A Medical Diagnosis

"Intermittent Explosive Disorder" Affects Millions In The U.S., Survey Finds

To you, that angry, horn-blasting tailgater is suffering from road rage. But doctors have another name for it – intermittent explosive disorder *– and a new study suggests it is far more common than they realized,* ***affecting up to 16 million Americans*.** **[That should open a whole new market of millions that can now be drugged into submission!]**

"People think it's bad behavior and that you just need an attitude adjustment, but what they don't know…is that there's a biology and cognitive science to this," said Dr. Emil Coccaro, chairman of psychiatry at the University of Chicago's medical school.

By definition, intermittent explosive disorder involves multiple outbursts that are way out of proportion to the situation. These angry outbursts often include threats or aggressive actions and property damage.

For a couple of decades, intermittent explosive disorder, or IED, has been included in the manual psychiatrists use to diagnose mental illness, *though with slightly different names and criteria. That has contributed to misunderstanding and **underappreciation of the disorder**, said Coccaro, a study co-author.*

Coccaro said the disorder involves inadequate production or functioning of serotonin, a mood-regulating and behavior-inhibiting brain chemical. ***Treatment with antidepressants, including those that target serotonin receptors in the brain, is often helpful,*** *along with behavior therapy akin to anger management, Coccaro said.*

The study was funded by the National Institute of Mental Health.

The findings were released Monday in the June issue of the Archives of General Psychiatry (http://www.msnbc.msn.com/id/13152708/).

To me, it appears that a great deal of creativity, along with a considerable amount of financial incentive, would likely be necessary to "create" that many mental conditions. Then to justify every single one, and to convince anyone that it is actually based on true science, would in my opinion be the greatest challenge of all. Incidentally, you will later discover what Dr. Coccaro's motivation really was, as he was actually paid by more than one of the pharmaceutical companies who just happened to be producing the SSRI antidepressants he was promoting.

With the latest and greatest new discovery, many people would no longer be held accountable for their actions, if it was somehow deemed the result of an uncontrollable temper (IED). Could you imagine what all the defense attorneys could do with this one? **It's now a "proven scientific fact" that IED is considered an uncontrollable mental condition.** You can rest assured that most criminals would have suddenly lost their "uncontrollable temper," or they obviously wouldn't commit such violent crimes.

It appears that we now have a perfect plan to begin emptying our prisons. Soon, people would not even be held responsible for their own actions, as **the uncontrolled rage, or urge, would be either due to an untreated mental condition, or the result of the medication for treating the condition!** That would also reduce the demand for criminal attorneys. As a result, they might be required to change specialties, (divorce attorneys are always in demand). And finally, we can't forget that some people seem to have a sudden urge to steal. I'm not sure if that's one they somehow overlooked, or possibly that has already been diagnosed as kleptomania. Although at this point anyway, I believe people are still being prosecuted for stealing, (at least the executives with Enron recently were).

I can already see one condition they might have somehow overlooked. I hate to mention it, because some psychiatrist might pick up on it and add it to the extensive list, although it actually makes just as much sense. It might possibly be labeled Uncontrollable Sexual Urge ("USU"), although it might possibly be confused as being an abbreviation for some University, such as "OSU" for Oregon State University, (sounds very similar, although definitely different). It does seem logical that if we can't control our temper, then maybe we can't control our sexual urges as well. The question then is: Are we really in control of anything? Before long, everyone would likely be taking some mind-altering drug to control whatever. Once the door is opened, who's to say that we have control over anything that we might do in life? Sounds a lot like Satan's plan to me.

Incidentally, the National Institutes of Health (NIH) funded the study that lead to the creation of "Intermittent Explosive Disorder". And I'm certain it's not just a coincidence that the conclusion was that SSRI antidepressants just happened to be an appropriate solution. Even though we likely can't resolve our broken health care system overnight, addressing the immediate threat we're currently facing just can't wait.

What Will They Think Of Next? Would You Believe, Your Vet Can Now Prescribe Prozac™ For Your Pet!

That's right! Your pet has now become their newest target! It appears that drugging every single human being, from 18 months until the day they drop dead, was just the first stage of a very aggressive marketing plan. And finally, it's now your pet, which veterinarians are currently prescribing antidepressants for. Now, as with humans, **your dog or cat (or whatever), can have any number of mental, or behavioral conditions,** which Prozac™ can somehow "resolve".

With 374 different mental conditions for humans, in the current *Diagnostic and Statistical Manual of Mental Disorders* (*DSM*), I would guess that the American Psychiatric Association has just about exhausted their creative capacity. But guess what, we now have a new challenge for them. A new *DSM* for pets, or possibly that might be a job for the Pet Psychiatrists. Although it might sound a little ridiculous, there are such creatures. And yes, they can prescribe Prozac™ for your pet! And incidentally, **they now have "triple-fish flavored" Prozac™ for your cat,** and in case I forgot to mention it, Eli Lilly also attempted to provide a mint flavored Prozac™ for your child, (they're so thoughtful). Fortunately, the FDA decided against that one. Otherwise, you might have had to hide the mint flavored Prozac™, or your child could possibly "down" the whole bottle, and if he did he likely wouldn't survive. That could very well have been a concern if your child just happened to like the flavor, (apparently something Eli Lilly wasn't too concerned about). Everything, to them, is just one more marketing strategy, and something they have become very proficient at.

Unfortunately, although there is always a good explanation for any child's (or pet's) unusual behavior, or depression, it is seldom considered. Sometimes, what might be considered as inappropriate by some therapist might actually be quite normal for a child who is intelligent, and basically bored from the lack of any real challenge. In fact, just an improper high-sugar diet is known to contribute to hyperactivity. I believe that our children are worth the time and effort necessary to identify the underlying problem, which is normally quite easy to resolve without any drugs. Even in difficult cases, there is always a solution, (and it won't be found in drugs).

Once you learn all the implications from long-term use of these "dangerous drugs," you will better understand why they should never be considered as an option for any child (or adult). As I previously mentioned in the Introduction of this book, Dr. Julian Whitaker is an M.D. that believes as I do, and claims that although nearly 40,000 people have come through his clinic over the years, he has "never once" placed anyone on an antidepressant medication, and in my opinion, there's absolutely no valid reason for any doctor doing so! He repeats an interesting and very appropriate quote from the *LA Times*, saying, ***"I think the pharmaceutical industry is looking at our children the way the logging industry would look at the Redwood forest."*** I concur, and very aptly stated I might add. Although, we have been quite successful in saving the Redwood forest to date, our children are still at risk. Unless someone comes to their aid, (and soon), they could very well begin experiencing major diseases, such as diabetes and cancer, (and even dementia), at an unbelievably young age. Although those statements might possibly seem questionable to the uninformed, you will soon discover there is ample scientific proof that it's actually true. We are also beginning to see statistics proving that is exactly what is already happening.

My guess is that few doctors prescribing Prozac™ are even aware of many of the serious risks associated with its use. You can rest assured that the doctor's pharmaceutical representative is not about to discuss the many risks associated with a drug such as Prozac™. That's just not what they do. And you could imagine what it would do to their sales if they did. You are about to learn many major concerns regarding Prozac™ for instance, that most doctors likely never heard of. If they had, (and had a conscience), they would in no way be prescribing it for their patients!

Some Things To Consider

It might be helpful to first consider where you are at personally, and what your concerns might be. My very first question is: Are you or your loved one either taking or considering taking an antidepressant (or Ritalin™)? No - not just children, but also many adults are also taking Ritalin™, and in increasing numbers. Or possibly are your children or grandchildren taking either Ritalin™ or one or more mind-altering medication? If not, they could very well be in the near future, due to a very aggressive campaign via a new program called "TeenScreen", promoted by the pharmaceutical giants, to place as many children as possible on their "highly profitable" drugs. Exactly how, I will be discussing in considerable detail. That is something you, as parents or grandparents, must become aware of, so your children or grandchildren do not become their victims! Although, to them it's just money, to you it's their physical and mental health, (and thus their future), that's at stake.

For Parents Whose Children Might Be At Risk

Although your children might be the ones who are at risk, their welfare is your ultimate responsibility, (not their teacher's or counselor's). And this new TeenScreen program is currently spreading like the plague, from state to state, and school district to school district. The promoters have even attempted to either circumvent parental consent, or find ways to entice children with bribes to get their parents' consent if necessary. **If faced with that decision, "just say no"!** Legal mind-altering drugs can be every bit as dangerous as illegal drugs. Not only that, but many doctors are all too quick to prescribe them, without any real justification. It's amazing just how little doctors actually know, regarding the many dangers associated with the drugs they prescribe daily, (or how to withdraw them safely when necessary). Proper supplementation with nutrients during withdrawal reduces the potential for reactions, or the associated risks that can sometimes result. Our brain can at times react to sudden changes, (good or bad), thus the proper transition during withdrawal can be critical, (especially after long-term use). Unfortunately, as the majority of traditional medical doctors were never trained in nutrition, they are ill equipped to assist their patients in the withdrawal process. To find out if TeenScreen is being conducted in your school, you can visit http://www.teenscreen-locations.com/index.htm.

Knowledge is power, if properly applied. The information in this book is especially critical for anyone who is currently taking, or is considering taking, any of these mind-altering drugs, or whose children might have been placed on them. They pose the very same risks for everyone, young or old. For example, they can either lower your child's IQ, or increase your risk of prematurely developing dementia or Alzheimer's disease. And they increase everyone's risk of developing diabetes or cancer, (or both).

The Deceptive Pharmaceutical Tactics Of Manipulating Medicine (Backed By Our Government – Forced On Our Children)

You are about to learn how drug companies have recently shifted their focus from adults, to our children, who are now being targeted as potential "profit centers" for their outrageously inflated and highly profitable drugs, (and worst of all, they are very dangerous)! Their obvious success has been based on a well-planned and structured strategy. First and foremost, due to their huge financial resources, along with the obvious support from the FDA, they carry a tremendous amount of clout.

The pharmaceutical industry has very tactfully, and I might add, quite effectively manipulated medicine to promote the sale of their drugs for decades. They have done so by interspersing doctors on their payroll, (those with absolutely no conscience or ethics), into key positions in various organizations, in order to influence important medical decisions and announcements. One objective is to create more conditions or diseases, (both physical and mental), so that new drugs can then be developed, and eventually promoted for them. They then assure that announcements will be made by organizations such as the NIH, or the NIMH (National Institute of Mental Health), who just happen to have enough of their "plants" to influence the "official announcements", often made through the national news, touting some new drug, supposedly with tremendous potential, (although tremendous risk is much more likely). That's by far the most effective advertising strategy there is. It then appears, to the general public, as though it's a "medical breakthrough," rather than the promotion of a new drug, which it actually is.

Once pharmaceutical companies saturate the market with drugs for existing conditions, the objective is then to create new diseases. For example, the "acid reflux disease," which is not actually a disease at all, but just an easily resolvable condition, (and without the use of drugs)! The same applies to **all the new psychiatric disorders, which have been conveniently "invented". And one study, from the Public Library of Science Medicine, confirms this,** as follows:

> ***Pharmaceutical companies are systematically creating diseases in order to sell more of their products, turning healthy people into patients and placing many at risk of harm,*** *a special edition of a leading medical journal claims today.*

The practice of "disease mongering" by the drug industry is promoting non-existent illnesses or exaggerating minor ones for the sake of profits, according to a set of essays published by the open-access journal Public Library of Science Medicine.

The special issue, edited by David Henry, of Newcastle University in Australia, and Ray Moynihan, an Australian journalist, reports that conditions such as female sexual dysfunction, **attention deficit hyperactivity disorder (ADHD)** *and "restless legs syndrome" have been promoted by companies hoping to sell more of their drugs.*

"Disease-mongering turns healthy people into patients, wastes precious resources and causes iatrogenic (medically induced) harm," they say.

Disease-awareness campaigns are often funded by drug companies, *and* ***"more often designed to sell drugs than to illuminate or inform or educate about the prevention of illness or the maintenance of health",*** *they say.*

Ordinary shyness is routinely presented as a social anxiety disorder and treated with antidepressants, *while newly identified conditions such as "restless legs syndrome" are presented as being much more common than they really are.*

Richard Ley, of the Association of the British Pharmaceutical Industry, rejected the accusations, pointing out that Britain has firm safeguards against disease-mongering. Many of the authors' criticisms, he said, were aimed squarely at countries such as the United States, where pharmaceuticals can be openly advertised directly to patients (http://www.timesonline.co.uk/article/0,,3-2128371,00.html).

Creating all these new mental disorders has provided the pharmaceutical industry with the perfect vehicle for tapping into a whole new market, (our children).

Over the last few years, the pharmaceutical industry has successfully created many "brand new" conditions or diseases (both physical and mental) that were never heard of a few years ago. Even common traits such as shyness, being overactive, or inattentive, are now considered as identifiable and "treatable" conditions (with drugs of course). **When did a child's personality and individuality suddenly turn into inappropriate behavior? And how do the "experts" arrive at their conclusions as to what is acceptable behavior and what is not?** Are we basically creating a generation of easy-to-manage zombies, void of any emotion or unique personality? On March 20th, 2000, Hillary Clinton brought to our attention, in a meeting of health and education officials at the White House, regarding a study on the use of Ritalin™, how ***"Some of these young people have problems that are symptoms of nothing more than childhood or adolescence."*** I believe we've all heard the term "the terrible twos" or "just a typical teenager". They eventually grow out of it, if given the opportunity.

And in 1999, the US Surgeon General also noted ***"The normally developing child hardly stays the same long enough to make stable measurements... the signs and symptoms of mental disorders are often also the characteristics of normal development"*** (http://www.sierratimes.com/06/07/22/71_158_154_172_87990.htm).

In fact, according to a March 16, 2007 press release by the Citizens Commission on Human Rights (CCHR), ***"even the pioneer of psychiatry's billing bible [the DSM] and 'godfather of ADHD,' Dr. Robert Spitzer, has now admitted that normal children are being labeled."*** The article continues:

> *Spitzer, a Columbia University psychiatrist, told BBC2 that **children experiencing perfectly normal signs of being happy and sad are being labeled as mentally ill.** While admitting this, he stopped short of informing BBC viewers that there is no scientific evidence that any of the millions of children so diagnosed have any physical abnormality that justifies the diagnosis. Nor that because of this, **psychiatrists cannot agree on who is sick and who is well.** Yet despite this fallible "science," worldwide sales of psychotropic drugs prescribed to treat "mental disorders," including stimulants antipsychotics and antidepressants, now exceed $80 billion annually.*
>
> *Psychiatrists have been using the DSM to fraudulently claim that mental disorders are the same as physical disorders, and thereby justifying the prescription of powerful, psychotropic drugs, including to very young children.*
>
> ***Despite FDA warnings that psychiatric drugs cause heart attack, stroke, suicidal and homicidal behavior, diabetes, psychosis and sudden death, Spitzer stated that psychiatric drugs "don't have serious side effects"*** (http://www.cchr.org/index.cfm/9027/19686).

DSM – The Psychiatrists' Diagnostic Bible A Major Marketing Tool For Dangerous Mind-Altering Drugs

Psychiatrists connected to major pharmaceutical companies have managed to "create" literally hundreds of mental conditions, with "absolutely no science" to back up any of them. Due to the drug companies' infiltration, and tremendous influence on psychiatry at the highest level, it has become an **"institute of deception"**, with no scientific basis or validation whatsoever. **They have allowed themselves to become the basis of a major "drug trafficking scheme", designed to promote the "totally unnecessary" use of extremely dangerous mind-altering drugs.** The only difference between these drugs and illegal drugs is, "they are still legal", although once you learn all the facts regarding their potential dangers, you will likely wonder why, (as I now do).

According to a study published in the January 2006 issue of *Psychotherapy and Psychosomatics*, the American Psychiatric Association's "billing bible" (the *Diagnostic and Statistical Manual of Mental Disorders* or "*DSM*"), is actually a "vindication". The study, by psychologist Lisa Cosgrove, and Tuft University professor Sheldon Krimsky, documents the following:

> ***The manual is used in decisions to remove a child from the custody of his or her parents, to deprive a person of his or her right to vote in some countries, decide if a defendant is fit to plead "guilty" in a criminal trial or to excuse***

***criminal conduct*, and has been used to invalidate a person's will, break legal contracts and override a person's wishes regarding business or property.**

***Schools and Child Protective Services can receive additional funds for a child labeled with a DSM disorder* while *parents have been forced* to administer violent- and suicide-inducing drugs to their children and *threatened with criminal charges if they refused*—all because the child was said to be "disordered" based on the DSM** (http://www.cchr.com/index.cfm/13106).

And they devised a perfect strategy for effectively doing so, using a new screening process called TeenScreen, which boasts a 10-minute self-administered questionnaire to diagnose mental disorders, as passed by the following legislation:

Bush-Backed Drug Marketing Scheme

At an FDA hearing on the safety of psychotropic drugs on Feb 2, 2004, ***dozens of tortured parents testified that their children had committed suicide or other violent acts after being prescribed the same drugs that are being marketed in the Bush-backed pharmaceutical industry schemes aimed at recruiting the nations 52 million school children as customers.***

In July 2003, the Bush-appointed New Freedom Commission on Mental Health (NFC), recommended screening all children for mental illness and designated TeenScreen as a model program to ensure that every student receives a mental health check-up before finishing high school.

The NFC also has a preferred drug program in place modeled after the Texas Medication Algorithm Project (TMAP), that lists what drugs are to be used on children found to be mentally ill.

The list contains every drug that people complained about at the FDA hearing, including Paxil, Zoloft, Celexa, Wellbutrin, Zyban, Remeron, Serzone, Effexor, Buspar, Risperdal, Zyprexa, Seroquel, Geodon, Depakote, Adderall, and Prozac.

There is little if any evidence that these drugs work on children but nevertheless, an estimated 10 million children in the US are now taking these mind-altering drugs even though they have documented side-effects including suicidal ideation, mania, psychosis, and future drug dependence.

In a report, Allen Jones, former investigator Penn Office of Inspector General Bureau of Special Investigations, points out that ***there has been a 500% increase in children being prescribed drugs during the past 6 years.***

Jones says the NFC call for mandatory screening of all students, with follow-up treatment as required, translates into putting more kids on mind-altering and potentially lethal drugs.

"TeenScreen is purely and simply a marketing scam to sell psychotropic drugs," *according to anti-child drugging advocate Ken Kramer, "When they use 'even if we save one life' as an argument to arouse emotions in parents that truly care, they are lying," he warns* (http://www.sierratimes.com/05/04/26/pringle.htm).

The above list of 16 drugs on the "preferred drug program" was approved for children's use by the companies who produce them, (not the FDA)! Why are we allowing the companies to determine the safety of their own drugs for children's use? Incidentally, the FDA "hearing" referred to, involving the testimonies of "dozens of tortured parents," took place on February 2, 2004, with many of the tragic stories, as relayed to officials during the hearing, posted at http://www.sierratimes.com/05/08/13/24_164_252_187_48525.htm.

How Do They Keep Getting Away With it?

Judith Graham of the *Chicago Tribune*, April 20, 2006, reported the following:

Most of the experts who prepared the world's leading medical guide to mental illness had undisclosed financial relationships with drug companies that presented potential conflicts of interest, *according to a report published today in the journal Psychotherapy and Psychosomatics.*

"The more lucrative the drug market, the higher the percentage of experts with financial ties. That has to raise serious questions about these panels' objectivity," said David Rothman, professor of social medicine at Columbia University.

The DSM, as it's commonly called, defines all the mental illnesses recognized by psychiatry and outlines the criteria used to determine whether a person has one of these conditions. Medical professionals refer to it as the "bible of mental health" in the U.S. The current version, the DSM-IV, was published in 1994 and modified in 2000.

The manual is of enormous importance to pharmaceutical firms, as the Food and Drug Administration will not approve a drug to treat a mental illness unless the condition is in the DSM.

Drug companies then can market approved medications to physicians and consumers. And the broader the criteria for disorder, the more people who might be considered candidates for treatments.

According to his calculations, *the original 1952 DSM manual contained 107 mental health disorders.* ***By the fourth edition in 1994, the number had more than tripled to 365.***

Dr. Thomas Szasz, Professor of Psychiatry Emeritus at the State University of New York, has strongly opposed the entire notion, as follows:

There is NO biological basis for DSM's mental disorders.

The designation disease can only be justified when the cause can be related to a demonstrable anatomical lesion, infection, or some other physiological defect. As there is no such evidence for any mental disorder, the term disease is a misnomer; in fact, it is fraudulent (http://www.ritalindeath.com/ADHD-Controversy.htm).

Physician and Texas Republican Congressman Ron Paul has also strongly opposed this mandatory mental-health screening on our children. Following are a few of his thoughts:

> ***A presidential initiative* called The "New Freedom Commission on Mental Health" has issued a report *recommending forced mental health screening for every child in America, including preschool children*.** *The goal is to promote the patently false idea that we have a nation of children with undiagnosed mental disorders crying out for treatment.*
>
> ***One obvious beneficiary of the proposal is the pharmaceutical industry, which is eager to sell the psychotropic drugs that undoubtedly will be prescribed to millions of American schoolchildren under the new screening program.*** *Of course a tiny minority of children suffer from legitimate mental illnesses, but* ***the widespread use of Ritalin and other drugs on youngsters who simply exhibit typical rambunctious, fidgety, and impatient behavior is nothing short of criminal. It may be easier to teach and parent drugged kids, but convenience is no justification for endangering them. Children's brains are still developing,*** *and* ***the truth is we have no idea what the long-term side effects of psychiatric drugs may be.*** *Medical science has not even exhaustively identified every possible brain chemical, even as we alter those chemicals with drugs.*
>
> ***The real issue is whether the state owns your kids. When the government orders "universal" mental health screening in schools, it really means "mandatory"***... *How in the world have we allowed government to become so powerful and arrogant that it assumes it can force children to accept psychiatric treatment whether parents object or not?* (http://www.lewrockwell.com/paul/paul203.html)

I might add that although congressman Paul, as well as the majority of parents in the nation, have no idea what the long-term side effects of psychiatric drugs might be, "I do", (and you soon will as well). All I can say is, they are rather scary, and as you will soon learn, they are rapidly destroying our children's physical and mental health!

As you can easily see, **this is obviously "not" a partisan issue, as president Bush, and congressman Paul, are both republicans, although with an opposite point of view.** I believe there are people in both parties, who always vote their conscience, and then there are those who are all too easily influenced by lobbyists willing to make a donation to their campaign fund. You will soon see exactly what I am talking about, and how the lobbyists tend to go as high up the ladder in the government as they possibly can, in order to achieve their goals.

The Rutherford Institute, (which has nothing to do with politics), is a nonprofit, conservative, legal organization, which proudly states on its website, that it is *"dedicated to the defense of civil liberties and human rights"* (http://www.rutherford.org/). Attorney and author John W. Whitehead, is founder and president of the Rutherford Institute. Following is a portion of the commentary he posted, titled ***"America's Schoolchildren Are Treated Like Lab Rats"***, as follows:

American's schools are beginning to resemble laboratories, and our children are the lab rats. ***In almost every state across the nation, schoolchildren are being subjected to behavioral exams and mental health tests, often without their parents' knowledge or consent.***

One such program is the Youth Risk Behavior Surveillance System (YRBSS). ***Currently used in at least 45 states.*** *YRBSS is similar to other mental health screening programs that have been creeping into the classroom since President Bush's New Freedom Commission on Mental Health recommended* ***mental health screenings for all school-aged children, including those in preschool.***

Critics of these risk assessment tests insist that they're aimed at pushing antidepressant drugs on teenagers. *For example, TeenScreen, which is similar to YRBSS in its intent to identify suicidal tendencies and social disorders, has been labeled by* ***the Alliance for Human Research Protection as a "duo-drug promotion scam" that declares "otherwise normal children to be mentally ill."***

Legitimate questions remain about whether such tests really help students achieve healthier lifestyles. ***TeenScreen, for example, has an 84% false-positive rate. This means that 84% of teens diagnosed as having some sort of mental health or social disorder are, in fact, perfectly normal teenagers.***

It's time for parents to stand up for their rights. *After all, it is still the job of the parents – not the schools – to parent.*
(http://www.rutherford.org/articles_db/commentary.asp?record_id=453)

One parent, voicing his opinion on how the TeenScreen program is being used to *"push drugs to students"*, made some particularly strong statements in a letter to the editor of *The Post-Standard*, Syracuse, New York (January 22, 2007), including the following:

TeenScreen promoters have stated that suicide is a leading cause of death among teenagers.

According to the U.S. Centers for Disease Control, ***the suicide rate among children, including teens, actually dropped 25 percent in the last decade.*** *A May 2004 Preventive Services Task Force concluded* ***that there is no evidence that screening for suicide reduces suicide attempts. In essence, the program is unwarranted and unproductive.***

> ***TeenScreen is simply a front for the pharmaceutical industry to peddle their drugs to our children.***
>
> ***Additionally, nine out of 10 children who go to see a psychiatrist leave with a psychiatric drug prescription. When this frightening statistic is combined with the fact that 100 percent of the 10th graders tested under TeenScreen at Hoover High in Fresno, Calif. Had "positive diagnostic impression," you are looking at some terrifying results.***
>
> *Todd Wilson*

What Is TeenScreen's Real Motive?

The entire premise for TeenScreen, as presented to the public, is to be a "suicide prevention tool." However, its purpose is highly debated, as you will discover from the following article by investigative reporter Evelyn Pringle:

> ***By far, TeenScreen has become the most controversial of all screening programs,*** *and critics are quick to point out a number of reasons. According to the June 16, 2006, Washington Post,* ***there were only 1,737 suicides by children and adolescents in the US during 2003, the last year for which national statistics are available.***
>
> *In perhaps one of their best arguments against TeenScreen, critics are asking* ***how such a low suicide rate, when measured against the total student population, can possibly justify subjecting 52 million children to mental health screening and the distinct probability that a high number of children will end up on psychiatric drugs with side effects that cause many more deaths each year than the number of child suicides.***
>
> *In fact, overall,* ***the statistics for people injured or killed each year due to prescription medications are extremely high.*** *According to a study published by Adverse Drug Reactions,* ***more than 1.5 million people are hospitalized each year and more than 100,000 die from largely preventable adverse reactions to drugs that should not have been prescribed in the first place.***
>
> (http://www.sierratimes.com/06/07/10/75_8_41_234_97438.htm)

One government-sponsored study published in the *Journal of the American Medical Association* (*JAMA*), surveyed 9,708 people aged 18 to 54, and compared the suicide data from the 1990 -1992 National Comorbidity Survey and the 2001-2003 National Comorbidity Survey Replication and found: ***"Despite a dramatic increase in treatment, no significant decrease occurred in suicidal thoughts, plans, gestures, or attempts in the United States during the 1990s,"*** ("Trends in Suicide Ideation, Plans, Gestures, and Attempts in the United States", 1990-1992 to 2001-2003, *JAMA*. 2005;293:2487-2495).

Not only do SSRIs not prevent suicide, but on July 21, 2004, *JAMA* again reported that **during treatment with SSRIs, there was actually a *"significantly higher risk of suicide and suicidal thoughts ... during the first nine days of treatment"*** (*JAMA*, 2004;292:338-343), and that **children first starting treatment were four times more likely to think about suicide, and 38 times more likely to commit suicide. In fact, children as young as five have committed suicide while taking these drugs,** the study found. As noted by one mother, whose daughter **stabbed herself to death after taking Paxil™ for just two weeks**, ***"Untold thousands have died because of the drug companies and the FDA's failure to heed the evidence over the past years"*** (http://www.sierratimes.com/05/08/13/24_164_252_187_48525.htm).

According to TeenScreen's Executive Director, Laurie Flynn, **TeenScreen's goal is to find students and *"link them with treatment,"*** and in 2004 she was proud to announce:

> *In 2003, we were able to screen approximately 14,200 teens at these sites; among those students, we were able to identify approximately 3,500 youth with mental health problems and **link them with treatment. This year, we believe we will be able to identify close to 10,000 teens in need, a 300 percent increase over last year*** (http://www.sierratimes.com/06/08/02/75_8_33_58_96580.htm).

Unfortunately, what this really means is that these teens are being "linked" to dangerous prescriptions. As pointed out by investigative reporter Evelyn Pringle, ***"TeenScreen's underlying motive is to recruit customers to funnel money to Pharma by drugging kids"*** (http://www.sierratimes.com/05/07/30/pringle.htm).

She also reveals the following:

> *Experts say **there is no evidence to support that TeenScreen does anything other than guarantee that a large number of children will end up on drugs.** In May 2004, after an indepth investigation, the United States Preventive Services Task Force issued a report with findings that:*
>
> ***(1) There is no evidence that screening for suicide risk reduces suicide attempts or mortality;***
>
> ***(2) There is limited evidence on the accuracy of screening tools to identify suicide risk; and (3) There is insufficient evidence that treatment of those at high risk reduces suicide attempts or mortality.***
> (http://www.sierratimes.com/06/07/22/71_158_154_172_87990.htm)

Following is part of an article by Texas Eagle Forum president Cathie Adams, published in the February 2007 issue of their *Torch* newsletter:

> ***"Have you often felt very nervous when you've had things to do in front of people?"***
>
> ***"Has there been a time when you had less energy than you usually do?"***

"Has there been a time when you felt you couldn't do anything well or that you weren't as good-looking or as smart as other people?"

If you would answer, "yes" to any of these questions, then you are either crazy or at least have mental health problems according to a Columbia University based program called TeenScreen. TeenScreen labels 15% of the students screened as having mental health problems, a diagnosis that leads to the use of powerful and sometimes hazardous medications.

What child or teen (or even adult, for that matter) hasn't felt at least one of these ways at one time or another? More than one is even more likely. And once they "label" your child, and mandate what drugs your child must begin taking in order to "help them", and even threatening you if you don't – there often seems to be no way out!

The article continues:

A January 2006 Brandeis University study found that ***psychotropic drug prescriptions for teens surged 250% from 1994-2001. One in every ten doctor-office visits by teenage boys led to a prescription for a psychotropic drug.*** *A diagnosis of Attention Deficit Hyperactivity Disorder, ADHD, a malady that was first defined in 1980, has grown to epidemic proportions. The subjective* ***diagnosis of ADHD was given to about one-third of the office visits during the study period. Last year 15 million antidepressant prescriptions were written for teens and children, but such medications may in part account for the doubling of suicide rates over the past 20 years for children 5-14 years old.***

Financial incentives such as Medicaid funding to the family of a child diagnosed with ADHD as much as $450 a month and funding to schools $400 a year for each ADHD child probably increases the number of diagnoses. It is insidious that this government-driven scheme puts children at risk while it profits pharmaceutical companies at taxpayer expense.

Even though pharmaceutical companies will profit from the Medicare Drug Package that was originally estimated to cost taxpayers $400 billion, but has now grown to $1.2 trillion, they want more. ***The industry's aim is to not only collaborate with the schools, but to also coax government into requiring mental health screening for every man, woman and child.***
(http://www.texaseagle.org/torch/NewTorch/2-2007Torch.pdf)

And The Numbers Just Keep Going Up

As noted in *Breaking Your Prescribed Addiction* (Sahley & Birkner, 1998, p. 16):

Today millions of children are targets of the pharmaceutical giants and their magic pills. *According to a story in U.S. News and World Report, August 18,*

> *1998, by Arianna Huffington, "At least 580,000 children are being prescribed antidepressants – and those numbers are likely to* ***increase dramatically****."* ***Eli Lilly already markets a peppermint-flavored Prozac.*** *Everyone knows where Prozac leads – to other antidepressant pharmaceuticals such as Zoloft and Paxil.* ***Huffington's story describes the future treatment of children in America.***

And that certainly seems to have come true! **Those numbers did "increase dramatically,"** as **there are now an estimated 10 million children taking some sort of mind-altering drugs (which included the SSRI antidepressants), thanks to advertising and programs like TeenScreen!**

Linda Hurcombe, an American citizen who resides in the UK, lost her 19-year-old daughter, Caitlin, to suicide as a result of Prozac™ advertising. She shares her story, as follows:

> [Linda] *describes how 8 years ago,* ***her "undepressed daughter saw an ad for antidepressants on television while visiting the US."***
>
> *"Caitlin decided she wanted this pill," Ms Hurcombe explains,* ***"because she was nervous about final exams and had heard at the university too that Prozac made you lose weight and feel great."***
>
> ***Caitlin got a prescription from the doctor, she said, with no problem.***
>
> ***"After 63 days on this medication," Ms Hurcombe says, "during which time her behavior descended into chaos, Caitlin hanged herself from a beam in the guest bedroom of our home."***
> (http://www.lawyersandsettlements.com/articles/pharma_lawsuits.html)

Healthcare analyst Thomas J. Moore, who analyzed the FDA data in 1997, posted the following comments in an article for the Alliance for Human Research Protection (AHRP) (http://www.ahrp.org/testimonypresentations/BestPharmaAct0803.php#r29):

> *It is astonishing that these drugs are being widely prescribed for children despite the absence of any scientific basis for even diagnosing depression in children - especially as a credible body of evidence exists showing the drugs pose serious, even life-threatening risks of harm.*
>
> ***This is evidence of the power of advertising*****: *"Like tobacco and beer companies, the pharmaceutical industry spends more for advertising and promotion than for manufacturing or research."***

Advertising is often very extensive, as well as deceptive, and it's not only through TV commercials.

For example, in the August/September 2006 issue of *Girls' Life* magazine, a magazine specifically aimed for girls, ages 10 – 15, a feature article regarding ADHD titled *"Out of Focus,"* supplies the reader with a suggested list of ADHD symptoms to check for, as follows:

Usually, someone with ADHD will have several of the following symptoms:

- *Constantly fidgeting, can't sit still for long.*
- *Trouble taking turns*
- *Doesn't finish things*
- *Easily distracted*
- *Gets bored easily*
- *Daydreams often*
- *Interrupts people*
- *Gets easily frustrated with school work*
- *Acts and speaks quickly without thinking*
- *Often sidetracked by what's going on around her*
- *Loses and forgets things*
- *Disorganized*
- *Low self-esteem*
- *Trouble with friendships*
- *Poor grades*

This is beyond a doubt, an outright attempt to convince children that their behavior, (which is often quite typical of many young children, or even teens for that matter), is somehow abnormal. Then of course, **there just happens to be drugs that will help fit you into their "normal" mold (a Stepford child, or a child that is perfect in every respect).**

Some of the symptoms on the list, which **"someone conveniently created"**, could easily describe a child on a high sugar diet. Others are possibly symptoms of children who are intelligent, although not adequately challenged, and are thus bored and distracted easily. Then some children might be overweight or possibly unattractive, and would thus have low self-esteem. Then some children get poor grades (another symptom) because they don't have as high an I.Q. as others. Possibly their mother had been taking Prozac™ during her pregnancy. That would assure that his or her I.Q. would be lower than it could have otherwise been, (you will soon learn exactly why that would be true). Even their mother's thyroid function, and diet during pregnancy, can play a part regarding a child's I.Q. Most importantly, it's not the child's fault, or something any drug can possibly fix, (although something drugs can instead create), and unfortunately it's just something the child must learn to live with for the remainder of their life.

This is where the psychiatrists "bible", the *DSM*, comes in, which includes 374 mental conditions that are now considered as abnormal! They just wanted to assure that no one would be left out, (very thoughtful of them), and a very creative endeavor, I might add. It's definitely a very effective marketing tool, and hopefully people will begin recognizing it for what it is, so they won't be deceived into believing that these dangerous mind-altering drugs are somehow a panacea, as portrayed in the next article.

Pretend for a moment that you're a typical teenage girl (whom this magazine is targeting), and see if it's not rather enticing. Although the characters portrayed are likely fictional, and the results just fantasy, they are playing with real (not make-believe) lives. Their drugs can easily destroy lives, and there are many "true stories" to prove how potentially dangerous they truly can be. So, we'll leave the real world for a moment, and step into the fantasy world, and learn of a panacea that would be rather difficult to resist.

The following *Girls' Life* magazine article describes one girl's "wonderful" experiences after taking the latest ADHD prescription medication Concerta, as follows:

> ***Right away, everything changed. I immediately got better grades, and my homework was getting in on time. By the end of the year, I had all A's and B's. I went from flunking Spanish to winning the Spanish Award.***
>
> ***I felt so good that I lost 20 pounds in a year and have since lost 13 more.*** *I jointed swim team and drama club, and* ***my social life is great.*** *At first, I didn't tell anyone except my best friend about my ADHD. But the more I talked to people about it, the more I realized having ADHD was no big deal.*
>
> *For the first time, I don't feel so different from everyone.* ***I'm more active, open and confident. I'm no longer the one everyone picks on*** *– and I love that!* (August/September 2006, Vol. 13, p. 90).

And would you believe, at the end of the entire article is **a list of websites to visit, for *"great info on teens with ADHD"*, all sponsored by the NIMH and the CHADD organization.**

According to *Freedom* magazine, it just so happens that CHADD (Children and Adults with Attention Deficit/Hyperactivity Disorder) *"found itself under scrutiny in 2002 at a hearing of the Government Reform Committee, where Committee Chairman Dan Burton (R-IN) lambasted CHADD and its CEO, E. Clarke Ross, for the group's ties with drug companies, noting that it had received $848,000 from one methylphenidate* [Ritalin™] *manufacturer alone."* Furthermore, educator and author Beverly Eakman told *Freedom* that ***"the whole thing is driven by money,"*** and calling **the connections between the NIMH, CHADD, and the pharmaceutical companies *"incestuous"*** (http://www.freedommag.org/english/vol36i1/page06.htm).

In fact, in the 2004-2005 financial year (ending 30 June 2005), it was reported that the pharmaceutical industry provided twenty-two percent of CHADD's total revenue! (http://medicine.plosjournals.org/perlserv?request=get-document&doi=10.1371/journal.pmed.0030182).

Both the United Nations International Narcotics Control Board (INCB), and the U.S. Drug Enforcement Administration (DEA), have also severely criticized CHADD's financial ties to the manufacturers of ADHD drugs. Coincidentally, more than half of the drugs promoted and endorsed on the CHADD website are manufactured by companies that fund CHADD. **Another coincidence, members of the American Psychiatric Association voted ADHD to be a mental disorder and to be included in its *Diagnostic and Statistical Manual of Mental Disorders* (*DSM*) in 1987, which is the same year CHADD was formed. Then, thanks to a financial boost from pharmaceutical interests, the number of CHADD chapters boomed from 29 to 500!** As noted by author of *Blaming the Brain* (1998), Dr. Elliot S. Valenstein, Ph.D., such funding *"enables the groups to increase newspaper and magazine advertising and the information they distribute by other means"* (http://www.cchr.com/index.cfm/9424).

An Overt Conspiracy To Promote Drugs At The Very Highest Level – Our Federal Government (Beginning With Our President)!

So, who's the one person with the very most influence in the nation? Obviously, our president! Thus the major drug manufacturers just needed to find someone with presidential potential, such as a governor with name recognition. Especially an individual who would like very much to become president, and who would be beholden to them if they provided the financial support to see that his wishes became realty. Once they found an appropriate candidate, they then proceeded to scope out as many senators and congressman via their lobbyists (some prior legislators), to see how many would respond to their lobbyist's requests. Just having the president on their side was obviously a distinct advantage. Many legislators were already obligated, due to prior campaign donations, and future commitments. The industry has been very successful in the past, as they have more lobbyists than congressman and senators combined.

I couldn't help but wonder why president Bush seemed to be promoting legislation that would not only increase the number of seniors placed on drugs, (with the new prescription drug benefit plan), but also assure that many more children would be as well. You would think he was in the pharmaceutical business, although that would obviously be a conflict of interest. It was about that time that I came across the answer. Although he wasn't in the business, both he and his father had many longtime friends who were, and he eventually owed them, big time. So, I'll share with you what I uncovered, which helps puts things in perspective, and explains the likely motivation behind the passage of recent legislation, which is obviously not in our best interest, (or our children's):

> *The NFC* [New Freedom Commission on Mental Health] *specifically calls for all screening programs to be linked to* ***"state-of-the-art treatments" using "specific medications for specific conditions."***
>
> *The Texas Medication Algorithm Project (TMAP) is the centerpiece of the NFC's recommendation for "specific medications." Algorithms are lists of drugs with guidelines that medical professionals must follow when prescribing medication to patients for specific mental illnesses, and contain flow charts that illustrate step-by-step prescribing process.*
>
> ***The TMAP drug lists and guidelines were developed and approved in Texas while Bush was Governor, through an "expert opinion consensus" by a panel of medical professionals chosen by the pharmaceutical sponsors of the program*** *that included Janssen Pharmaceutical, Eli Lilly, Johnson & Johnson, AstraZeneca, Pfizer, Novartis, Janssen-Ortho-McNeil, GlaxoSmithKline, Abbott, Bristol Myers Squibb, Wyeth-Ayerst and Forrest Laboratories.*
>
> ***The way the NFC scheme is set up, tax dollars not only fund the implementation of the screening programs, but also a large portion of the costs for "specific medications"*** *that are prescribed to patients to treat mental disorders detected by the screenings* ***through government health care programs like Medicaid.***
>
> ***The fact is, when Bush took office, he owed Big Pharma a lot favors in return for all the money he raked in from the industry and the mental health screening scheme represents a major part of his efforts to cover those debts.***

The financial backing that Bush received from Big Pharma is legend and it's safe to say that he would not be sitting in the White House today without it. *In 2004, a report by the advocacy group, Public Citizen, listed* ***21 drug industry and HMO executives or lobbyists among Bush's Rangers and Pioneers – titles given only to those people who have raised at least $200,000 or $100,000, respectively, for one of his presidential campaigns.***

The list includes 5 executives from drug companies, 6 officials from HMOs, the CEO of a pharmacy services company, the head of a direct-mail pharmacy, and 8 lobbyists who represent drug companies and HMOs at the time.

Eli Lilly, a manufacturer of many of the "specific medications" chosen for the lists, has multiple ties to the Bush family dating back decades. Before becoming President Reagan's Vice President, the first President Bush was a member of Lilly's board of directors and the current President Bush appointed Lilly CEO, Sidney Taurel, to the Homeland Security Council.

In the year 2000, eighty-two percent of Lilly's $1.6 million in political contributions went to Bush and the Republican Party.

Another industry big-wig, retired Bristol-Myers Squibb Vice-Chairman, Bruce Gelb, was a Bush Pioneer who also had longstanding ties to the Bush family. *Gelb was appointed chief of the US Information Agency, and ambassador to Belgium, by the first President Bush.*

Before the 2000 election, Bristol-Myers executives reportedly were pressured to make maximum donations to the Bush campaign and reluctant donors were warned that CEO, Charles Heimbold Jr, *whom Bush later named ambassador to Sweden,* ***would be informed if they failed to give, according a September 5, 2003 New York Times article.***

Pfizer CEO, Hank McKinnell, was a 2004 Bush Ranger and until 2003, served as chairman of the board of Pharmaceutical Research & Manufacturers of America, the industry's gigantic trade group, *until Republican lawmaker, Billy Tauzin, quit Congress and took over the position that came with a multi-million dollar package in combined salary and perks.*
(http://www.lawyersandsettlements.com/articles/pharma_business.html)

Then as a special bonus, **Bush set up the whole scheme in a way that taxpayers will foot the bill for the implementation of the TeenScreen program,** by signing a bill on October 21, 2004, which authorized $82 million to be used over 3 years for programs like TeenScreen (http://www.sierratimes.com/06/08/02/75_8_33_58_96580.htm).

By the time President Bush was elected, it appears that the stage had already been set. The plan would be to convert a program called "Texas Medication Algorithm Project" (TMAP), which several major drug manufacturers helped Bush establish for the state of Texas, (while he was still governor), into a nationwide program called the "New Freedom Commission on Mental Health" (NFC). One can easily see that Bush would thus have, by far, the greatest potential for helping them establish a nationwide program to promote the placing of millions of children on their psychiatric medications. As billions of dollars in profit were at stake, they were highly motivated to assure that governor Bush became president. It seems as though they pulled out all the stops, as huge financial resources were soon invested, and unfortunately, it paid off. It appears as though their extensive marketing plan is now in place, and our children have become their primary targets.

The Plot Just Thickens!

I couldn't help but wonder **why in the world President Bush would decide to appoint "Eli Lilly's CEO," Sidney Taurel, to the Homeland Security Council!** What part could a major drug company's CEO possibly play regarding our country's security? Then, the answer soon became obvious, and it had absolutely nothing to do with our security. I discovered the answer in an article in the September 2006 issue of the *AARP Bulletin* (Vol. 47, No. 8), titled *"Where's My Medication?"* As we are fully aware, the U.S. drug companies have been aggressively fighting any effort to import much cheaper, (but just as safe), medications from Canada. Something many seniors have continued doing, due to their overly stretched budgets, and our highly inflated drug prices, just to help make ends meet.

Guess what many soon began receiving in the mail, instead of their medications? **Not only had the drugs they ordered and paid for been confiscated, but they also received notice from the U.S. Department of Homeland Security, stating that they were violating federal law!** What could seniors, attempting to save money on their medications, possibly have to do with our security? Obviously, nothing! **The "only thing" they are protecting is the U.S. pharmaceutical's highly inflated drug prices.** Worst of all, the Department of Homeland Security can't as effectively protect the nation against the true threat of terrorists, when they are now assuming additional responsibilities that have absolutely nothing to do with our security! And worst of all, we the taxpayers are supporting Homeland Security with our hard-earned tax money, just so they can take away our God-given right to save money on our medications, (a right we should all enjoy)!

Is the picture becoming clearer? **Once they have the president of the United States, and the majority of legislators on their side, anything is possible.** And I'm sure they are fully aware that in just a few years the children will be acquiring adult diseases such as diabetes, cardiovascular disease, and even cancer, caused by the long-term use of their drugs. They are basically establishing a whole new market, for additional drugs that would eventually follow. Everything to them is based on numbers, and each child is just another number, or potential profit center, similar to a lifetime annuity policy. To them, they have no name or face, spirit or even potential future, (they're just another statistic). **One can't help but wonder who managed to steal their conscience, or sense of moral values, and at what price?** I could never imagine placing a value on money (no matter how much), over even one child's life, and **we're talking about millions of innocent children's lives!**

CHAPTER TWO

The Role of Big PhRMA

A Whole New Industry Created To Promote Misinformation

As defined by the online encyclopedia *Wikipedia*: ***"The phrase 'Big Pharma' is often used to refer to pharmaceutical companies with revenue in excess of $3 billion, and/or companies with research and development (R & D) expenditure in excess of $500 million."*** This is not to be confused with PhRMA, whose definition is as follows: ***"[The] Pharmaceutical Research and Manufacturers of American (PhRMA) is a trade group, representing the pharmaceutical research and biotechnology companies in the United States."***

In my opinion, PhRMA is a "well-financed" institution, whose primary goal is promoting the use of drugs, and discrediting any benefit associated with supplements, or natural therapies. PhRMA basically represents the pharmaceutical industry, (more than 100 brand name drug companies), and are thus looking out for their "financial interest." To them, the fact that more and more people have been turning to natural solutions, due to the poor health they had been experiencing by following their doctor's recommendations, is an obvious threat to the industry they represent. When you hear announcements that in any way attempt to convince you that supplements such as vitamin C or vitamin E, (or possibly DHEA), have been proven to have no real benefit, you can rest assured it originated with PhRMA, irrespective of where the announcement might have been made.

Their influence is extremely widespread, from the FDA, the AMA, the NIH, and The American Psychiatric Association, to the medical journals and the news media, (and of course our legislators). They want you to believe that you normally don't really need any vitamins, and if you do, just a cheap once-a-day vitamin/mineral (basically a placebo) should be adequate. Also, that anything in excess of the established recommended daily allowance (RDA) is a total waste of your money, and could even be dangerous. Actually, nothing could be further from the truth. I have taken all kinds of vitamins and minerals, as well as amino acids and herbs, plus many different plant extracts, for over four decades, and the only reaction I got is "excellent health at 73"! If vitamins are somehow dangerous, or don't seem to have any real benefit, maybe I'm just extremely lucky.

A nutritional deficiency is especially a concern for anyone taking all the drugs they recommend, as drugs are notorious for depleting critical nutrients, (for example, Prozac™ depletes 16). Then by far the majority of adults in the nation are taking several nutrient-depleting drugs. We spend more on our healthcare than any other nation, yet we have the poorest health of any developed nation in the world, (although there is an obvious explanation). We consume far more "highly inflated" drugs than any other nation in the entire world.

You can't always blame your doctor, because all traditionally trained M.D.s were taught in medical school, that the only viable solutions are symptom-suppressing drugs or surgery. Not only that, but those are the very procedures that M.D.s are often required to follow, by the AMA. By following AMA-approved guidelines, (regardless of the results), a doctor is not risking their license to "practice" medicine, but unfortunately, they are still "practicing" on you. It's also obvious that most doctors must be following their own advice, as in a recent study it was discovered that the average doctor lives a total of 56 years! Incidentally, that's not much older than my daughter, who is actually 51. It's likely difficult to pass up all those "free samples" that your doctor's pharmaceutical rep is so generous with. Not only would I **not** pay two cents for any of them, but, (knowing what I know), you couldn't even pay me enough to take any of them! They are basically toxins, (which our liver is fully aware of), and as I often state, by far the greatest contributor to most people's poor health. In a recent survey, it was found that only **4% of medical doctors were very familiar with natural therapies!** That absolutely must change if our nation's health is ever going to improve.

A Deliberate Attempt To Deprive Everyone Of Their Health Freedom

There's a concerted all-out effort, orchestrated by Big PhRMA, with the full support of the FDA, to basically legislate Natural Practitioners out of business, and take away your free access to supplements in sufficient strength to be truly effective.

According to Gwen Olsen, a pharmaceutical insider-turned-informer, *"The FDA and the drug companies are working very hard to eliminate the competition of natural health care.* ***Right before I left the pharmaceutical industry we were told that, 'If we can't beat them, we'll buy them... If we can't buy them, we'll put them out of business.'*** *"*

Then according to an email *Action Alert*, sent out by The Natural Solutions Foundation, Medical Director Dr. Rima E. Laibow, M.D. states the following:

> ***The FDA is using a legal ploy to make all natural health criminal in either one way or another.*** *You can't engage in it if you are not a physician and you cannot use the products even if you are.* ***That's very similar to the laws recently introduced in Australia (5 year prison sentence for using, providing to another person or teaching the use of nutrients) and India (illegal to practice or teach acupuncture, energy healing, sound therapy, etc., etc.). Neither law passed but they will be back in Parliament again.*** *It's the same process:* ***marginalize, then criminalize all competition*** *to the deadly, expensive and oh-so-useful drugs!*

For decades, they have taken away any access to Natural Practitioners, or the use of natural supplements, from the poor especially, (they are conveniently not covered by your insurance). Although, medications (appropriate or not), and at times surgeries (which at times are unnecessary), are covered without question, and often without any justification. Thus the poor are deprived of much safer natural therapies, even if they are less expensive, and proven to work, (they basically don't have a choice).

If there's any freedom that we should all enjoy, it's the choice regarding our healthcare. Their next step is to assure that "absolutely no one" can any longer make that choice, (a joint effort by PhRMA and the FDA), along with a movement in Europe called "Codex", (backed by the pharmaceutical industry), which have been attempting to restrict your access to supplements for years. Every single initiative has been promoted, either directly or indirectly, by the pharmaceutical industry, using devious, underhanded, mafia-like techniques of corruption, deception, and bribery.

Our Latest Gift From President Bush

As of January 2006, the Bush administration announced that ***"people who believe they have been injured by drugs approved by the FDA should not be allowed to sue drug companies in state courts"*** (http://www.sierratimes.com/06/05/14/71_158_158_30_69115.htm).

Then, the FDA's deputy commissioner for medical and scientific affairs, Scott Gottlieb, backed this up by stating: *"You should not be second-guessed by state courts that don't have the same scientific knowledge* [as the drug companies]*."*

As the argument continues, columnist and investigative journalist Evelyn Pringle, reports the following:

> *In response to the FDA's statement, Senator Edward Kennedy (D-MA) issued a statement of his own that said:* ***"It's a typical abuse by the Bush Administration – take a regulation to improve the information that doctors and patients receive about prescription drugs and turn it into a protection against liability for the drug industry."***
>
> ***The ploy was also readily recognized by state lawmakers and trial lawyers as another ploy to reduce the public's ability to hold Big Pharma accountable. "Eliminating the rights of individuals to hold negligent drug companies accountable puts patients in even more danger than they already are in from drug company executives that put profits before safety,"*** *said Ken Suggs, president of the Association of Trial Lawyers of America.*
>
> ***"The fact that the drug industry can get the FDA to rewrite the rules so that CEOs can escape accountability for putting dangerous and deadly drugs on the market is the scariest example yet of how much control these big corporations have over our political process,"*** *Mr. Suggs told the Washington Post* (http://www.sierratimes.com/06/05/14/71_158_158_30_69115.htm).

Actually, just passing the prescription drug coverage program, insuring that many seniors would soon be placed on even more medications, (especially the poor, who couldn't afford them in the past), when we are already experiencing a crisis with maintaining the funding of both Medicare and Medicaid, is obviously financial suicide, and shows just how much influence they actually have. Then, to assure that there would be no negotiated discounts for their highly inflated drugs, a responsibility the taxpayers would now be assuming, is ludicrous. The government somehow managed years ago to negotiate a discount on veterans' medications, although that's a much smaller group than those currently on Medicare and Medicaid. Then in a few years, when approximately 75 million baby boomers begin qualifying for Medicare, the number of recipients will increase dramatically.

The fact that the very same drugs are sold for much less in Canada and other countries, should be a clue that drugs in this country are obviously over-priced. Just how highly inflated, is reflected by one study conducted by the non-profit *Life Extension Foundation* (April 2002), listing just a few of the more common medications on the market as follows:

What Drugs Really Cost

BRAND NAME	CONSUMER PRICE (For 100 tabs/caps)	COST OF GENERIC (For 100 tabs/caps)	PERCENT MARKUP
Celebrex 100 mg	$130.27	$0.60	21,712%
Lipitor 20 mg	$272.37	$5.80	4,696%
Paxil 20 mg	$220.27	$7.60	2,898%
Prevacid 30 mg	$344.77	$1.01	34,136%
Prilosec 20 mg	$360.97	$0.52	69,417%
Prozac 20 mg	$247.47	$0.11	224,973%
Xanax 1 mg	$139.79	$0.024	569,958%
Zocor 40 mg	$350.27	$8.63	4,059%
Zoloft 50 mg	$206.87	$1.75	11,821%

Absolutely no industry in the world has that kind of profitability. **They could easily charge half as much for their drugs and still realize exorbitant profits.** If they did, the cost of Medicare and Medicaid would be reduced dramatically as well.

Something PhRMA Would Rather You Were Unaware Of – Most Of Your Medications Are Totally Unnecessary (and Unhealthy)

It is important that we now address the issue that few medications the seniors are being placed on are actually even necessary, giving us an even greater potential for savings. According to an article in the *AARP Bulletin* (Sept 2004), **pharmacist Armon Neel indicated that nearly 100 percent of the people he saw as out patients were overmedicated.** He also noted that even in a long-term care environment, it is still about 80 percent. **According to Neel, medication levels in nursing homes could, in his opinion, be cut in half or even better. Neel stresses that: *"If I can get the drug therapy management correct, there are fewer hospital stays, fewer hospital admissions, lower labor costs involved in care and a better quality of life for residents."*** Certainly a tremendous benefit, if he could just get the doctors' cooperation, which according to Neel seldom happens.

I have come to realize that **most, if not all of many people's medications are actually inappropriate, as well as totally unnecessary.** A prime example is Mary Lou, who you will learn about later in this book. She went from nine medications to none, in only 60 days, (including a 16-year dependence on Prozac™). Not only that, but she felt much better off, than on, her medications. Proof positive they were inappropriate.

Another example is a lady I know named Shirley, who works at the local grocery store. She said she never really believed in taking medications, although her husband did, and according to Shirley, he always seemed to be taking a drug for something. The problem was, they were getting expensive, and he wanted to retire, but if he did, they could no longer afford his medications. Together the decision was made that as each prescription drug ran out, he would just stop taking it, which he proceeded to do. Then, to his amazement, he not only began feeling much better, and having more energy, but he also began losing unwanted weight.

One potential problem associated with **over half** of the medications on the market, is that they often contribute to weight gain. Incidentally, Shirley's husband eventually lost a total of 50 unwanted pounds, and did so with no other changes to either his diet or life style. According to Shirley, he is currently 69 and doing great without all those medications. I believe it bears repeating that if you feel better off your medications, it's quite obvious they were inappropriate and totally unnecessary to begin with, (something you might discover as well, if you just give it a try). Many have indicated that they were required to stop all medications prior to surgery, and when they did they actually felt much better. Maybe we should pay more attention to what our body is trying so desperately to tell us: "These drugs are toxins!" Then, if you begin taking supplements to restore any damage and nutrient depletion caused by your medications, you should begin feeling even better.

How can we start fighting back against such outright corruption? Actually, it's quite simple. Just begin withdrawing from your unnecessary medications, and encourage your friends and family to do so as well! In my opinion, most (if not all) medications people continue taking are not only totally unnecessary, but by far the greatest contributor to their poor health as well. This was the primary focus of my first book, *A Drug-Free Approach To Healthcare*, (which is now available in the 2007 *Revised Edition*), along with drug-free solutions for 18 of the most common conditions many are unnecessarily dealing with.

QuackWatch℠ (an organization established by PhRMA)

Just to prove how devious and fraudulent PhRMA's claims can be, I'll now show you a typical example of just one **"obvious deception"** they portrayed! First, we will see what QuackWatch℠ has reported about Dr. Royal S. Lee, and a natural supplement that he produced way back in 1929, called Catalyn. It's still sold today by the company called *Standard Process™, Inc.*, which Dr. Lee established. **Following is what QuackWatch℠ "somehow concluded" from their "research"**:

> *Lee's first product was* ***Catalyn, a patent medicine composed of milk sugar, wheat starch, wheat bran, and other plant material.*** *During the early 1930s, a shipment of Catalyn was seized by the FDA and destroyed by court order because it had been marketed with false claims of effectiveness against goiter, hardening of the arteries, heart trouble, high blood pressure, insomnia, prostate trouble, and other serious ailments.*
>
> *In 1945, the FTC ordered Lee and the Vitamin Products Company to discontinue illegal claims for Catalyn and other products. In 1956, the Post Office Department charged Lee's foundation with fraudulent promotion of a book called Diet Prevents Polio. The foundation agreed to discontinue the challenged claims.*

In 1962, Lee and the Vitamin Products Company were convicted of misbranding 115 special dietary products by making false claims for the treatment of more than 500 diseases and conditions. Lee received a one-year suspended prison term and was fined $7,000. Lee also consented to a permanent injunction prohibiting his use of claims for the products as well as claims such as "Arthritis and tooth decay are caused by eating the cooked foods" and ***"Some 700,000 people a year die of preventable and curable heart disease caused by deficiency of natural vitamins."***

In a speech on the day after the seizure had been made, Kenneth Milstead, Deputy Director of the FDA Bureau of Enforcement, described Lee as "probably the largest publisher of unreliable and false nutritional information in the world" (http://www.quackwatch.org/11Ind/lee.html).

If you noticed, they made it sound as though Dr. Lee was somehow a criminal, with the FDA and FTC doing their utmost to discredit all the claims he made regarding any benefits his supplements might have, and basically attempting to put him out of business. Fortunately, they were not successful. It should be obvious, to anyone who follows the actions of both the FDA and FTC, whose interest they are unquestionably protecting.

We will now look at a very small part of Dr. Lee's history, and his tremendous contribution to society, which proves beyond a doubt that his motivation in life was definitely not making a lot of money, although with his tremendous talents, that is something that Dr. Lee could quite easily have done, had he chosen to. In fact, a great deal of his financial resources were unfortunately depleted while attempting to defend himself, and continue his work, which he strongly believed in. Below you will find the **unbiased true story**, as follows:

Those of us who have made the transition into the 21st century are fortunate as we benefit from the numerous inventions and creations from the past that make our daily existence so much more rewarding and enjoyable. ***One of the intellectual giants who contributed to our contemporary high standard of living and knowledge of human nutrition was Dr. Royal Lee. Even though his name is known to only a small number of Americans, Dr. Lee was a researcher, inventor, scientist, scholar, statesman, businessman and philanthropist of the first order.***

One of Dr. Lee's most important inventions was a speed governor for electric motors, patented on May 31, 1927. These are needed wherever precise time intervals or constant speeds must be maintained for such equipment as radar, calculating machines, food mixers, flame-cutting machinery, fusion welding equipment, drill presses, telephone equipment and motion picture sound equipment. When talking pictures came out, ***Bell Telephone Laboratories had a speed governor selling for $1,200 – Dr. Lee sold his to them for $3.50. Through the years he acquired close to one hundred patents in the electrical field.***

As far back as 1911, Dr. Lee had begun a systematic search of medical literature to assemble facts that could help to establish a rational theory of function of the ductless glands or endocrine system, a subject that was almost totally ignored at that time. The culmination of his project came in 1929 when he was able to produce a food-based, natural state package of nutrients in the most potent and "bioavailable form" which he named Catalyn. It was derived from the following whole foods: defatted wheat germ; carrots; nutritional yeast; bovine adrenal, liver, spleen, and kidney; bovine spleen; dried pea (vine) juice; dried alfalfa juice; mushroom; oat flour; soy bean lecithin; and rice bran extract. At the outset his product was provided at no charge solely for the health and welfare of his mother and intimate friends. *However, because of the remarkable results the product achieved, the fame of this food concentrate spread rapidly. The volume of demand reached such proportions that he had to create a new company, the Vitamin Products Company.*

In 1941 Dr. Lee organized the Lee foundation for Nutritional Research under a state charter as a nonprofit organization. The purpose of the Lee Foundation was to engage in research and to coordinate and communicate nutritional breakthroughs from laboratories around the world. The Foundation was the world's largest clearinghouse for nutritional information for doctors, agriculturists, and homemakers. During its existence the Lee Foundation disseminated millions of pieces of literature and hundreds of thousands of books on health and nutrition.
(http://www.westonaprice.org/nutritiongreats/lee.html)

I found it quite interesting that Bell Telephone Laboratories sold a speed governor for $1,200, which Dr. Lee sold to them for only $3.50! Then, one thing not discussed in this article, is that over a period of 30 years, Dr. Lee only averaged 5% profit, yet according to the research by the *Life Extension Foundation*, (found under "What Drugs Really Cost"), the average markup on some of the more popular medications on the market, (comparing the list price versus the cost of ingredients), was found to be over 65,000 percent! Not only that, but the FDA once confiscated thousand of dollars worth of *Life Extension*'s supplements, basically attempting to put them out of business, which fortunately they were again unable to do. They just happen to have a very good attorney, (although it's unfortunate that is necessary). Far too often, many are unnecessarily forced to defend themselves, when they have done absolutely nothing wrong, unless being a threat to the pharmaceutical giants is somehow a crime. Worst of all, our tax dollars are being wrongfully employed by the FDA to provide protection to a very profitable industry, who could easily afford their own defense.

Of particular interest was how Catalyn was portrayed, as a "patent medicine", although it's instead a "natural supplement". Then I would like for you to consider an obvious deception, when comparing the ingredients that they claimed Catalyn contained, versus the "actual ingredients". They never even came close! It just so happens that Catalyn is just one of their products I have taken for years, yet if it contained the ingredients they wrongfully claimed it did, I definitely wouldn't be taking it. The supplements I personally do take are based on more than four decades of nutritional research. One thing I have learned over the years is, concentrates of "God's creations" (which applies to Catalyn) are both the safest, and by far the most beneficial of all.

Dr. Bruce West claims that *"Kids respond better to nutritional therapy than adults. And if they are given a good start, without being overwhelmed with invasive high-tech birthing and powerful drugs, they truly flourish"* (*Health Alert* newsletter, March 2007, Vol. 24, p. 4). He then goes on to say that ***"Catalyn by Standard Process is the best of all supplements for children"*** (p. 6). Incidentally, that's the "very same Catalyn" that PhRMA, under the guise of QuackWatch[SM], attempted to discredit, by deliberately misrepresenting its ingredients. If there is anything that troubles me, it's deliberate deception, especially when millions of lives are at stake.

If you're still unsure, just consider a few of the following facts for a moment:

1. First, consider who is motivated by money: Dr. Lee, or the pharmaceutical giants, (5% versus 65,000%)?
2. Why would any organization deliberately attempt to portray Dr. Lee, (an individual that contributed so much to society during his lifetime), as some common criminal?
3. Why would they then "totally misrepresent" the ingredients in Catalyn, and thus portray it as being basically useless, although quite the contrary is true, (which I can personally attest to).
4. Why does our body consider the "inorganic chemicals" called "medications", (that cost so little to produce, yet sell for so much), as toxins that must be eliminated? It obviously knows difference between nutrients and toxins!
5. Why is it that the healthiest, longest-living people in the world never take drugs (legal or illegal, prescription, or over-the-counter)?

We should stop ignoring the facts, and consider the obvious. We all know our body is organic, so why should we expect any "inorganic chemical" to possibly be of any benefit? The answer is, they are not, which is something that our liver is fully aware of, (as is Our Creator). Then if you still don't believe me, I suggest you pray about it, (something I depend upon on a regular basis). I would assume that we should both receive the very same answer.

Incidentally, Dr. Bruce West has used *Standard Process*™ supplements almost exclusively in his practice for decades, and has proven the claims Dr. Lee made years ago, to be true, that: *"some 700,000 people a year die of preventable and curable heart disease caused by* [a] *deficiency of natural vitamins,"* (just part of the information the FDA referred to as false, but was proven by Dr. West to be true), yet the number is far greater today. Dr. West claims he has been successful in curing "tens of thousands" of those suffering with cardiomyopathy, congestive heart failure, and even mitral valve prolapse, (basically heart disease, in general), using their complete vitamins that were derived from a natural source. He claims that it's impossible to achieve the same results with most vitamins. One important ingredient found in Standard Process's natural vitamin B complex called Cataplex B™ is vitamin B_4, which you likely never heard of before, and will not be found in other B-complex formulas.

In my book *A Drug-Free Approach To Healthcare*, (which is now available in the 2007 *Revised Edition*), I explain how these heart conditions can be, and have been, resolved. Both the heart and liver are very resilient, and can often be restored back to normal, by using the proper supplements. Medications are most often the greatest contributor to both heart and liver damage. Once you get off the drugs that are creating the damage, you can then begin the restoration process. Many of Dr. West's patients were those whose cardiologists had basically given up on them. Not only that, but it was often the medications their prior doctors had placed them on that actually contributed to their problem in the first place! Why must we continue making the very same mistakes in medicine, when we have ample proof there is a much better way, (one that PhRMA would prefer you were unaware of)? Thus they were formed, to promote false information, and now you know their mission!

The Long History Of Corruption

There's so much corruption connected with the major drug companies, that it's rather difficult to keep up with it all. And it's been going on for years!

15-Year History of SSRI Litigation

Unbeknownst to most people, hundreds of SSRI suicide lawsuits have been ongoing behind the scenes for more than 15 years and Baum Hedlund has been involved from the start. ***The drug makers have done everything in their power to keep these cases from going to trial.***

In one of the only three cases to ever go to trial, <u>Eli Lilly was caught corrupting the judicial process</u> by making a deal with the plaintiff's attorney to throw the case, in part by not disclosing damaging evidence to the jury.

The case involved a Kentucky man on Prozac, who went to his workplace and opened fire with an assault rifle killing 8 people, and injuring 12 others before turning the gun on himself. The jury returned a 9-to-3 verdict in favor of Lilly.

In the media, Lilly touted the verdict as a vindication for Prozac, but the judge in the case figured out what had happened and was outraged that a secret settlement occurred behind his back. He complained to a reporter from the British Broadcasting Company, stating:

"After the verdict came in, Eli Lilly gave it a great deal of publicity and various people went on television and on the radio and in newspapers proclaiming that this was a vindication of Prozac. *I think the public has a right to expect that a trial is a bona fide contest and not some sort of show that one side puts on with the consent of the other to influence public opinion. Because* ***it was done to discourage other plaintiffs and to help settle the pending lawsuits for less money than they might have been settled otherwise."***

The judge, in the end, took the matter to the Kentucky Supreme Court, which found that "there was a serious lack of candor with the trial court and ***there may have been deception, bad faith conduct, abuse of judicial process and, <u>perhaps even fraud</u>."***

> ***The judge later revoked the verdict and instead, recorded the case as settled. The value of the secret settlement deal has been reported to be over $20 million*** (http://www.sierratimes.com/06/12/28/75_7_240_61_62632.htm).

The tremendous profits involved have to be obvious, when you consider that Eli Lilly has been settling thousands of lawsuits for damages, **caused by the very same drugs that not only remain on the market today, but are even continuing to be aggressively promoted for pregnant women, and young children**!

How President Bush Contributed To The Corruption

The obvious question is, **what ever happened to the FDA?** Investigative reporter Evelyn Pringle shares even more, in another one of her online articles, titled **"The Bush Administration's FDA"**, as follows:

> ***Since the Bush administration took control of the FDA,*** *editorial pages in the major newspapers, along with respected medical journals, have broadcast* ***outrage over the agency's failure to protect the public from an industry focused on profits only.***
>
> *And a number of current and former FDA employees have come forward to say that* ***the politically appointed officials at the top of the agency have sold out to the very industry that it is supposed to regulate.***
>
> *One does not have look far back in history to substantiate that allegation.* ***Two months after the last FDA commissioner, Lester Crawford, was confirmed, MSNBC ran the headline, "Embattled Food and Drug Administration Commissioner Lester Crawford abruptly resigned Friday, telling his staff that at age 67 it was time to step aside."*** **[MY OBSERVATION: After two whole months, wow – he must really tire fast!]**
>
> ***"As late as 2004, former Food and Drug Administration head Lester Crawford or his wife owned stock in companies that make or distribute products regulated by the agency," the Wall Street Journal reported on October 26, 2005.***
>
> *Representative, Maurice Hinchey (D-NY), led the call last year for an investigation into* ***Mr. Crawford's sudden resignation with a focus on potential financial conflicts of interest.*** *On October 16, 2006, he released a statement saying,* ***"Senior officials at the FDA have led the agency down a dark road into a state of crisis."***
>
> ***"By blatantly ignoring the law on financial holdings and conflicts of interest,"*** *Rep. Hinchey stated,* ***"Lester Crawford used his position as the head of the FDA to send all the wrong signals to other FDA employees and the American public."***

"It is not possible for the FDA to fairly and impartially regulate the food and drug industries," he said, "when the commissioner of the agency has a vested financial interest in the results."

"The days of letting the FDA treat the pharmaceutical industry as a client rather than a regulated entity," Rep. Hinchey stated, "must come to an end."

After leaving the FDA, Mr. Crawford went directly to a new job with a firm called Policy Directions. On its Web site, the firm states, "PDI has longstanding relationships with key personal and committee staffs in Congress, as well as with critical players at important agencies within the Administration."

In February 2004, the FDA held an advisory committee meeting to discuss whether there was a link between SSRI antidepressants, and suicidality in children and Dr. Andrew Mosholder, the FDA's expert on the issue, conducted a study and reported that there was.

However, it has since been learned that ***his superiors suppressed his findings, canceled his presentation to the advisory committee,*** *and gave Dr. Moshlder a script to read if he were asked why he was no longer making a presentation before the committee.*

FDA employees brave enough to speak out about wrongdoing have formed a strong alliance with ***Senator Chuck Grassley (R-Iowa),*** *the outgoing chairman of the Finance Committee, who has been one of the FDA's most out-spoken critics since the Vioxx and SSRI debacles, and* ***has called for a "major overhaul and a culture change at the highest levels" of the FDA.***

In July 2006, the Senator even wrote a letter to Daniel Levinson, the Inspector General at HHS, asking for an investigation into whether Dr. Brian Harvey of the FDA, conspired against Dr. Graham by providing Merck with the details about his Vioxx presentation before the hearing in November 2004, to help Merck refute Dr. Graham's testimony.

"It is no secret that Dr. Graham was and is a critic of the FDA," Senator Grassley wrote. "However, ***that does not mean the FDA should scheme with drug sponsors to discredit its own employees,****" he said.*

Top FDA officials have not only disregarded warnings from the agency's own scientists, they have also pressured scientists to change their findings regarding the safety and efficacy of pharmaceutical products. Most notably, Dr. Mosholder and Dr. Graham, were pressured to alter their findings regarding SSRIs and Vioxx, but the practice appears to be more wide-spread than previously thought.

A July 20, 2006, report by the Union of Concerned Scientists (UCS) and the Public Employees for Environmental Responsibility (PEER), said that approximately one-fifth of the nearly 1,000 FDA scientists who responded to a survey stated that they had been asked, for nonscientific reasons, to alter or exclude technical information or conclusions.

And, ***one-fifth said that they have been asked explicitly by FDA decision-makers to provide incomplete, inaccurate or misleading information to the public, industry, the media and government officials.***

The UCS also cited an earlier survey by the HHS Office of Inspector General in which ***nearly one in five scientists said they had been pressured to approve or recommend approval of a new drug despite concerns about its safety, effectiveness, or quality.***

The UCS survey found that ***over one-third of the scientists said they could not openly express any concerns about public health within the FDA without fear of retaliation.***

Congressman Hinchey released a statement on June 24, 2006, in response to the report, which he said, "shed light on the serious and widespread problems at the FDA."

"One of the more disturbing findings of the study," he said, "is that ***more than half of the scientists at the FDA said their job satisfaction has decreased over the past few years during President Bush's time in office."***

"Under this president," he noted, "the FDA has decided to let politics overrule science."

We saw it with the way in which Vioxx, Bextra, and other drugs were mismanaged, Rep. Hinchey stated, and "in the agency's repeated efforts to preempt state law in order to minimize drug company accountability under former Counsel Daniel Troy."

"We must end the financial link and inappropriately close relationship between the drug industry and the FDA, eliminate conflicts of interest on FDA advisory committees, *and vastly improve the agency's post-market drug safety operations," he advised.*

"We must return the FDA to a time," he said, "when science was the only consideration for approving a drug, not politics."

(http://www.sierratimes.com/07/01/16/75_8_40_104_55147.htm)

Merck and The New Gardasil™ Vaccine - A Prime Example

The following testimony of Dr. David J. Graham, M.D., M.P.H., (November 18, 2004), exemplifies the tremendous influence that Merck wields with the FDA: ***"Prior to approval of Vioxx, a study was performed by Merck named 090. This study found nearly a 7-fold increase in heart attack risk with low dose Vioxx. <u>The labeling at approval said nothing about heart attack risks</u>"*** (http://www.senate.gov/~finance/hearings/testimony/2004test/111804dgtest.pdf).

It appears that Merck couldn't care less about the safety of a drug, as long as the profit potential was sufficient, and they could somehow get FDA approval. And now we have another prime example of Merck's tremendous influence with the FDA, by their ability to fast track the approval of their Gardasil™ vaccine, followed by their extensive lobbying power with state and federal legislators. If they achieve their goal, it will be mandated that every single pre-adolescent girl in the nation will receive three injections, at $120 each, (a total of $360 per child).

Some things to consider:

1. First, according to the National Cancer Institute, a small percentage of women (approximately 8 in 100,000) actually get cervical cancer. Although, by far the majority (92%) actually recovers when detected early.

2. Then, the vast majority of women who do acquire cervical cancer are over the age of 40, (not in the 16 to 26 year range, as those involved in the study conducted by Merck).

3. Merck claims that Gardasil™ can only prevent 70% of cervical cancers. So, if someone did get the series of injections, and later acquired cervical cancer, they would of course fall into the 30% not covered, with absolutely no accountability or liability whatsoever on Merck's part.

4. The following was reported in the *Orange County Register* (October 7, 2005):

> *The studies tested Merck's Gardasil vaccine for six months on more than 12,000 women in 13 countries.*
>
> *The latest Merck studies enrolled sexually active female volunteers age 16 to 26. They were given the recommended three doses of Gardasil over six months and then tested for either cervical cancer or precancerous cervical lesions.*
>
> *All of those who received the drug remained disease-free after being followed an average of 17 months, Merck said.*
>
> *But questions remain. Will girls vaccinated at age 9 remain protected into adulthood?*

5. If the study lasted just under 2 years, including the "average" 17-month follow up, and only 12,000 young women ages 16 to 26 were involved, what are the chances that any of them would have acquired cervical cancer to begin with? Even if the Gardasil™ vaccine was <u>totally</u>

ineffective, it's not that likely that any of them would actually acquire cervical cancer, (especially in that age group)!

6. It's interesting that the "average" follow up period just happened to be a total of 17 months – one month short of completing the two years' study period. The obvious question is: Were some studies deliberately terminated earlier due to some potential problems, while others' time might have been extended to make up the difference? Manipulating the results would be so easy under the circumstances.

7. One can't help but wonder why Merck chose to conduct their study in 13 countries. After traveling extensively over the years, I believe I know the answer. Although we definitely have more than our share of corruption in this country, believe me, it's far worse in other countries. You could easily buy whatever conclusion you might want, if you are willing to spend the money, (and Merck definitely has the financial resources to do so). Spending money in the right places is one way that Merck definitely excels!

8. Then we can't ignore the serious events (including **17 deaths**, discussed next), which is not typical for young women in that age group. Although life has very little value in some third-world countries, young girls in this country, (where life does have tremendous value), will now be getting the vaccine. We have absolutely no way of knowing what the long-term risks might be, or possibly if some condition they might later develop could have been associated with the Gardasil™ vaccine, which Merck would of course deny.

9. There is a major flaw in our current drug approval process, (and has been for quite some time), which is reflected in Merck's study. For instance, companies can now conduct their own studies, and could easily conduct parallel studies, and then choose the one with the most favorable results, for FDA approval, (an all too common practice). Conducting smaller studies in 13 different countries would provide a perfect opportunity for doing just that. And who would be the wiser if they did? It's a well known fact that when companies are allowed to conduct their own studies, the chances for FDA approval nearly doubles, and it's easy to see why. Then the obvious question remains: Why in the world was it necessary for Merck to go outside the US to conduct their studies to begin with, and then why would the FDA possibly allow them to do so? The FDA is "supposed to be in charge" of establishing the criteria for conducting a "reliable study", which in my opinion doesn't appear to be true regarding Merck's study.

When you look at the odds, and the potential risks involved, how can we possibly subject young girls to that kind of risk, while also greatly increasing the cost of our already over-burdened healthcare system in the process, especially with no real proven benefit, (except for Merck, of course)!

MERCK'S GARDASIL VACCINE NOT PROVEN SAFE FOR LITTLE GIRLS
National Vaccine Information Center Criticizes FDA for Fast Tracking Licensure

Washington, D.C. - The National Vaccine Information Center (NVIC) is ***calling on the CDC's Advisory Committee on Immunization Practices (ACIP) to just say***

"no" on June 29 to recommending "universal use" of Merck's Gardasil vaccine in all pre-adolescent girls. *NVIC maintains that Merck's clinical trials did not prove the human papillomavirus (HPV) vaccine designed to prevent cervical cancer and genital warts is safe to give to young girls.*

"Merck and the FDA have not been completely honest with the people about the pre-licensure clinical trials," *said NVIC president Barbara Loe Fisher. "This is not just about teenagers having sex, it is also about whether Gardasil has been proven safe and effective for little girls."*

The FDA allowed Merck to use a potentially reactive aluminum containing placebo as a control for most trial participants, rather than a non-reactive saline solution placebo. Merck and the FDA did not disclose how much aluminum was in the placebo.

Animal and human studies have shown that aluminum can cause nerve cell death and that vaccine aluminum adjuvants can allow aluminum to enter the brain. Nearly 90 percent of Gardasil recipients and 85 percent of aluminum placebo recipients followed-up for safety reported one or more adverse events within 15 days of vaccination*, particularly at the injection site. Pain and swelling at injection site occurred in approximately 83 percent of Gardasil and 73 percent of aluminum placebo recipients.* ***About 60 percent of those who got Gardasil or the aluminum placebo had systemic adverse events including headache, fever, nausea, dizziness, vomiting, diarrhea, myalgia. Gardasil recipients had more serious adverse events such as headache, gastroenteritis, appendicitis, pelvic inflammatory disease, asthma, bronchospasm and arthritis.***

Clinical trial investigators dismissed most of the 102 Gardasil and placebo associated serious adverse events, including 17 deaths, that occurred in the clinical trials as unrelated.

"Nobody at Merck, the CDC or FDA know if the injection of Gardasil into all pre-teen girls - especially simultaneously with hepatitis B vaccine - will make some of them more likely to develop arthritis or other inflammatory autoimmune and brain disorders as teenagers and adults. ***With cervical cancer causing about one percent of all cancer deaths in American women due to routine pap screening, it was inappropriate for the FDA to fast track Gardasil.*** *It is way too early to direct all young girls to get three doses of a vaccine that has not been proven safe or effective in their age group."*

The National Vaccine Information Center (NVIC), founded in 1982 by parents of vaccine injured children, has been a leading critic of one-size-fits-all mass vaccination policies and ***the lack of basic science research into biological mechanisms and high risk factors for vaccine-induced brain and immune system dysfunction*** (http://www.nvic.org/PressReleases/pr62706gardasil.htm).

One question is: Were any of the parents of the children in this study made aware that **they would "all be exposed to aluminum", which was proven in human studies to enter the brain and cause nerve cell death?** That is especially a concern regarding children on drugs such as Prozac™, which contains high levels of fluoride. And might they have possibly had fluoride in their drinking water as well? Fluoride doesn't always have to be added to drinking water, as we sometimes do in this country, (other countries know better). It is an environmental toxin, found in various countries with prior volcanic activity. In the next chapter, titled "Prozac™ and The Dangerous Fluoride Connection", we will discuss how just a small amount of aluminum, combined with fluoride, can contribute to chronic fatigue, by suppressing the immune system, and to major antioxidants, as well as depleting the energy molecule ATP, (a major concern), and for what?

Interestingly, sixty percent of those who received either Gardasil™ or the "aluminum placebo" actually had many of the very same side effects that parallel symptoms of those experienced by people just before coming down with chronic fatigue. Although the Gardasil™ recipients experienced some of the most serious adverse events, "including 17 deaths", the clinical trial investigators somehow dismissed them as "unrelated"!

I can't help but wonder how that determination was made! I would guess that most people would be totally shocked if they only knew how many medical opinions or conclusions were actually bought and paid for, although the fees in other countries are not nearly as highly inflated as ours are. Incidentally, if you noticed at the beginning of the previous article, the approval of this vaccine weighed heavily on recommendations from the Advisory Committee on Immunization Practices (ACIP). Research has uncovered the fact that the executive secretary for this advisory committee just happens to be Dr. Larry Pickering, M.D., the *"former Chairman of DLJMB Global healthcare Partners, with a distinguished background in various senior management positions for Johnson & Johnson"* (http://www.avistacap.com/industry-executives-pickering.html). It was also discovered that:

> ***During his more than three decades with Johnson & Johnson, Mr. Pickering held key positions in pharmaceuticals, including service as President of*** *Ortho Dermatology and* ***Janssen Pharmaceuticals****, and Chairman of Janssen North America*. ***In that role, he helped refocus the Janssen strategy and align its operations for a six-fold increase in revenues during his tenure.***

How convenient.

Why Does It Always Seem To Start In Texas?

And then somehow, according to the *Los Angeles Times*, ***"Texas on Friday became the first state to require school-age girls be vaccinated against a virus – typically transmitted through sex – that has been shown to cause cervical cancer"*** (*The Register-Guard*, February 3, 2007). And the article continues:

> ***Gov. Rick Perry signed an executive order mandating that most girls, starting in September 2008, receive the vaccination against the human papilloma virus, or HPV, prior to entering sixth grade.***

The federal government approved an HPV vaccine last year, and a government advisory panel has recommended that all girls get shots at age 11 or 12 – before they begin having sex. But the American College of Pediatricians, a socially conservative group, has opposed any vaccination requirement, calling that a "precedent-setting action that trespasses on the right of parents to make medical decisions for their children, as well as on the rights of the children to attend school."

By sidestepping the legislature, Perry** – a conservative Republican – **avoided a showdown with GOP lawmakers and Christian organizations** that oppose mandatory HPV vaccinations on the grounds that teaching young people to avoid premarital sex is a better solution. **The mandate would affect roughly 365,000 girls a year.

*The move drew immediate criticism from conservative groups, which noted that **the governor had accepted campaign contributions from Merck & Co., the drug company that manufactures the vaccine**.*

*"**All Merck wanted was a mandate so the insurance companies would have to pay for this**. Follow the money," said Cathie Adams, president of the Texas Eagle Forum, an organization that promotes socially conservative policies. **Merck has been pushing for laws mandating its Gardasil vaccine in numerous states**.*

The New Jersey-based drug company donated $6,000 to Perry's reelection campaign last year, Texas campaign finance records show. One of its top Texas lobbyists, Mike Toomey, is Perry's former chief of staff. Merck was paying Toomey between $25,000 and $50,000 to influence politicians, according to disclosure reports.

Apparently Merck has also funneled money through "Women in Government", an advocacy group made up of female state legislators around the country, sponsored by many pharmaceutical companies, including Abbott laboratories, AstraZeneca, Bristol-Myers Squibb, GlaxoSmithKline, Johnson & Johnson, Merck, Novartis, Wyeth, Pfizer, PhRMA, and Eli Lilly! In fact, their website boasts EIGHTY-ONE different "sponsors", including such contributors as ExxonMobil, Anheuser-Busch Companies, Inc., and Wholesale Beer Distributors of Arkansas, Inc., (clearly mentioned on their website at http://www.womeningovernment.org/home/)! And not only has Merck conveniently chosen women in government to promote their new vaccine, but another example of their craftiness was cited in an article in the local newspaper, the *Register Guard* (February 5, 2007), as follows:

*Dr. Audrey Garrett, a gynecological oncologist with Women's Care in Eugene, who also has a master's degree in public health, is a staunch supporter of Gardasil, and, since last fall, **Merck & Co. has paid her to be part of its speakers bureau, traveling around the Northwest talking to medical professionals about the vaccine.***

The Latest Discovery Regarding Gardasil™

Research published in the May 10, 2007 issue of the *New England Journal of Medicine* (Vol. 356, No. 19), has apparently raised "serious questions " about its effectiveness, as follows:

> *Although Gardasil blocked almost 100 percent of infections by two strains of HPV, it only reduced the incidence of cervical cancer precursors by 17 percent. One possible reason is that many of the women examined to obtain this information had already been exposed to the virus. But Gardasil may also, by blocking only specific strains, allow other varieties of HPV to flourish.*

I would assume there will likely be more discoveries in the future, regarding Gardasil™, just as there were regarding Vioxx™ (another of Merck's contributions to society).

This Kind Of Obvious Corruption Absolutely Must Be Stopped!

First it was Ritalin™, followed by Prozac™, and then other more potent SSRI antidepressants such as Paxil™ soon followed. Now there are the atypical antipsychotic drugs such as Zyprexa™, and finally, the mandatory injections with a new vaccine with no long-term studies to prove its safety! It took years to discover how dangerous Vioxx™ was, and you can rest assured that Merck is not about to do any future long-term follow-up studies on the girls in thirteen different countries, unless the FDA required them to! What in the world are they trying to do to our kids? And just for the sake of making a few billion! In fact, drug-industry analyst Steve Brozak of W.B.B. Securities has **projected Gardasil™ sales of at least one billion dollars per year,** (even billions more if states start requiring the vaccine), and comments: *"I could not think of a bigger boost,"* (http://www.msnbc.msn.com/id/16891832/).

It's obvious what Merck is now up to. They are just following the very same route, (via Texas), which has proven successful in the past, in getting their drugs approved for kids under the new TeenScreen program. They somehow managed to totally bypass the normal process of conducting studies on children, and requesting FDA approval for children's use. They had already established a successful route: First, start with Texas, and then go nationwide. It was obviously a deliberate attempt to fast track one of their most profitable creations ever, in president Bush's home state, and do so while he was still in office. At $360 per child, for the serious of three injections, the profit potential is huge, as is the added expense to our healthcare system, which is already under-funded!

There is absolutely no excuse for allowing such obvious corruption to continue any longer. It rather reminds me of the illegal drug cartels, with their huge financial resources – it's just legal. And worst of all, we the taxpayers, will be the ones supporting Merck, with our ever-increasing healthcare costs, which are already out of sight, (by far the highest in the entire world). Yet we have the poorest health of any of the developed nations in the world, (something is obviously wrong with that picture). Our federal government might soon be required to acquire a loan from Eli Lilly and Merck to help fund our escalating healthcare costs – something they would likely agree to, as they would just continue getting back a large percentage of our healthcare expenditures!

CHAPTER THREE

Prozac™ And The Dangerous Fluoride Connection

We will first take a look at what Prozac™ is chemically composed of. The generic name of Prozac™ is **Fluo**xetine hydrochloride, which gives us a clue as to its true identity, or chemical make up. Dr. Sherry A. Rogers, M.D., author of the book *Detoxify or Die* (2002), focuses on the many toxins we are all exposed to, and the concerns regarding each one, and points out that **every molecule of Prozac™ (fluoxetine) actually contains *"three molecules of the toxin fluoride"*!**

And as noted by Dr. Michael Schlachter, M.D., ***"Prior to 1945, fluoride was properly regarded as an environmental pollutant. This fluoride destroyed crops and animals,*** *leading to lawsuits."* Dr. Schlachter explains, as follows:

> ***Power tactics including threats, ridicule and frank censorship aimed at scientists and clinicians knowledgeable about fluoridation have prevented the truth about fluoride from being disseminated to the science world as well as to the public.***
>
> *Epidemiology research in the mid-1970s by the late Dr. Dean Bur, head of the cytochemistry division of the National Cancer Institute, indicated that* ***10,000 or more fluoridation-linked cancer deaths occur yearly in the United States.*** *In 1989,* ***the ability of fluoride to transfer normal cells into cancer cells was confirmed by Argonne National Laboratories.***
>
> ***Fluoride even at dosages of 1 part per million, found in artificially fluoridated water, can inhibit enzyme systems, damage the immune system, contribute to calcification of soft tissues, worsen arthritis and, of course, cause dental fluorosis in children*** (http://www.mbschachter.com/dangers_of_fluoride_and_fluorida.htm).

The Many Dangers Associated With Fluoride Exposure

In her book *Prozac: Panacea or Pandora?* (1991/1994), Dr. Ann Blake Tracy refers to Dr. Craig N. Karson, a professor of psychiatry and pathology at the University of Arkansas and Chief of Psychiatry at John McClellan Memorial Veterans Hospital, who discovered that **Prozac™ accumulates at high levels in the brain, which he learned was actually 100 times the level normally found in the bloodstream!** Dr. Karson indicates that **one woman had been on Prozac™ for one year, and off for two years, yet upon autopsy, it was discovered that the level of Prozac™ in her brain was much higher than he had anticipated.** This was confirmed by another study reported in *Neurotoxicology and Teratology*, ("Neurotoxicity of Sodium Fluoride", Muellenix, Denbesten, Schunior, Kernan, 1995, Vol. 17, No. 2, p. 176), stating ***"Fluorides accumulate in the brain over time to reach neurologically harmful levels."***

Dr. Tracy also points out that *"patients have reported consistently that other drugs cause a variety of adverse reactions for them long after their use of Prozac"* (p. 123).

The fluoride in Prozac™ is very efficient at undermining the liver's attempt to detoxify and remove it, (basically its self defense). Unfortunately, fluoride contributes to some serious conditions in the body and brain, as its characteristics allow it to basically bypass a great deal of the detoxification process in the liver, allowing it to accumulate at higher levels, (especially in the bones and brain).

Then we find **that whenever there is a deficiency of calcium, magnesium, and/or vitamin C, fluoride accumulates at higher levels,** making us more susceptible to its toxic effects. The problem is, **"Prozac™ actually depletes all three nutrients",** (aren't drugs fascinating?)! Only by truly understanding just how dangerous high levels of Prozac™, (and thus fluoride), in the brain can really be, can you fully appreciate the importance of avoiding them like the plague! They pose a "serious threat" to everyone's physical and mental health, (young or old).

Prozac™ (Fluoride) – Increasing the Cancer Risk

According to an article published April 2002 in the *Journal of the American Society of Hematology*, ***"Antidepressants in the class called SSRIs (Prozac, Luvox, Paxil, Zoloft, Celexa) could potentially increase the risk for brain cancer,** according to some researchers."* The article continues, as follows:

> *Professor John Gordon of Birmingham University found that SSRIs encouraged the growth of Burkitt's Lymphoma, a type of cancer, in test tube experiments.*
>
> *The mechanism of action for this increased risk is by blocking the body's natural ability to kill tumor cells. Gordon, whose results have been published online in the journal Blood, says that serotonin is a key player in stimulating apoptosis, a natural programmed cell death which brings into control runaway cell growth. Without this process to rein in these renegade cells, cancer may develop.*
>
> *The specific drugs investigated by Gordon were Prozac, Paxil and Celexa. Since the early 80s, Prozac has been the leading antidepressant prescribed worldwide, but recently overtaken by Paxil with $2.7 billion in sales in 2001.*
> (http://www.bloodjournal.org/cgi/content/abstract/99/7/2545)

At first, the above might appear to be a contradiction, as it was noted that serotonin stimulates apoptosis, or programmed cell death of renegade cells that can develop into cancer. What many fail to understand is: **The SSRI antidepressants "do not" produce serotonin!** They instead override the normal reuptake of "excess serotonin" in the synapses, so it could be used elsewhere, (such as controlling runaway cell growth). For example, according to Dr. F. Batmanghelidj, M.D., the late author of *Are You Sick Or Are You Just Thirsty*, another function of serotonin is storing energy.

Overriding the body's natural process with drugs can have unseen consequences. We can often find a logical explanation for all their seemingly unexplainable side effects, if we just do a little detective work, (my specialty). Drugs tend to create "far more" problems than they resolve, although they are not actually created to "truly resolve" anything, (that's not where the money is). Once you learn of all the chaos they create, in both the body and brain, I believe you'll agree as well. Then keep in mind that there might very well be some additional risks that even I am still unaware of as well! And just from what we do know, their potential for damage to both the body and brain are unbelievably extensive.

Dr. Rogers also notes that **fluoride is *"known to cause excessive calcification, not only in arteries but joints and ligaments, and contributes to many forms of cancer and osteoporosis."*** The arteries of greatest concern, regarding the brain are the carotid arteries, which supply the brain with oxygen and nutrients. So, this is just one of several ways that Prozac™ can have a negative influence on brain function. **And then the fact that fluoride (found in Prozac™) was also found to cause normal cells to convert into cancer cells, that is likely an explanation for the dramatic increase in the rate of cancer in children as well.**

Fluoride's Damage To The Liver

This becomes obvious in the following statement by Professor Dzulkifi Abdul Razak, from the National Poison Centre at University Sains Malaysia, issued September 2, 2001:

Poison Control: Fluorides, the deadly toxin within

> *According to a recently released commentary by a Canadian group,* ***Parents of Fluoride Poisoned Children* [PFPC], *a series of fluoride-containing drugs or so-called fluorinated drugs have been withdrawn from the market in the last 10 years due to their toxic effects on human beings*.**
>
> ***In the liver especially,* organic fluoride compounds undergo extensive transformation,** *mainly via oxidative demethylation, involving the thyroid hormone (T3) mediated P-450 enzyme system. And* ***the resulting metabolites may have higher activity and/or greater toxicity than the original compound.***
>
> ***The activity of organic fluoride compounds on the P-450 enzyme system is critical as it relates to the elimination of many other drugs. Inhibition of these enzymes can cause other drugs to accumulate to dangerous levels in the body, leading to hazardous drug-drug interactions.*** *In many cases fluorinated drugs are being implicated as documented in hundreds of well-established studies* (http://bruha.com/pfpc/html/malaysia/html).

If you noticed, Professor Razak posed another concern, regarding fluoride-containing drugs, (which includes Prozac™), and the potential for a greater toxicity of the metabolite of fluoride in the liver, (which is entirely possible). As there are many factors that could easily prolong the detoxification of fluoride, it could very well pose an even greater risk than the exposure to fluoride itself would. It would be interesting to know what the metabolite of fluoride might be, and what it's potential influence on the liver and brain might possibly be as well. The truth is, no one really knows exactly how he or she might respond to these very risky, and inherently unpredictable medications. And the more medications a person might be taking, the greater the risk for experiencing some of the more serious side effects. The particular antidepressant prescribed also comes into play, as does the prescribed dosage. That's why all drugs are potentially dangerous and inherently unpredictable, (especially the psychiatric drugs).

Prozac™ and The Chronic Fatigue Connection (Fluoride and Aluminum – Partners In Crime)

Although Prozac™ doesn't contain aluminum, at three molecules of fluoride for every molecule of Prozac™, it definitely contains more than its share of fluoride! Then you will find that aluminum is surprisingly ubiquitous, (it's amazing how many different things aluminum will be found in). You actually have to be very vigilant in order to avoid aluminum. As you already learned, fluoride alone is capable of creating havoc throughout the body and brain. Yet, once fluoride gets together with its partner in crime (aluminum), its potential for damage is even greater. The fluoride/aluminum combination can begin shutting down your immune system, depleting the two primary detoxifiers resulting in the accumulation of toxins, and greatly depleting your energy level. It's rather scary when you consider the many different ways, (directly or indirectly), that Prozac™ can destroy your health, (especially your mental health). And worst of all, doctors continue placing pregnant mothers, and even very young children on it!

As you might have guessed, **Prozac™ combined with aluminum, (even found in common table salt), is setting the stage for a condition called Chronic Fatigue Syndrome (CFS).** The condition was first identified, and labeled CFS, (or CFID) in the mid 1980s. Incidentally, that was about the time that Eli Lilly announced Prozac™, and in my opinion, at least one reason more and more people are being diagnosed with CFS. Most doctors claim the cause is unknown, and that there is no known cure for CFS. The first step is to identify the cause.

Dr. Paul Cheney is in my opinion, one of the most knowledgeable doctors regarding chronic fatigue syndrome (CFS), and was apparently the first to identify at least one cause of CFS, written about by Carol Sieverling, in an article posted on the "CFS and FM Support Group of DFW" website (http://www.dfwcfids.org/medical/cheney/heart04.htm), titled ***"The Heart of the Matter: Dr. Cheney on Chronic Fatigue Syndrome and Cardiac Issues".*** Dr. Cheney discovered that, in an area of South Lake Tahoe on the California and Nevada border, people were coming down with a mononucleosis-like illness, with flu-like symptoms that seemed to persist. That is an area of volcanic origin that can at times contaminate both water wells and the soil. If it's in the well water that you water your garden with, you will obviously be contaminating the soil and thus the food in your garden. Interestingly, **"elevated fluoride" is often found in the water in areas of volcanic activity**, which just happens to be found in some of the wells in South Tahoe. These people would not only be drinking water with elevated fluoride, (similar to taking Prozac™), but it would likely be found in some locally grown produce as well.

It appears that fluoride accumulates at the highest levels in both the brain, and bone tissue. In the back of this book, under "Additional Technical Information", I discuss how fluoride disrupts the iodine receptors throughout the brain, reducing the energy level, suppressing enzyme action necessary for conversion of neurotransmitters, and damaging the hormone receptors, reducing the efficiency of the hormones or neurotransmitters. If you recall, Dr. Tracy talked of one of Dr. Cade's patients who had been on Prozac™ for only one year, and then off for two years prior to her death. He was surprised to find an amazingly high level of Prozac™, (and thus fluoride), still in her brain upon autopsy.

One of the major antioxidants, glutathione, (depleted by the combination of fluoride and aluminum), is responsible for DNA repair. When that function doesn't take place as it should, either cell apoptosis (cell death) occurs, or normal cells could mutate and turn cancerous, both serious concerns. Millions in the nation have compromised immune systems, and when the fluoride in Prozac™ gets together with aluminum, it greatly increases the rate of various viruses, (such as the Epstein Barr Virus), that many seem to experience just before the symptoms of chronic fatigue begin to emerge. For many, it can be a dramatic life-changing experience. It's well known, by those whose research focuses on achieving longevity, and maintaining optimum health, (as mine has over the years), that two critical antioxidants in particular play a dominant role. They just happen to be the very same two that begin shutting down, due to the fluoride/aluminum combination, namely **s**uper**o**xide **d**ismutase (SOD), and glutathione. What a coincidence! So we now have a perfect "aging program", all too often beginning with the fetus. This is evidenced by the fact that, **of those who are exposed to fluoride in their well water, many are already disabled at only 40 years of age.**

According to Martin L. Pall, Ph.D., professor at the School of Molecular Biosciences, Washington State University, **our body can produce a highly damaging substance called peroxynitrite, from the two substances nitric oxide and superoxide, both essential for life.** Each have separate, although important, functions. The superoxide is normally found inside the mitochondria, (or powerhouse), of the cell, and the nitric oxide outside the mitochondria. It takes one molecule of superoxide, combined with one of nitric oxide, to produce the damaging peroxynitrite, which under ideal circumstances should not take place. It's **when the two toxic substances, fluoride and aluminum, combine forces and suppress the action of two extremely critical antioxidants, (the SOD and glutathione), which normally prevent the formation of peroxynitrite, that free radical damage begins.**

Professor Pall poses the question: ***"What do humans die of, usually?"*** He then goes on to explain:

> ***The top killer is Coronary Artery Disease [CAD], and the next is cancer. It turns out that CAD and cancer are also driven in part by peroxynitrite formation. Neurodegenerative diseases like Parkinson's and Alzheimer's are also suspected of being driven by free radical formation. Even suicide is increasingly thought to be generated by oxidative stress in the central nervous system.***
> (http://www.chronicfatiguesyndromesupport.com/library/showarticle.cfm/id/6679)

The very first thing most people experience when getting off Prozac™ is a gradual return of their emotions. They often claim that it's as though the fog is beginning to lift. Unfortunately, resolving the chronic fatigue that some experience, often takes considerably longer. Then to bring their IQ level back to where it should have been, would be rather difficult, (if not impossible). What a terrible travesty, due to the dramatic influence it can have on a child's future physical and mental health; something those promoting these dangerous drugs won't be forced to deal with, although it comes at a terrible cost to millions of innocent victims that, unfortunately will.

How Does The Fluoride In Prozac™ Cause Such Fatigue?

Many who have chronic fatigue, often experience adrenal fatigue as well. As we learned, due to the 200% increase of the stress hormone cortisol, which Prozac™ causes "on a daily basis", the adrenals eventually become exhausted. And we also discovered that even the fetus sometimes attempts to supplement the mother's cortisol when necessary, so that process can even begin before birth. Doctors claim that, by far, the most common complaint they hear from their patients is fatigue, (especially with women).

It often begins with overlooking a common low thyroid condition (hypothyroidism), or prescribing the wrong thyroid hormone. Two common symptoms associated with hypothyroidism are depression, and fatigue. Unfortunately, most doctors' solution is a prescription for an SSRI antidepressant such a Prozac™, which basically contributes to a worsening of fatigue by suppressing the thyroid and depleting the adrenals, eventually leading to fatigue.

As we discussed, fluoride combined with aluminum greatly reduces your energy level. According to Dr. Phelps, this combination causes the swelling of, and thus damage to, the mitochondria (energy powerhouses of the cell). Thus the number of mitochondria in the cells is reduced, as is the amount of the primary energy molecule ATP produced in the mitochondria, (a major contributor to chronic fatigue). According to Dr. Neil Rouzier, M.D., both the number and size of the crista in the mitochondria, (responsible for producing energy), are thyroid related. And the more thyroid hormone, the more dense the crista in the mitochondria will be. Then as the elevated cortisol in Prozac™ reduces the thyroid function, and fluoride disrupts the action of iodine in the thyroid hormone as well, we can easily see why Prozac™ would contribute to reduced energy output, and thus fatigue.

Anything such as peroxynitrite, that can disrupt the ability of cells to create and then store energy, is an obvious concern. It eventually results in what's referred to as Chronic (long-term) fatigue. All cells contain mitochondria, which produce energy that is in turn stored in the energy molecule called ATP. The number of mitochondria in a cell varies considerably, and depends primarily on a cell's function, and the demand placed on a particular cell.

An athlete's muscles, for instance, contain more mitochondria than the average individual, because they consume far more energy daily than a couch potato. Those who are less active would experience more fatigue, as they don't have any mitochondria to spare to begin with. Then, if they also have a low thyroid function, (and thus less crista responsible for producing energy in each mitochondria), they would experience even greater fatigue. Some of those with chronic fatigue even have difficulty getting out of bed in the morning, let alone walking around the block.

Dr. Cheney eventually discovered that all those with Chronic Fatigue who also experienced post exertion fatigue, (fatigue following physical exertion), seemed to have one thing in common, (low Q). The "Q" is basically the number of liters of blood per minute that the heart is capable of circulating. Although normal Q is about seven liters, those with chronic fatigue typically have a Q in the range of five liters. They basically have cardiomyopathy, (or a weak heart), and thus reduced circulation, and I believe there is a good explanation. The heart muscle is known to have far more mitochondria than any other muscle in the body. Then as the fluoride/aluminum combination damages and reduces the number of mitochondria, the most active muscle (the heart) would likely experience the greatest loss, which apparently holds true. Although I could explain in greater detail exactly how the process takes place, I will spare you the details and save that for an in-depth book on Chronic Fatigue. Sometimes I have to stop and remind myself that, although we're discussing just a few of Prozac's 575 potential side effects, we can't cover them all, or discuss each one in detail, or I'd never finish this book, and you would likely not to have time to read it all.

Prozac™ - The HIV Virus (AIDS) Connection

In case you're not aware, the HIV virus attacks the immune system, although fluoride, combined with aluminum, does as well. Due to their polarity, fluoride is highly attracted to aluminum. Then, although aluminum has difficulty crossing the blood-brain barrier, and gaining access to the brain, fluoride can assist it in that regard. A perfect way to set the stage for Alzheimer's disease, and lower your children's IQ, which fluoride was proven to do in many epidemiological studies on its own. Just another concern associated with Prozac™, although we are now focusing on immune suppression, and how it could increase the risk for acquiring the HIV virus.

It's thought that fluoride tends to accumulate over a lifetime, and that the total amount of the accumulation in the body depends on the amount you are exposed to daily, multiplied by your length of exposure. Just remember you can avoid fluoride exposure now that you know where it often comes from.

According to *"The Chronic Fatigue Syndrome Report"*, (2005), by J.E. Phelps, ***"The rise of fluorides in the body is the principle trigger for HIV infections.*** *Due to the fluoride in the bone mass upsetting the beneficial trace metal* [mineral] *concentrations for cellular enzymes"* (http://members.aol.com/doewatch/cfs.html). It's the bone mass that the immune system cells are formed from. **Fluoride also leads to the shrinkage of the thymus gland, greatly increasing the immune suppression.** Phelps discovered that: *"Regions in Africa* ***with the highest fluoride in well water and food have the largest problem with HIV transmission,"*** and that *"Many of the high fluoride regions follow the east African Rift Valley Zone that is line with volcano and seismic zones. In many of these areas the persons have frosty white teeth from dental fluorosis and* ***many are disabled by age 40."*** Phelps also notes that ***"Fluoride's affinity toward beneficial trace metals*** **[minerals]** ***damages literally hundreds of enzyme processes that lead eventually toward poor health, illness, and death."***

Any drug (such as Prozac™) that has the ability to drastically influence our perceptions, turning misconceptions into reality, and eventually leads to poor health, illness and death, is obviously a serious threat!

What Else Do We Know About Fluoride?
Opinions of Fluoride - By Some Knowledgeable Professionals

Robert Carlton, Ph.D., and former U.S. EPA scientist, strongly stated: ***"Fluoridation is the greatest case of scientific fraud of this century, if not of all time"*** *("Marketplace"*, Canadian Broadcast Company, Nov 24, 1992).

The following was obtained from a study, announced by Selwyn Johnston and the Queensland Independent Senate Team (http://www.johnston-independent.com/):

> ***Fluoride is, in fact, highly poisonous,*** *and the following outlines the long list of health problems associated with it, with copious scientific references.*

- *Fluoride is described by its manufacturers' safety data as a* ***"hazardous waste."*** *It is illegal to dump it at sea.*

[MY OBSERVATION: Although it's OK to put in our drinking water!]

- ***Fluoride consumption by human beings increases the general cancer death rate.***

- *Fluoride inhibits antibody formation in the body.*

- ***Fluorides have a disruptive effect on various tissues in the body.***

- ***Fluoride confuses the immune system and causes it to attack the body's own tissues, and increases the tumour growth rate in cancer prone individuals.***
- ***Fluoride kills red blood cells*** *and damages gastric mucosa, resulting in the symptoms of "Irritable Bowel Syndrome."*

- ***Fluorides are medically categorized as protoplasmic poisons, which is why they are used to kill rodents.***

- ***Fluoride is a cumulative poison****...we excrete about half what we ingest. The rest is stored,* ***mainly in the bones****, where it increases the density* ***but changes the internal architecture of the bone. This makes bones more brittle and prone to fracture*** *(Eight papers published in reputable medical journals have described the* ***increased risk of hip fracture in elderly people living in fluoridated areas).***

Fluoride is hexafluorosilic acid – a toxic industrial waste by-product *derived from the super-phosphate fertilizer, and aluminum, industries.*

The suppliers' Safety Data Sheet for hexafluorosilicic acid clearly states: ***"Do Not let the chemical enter the environment. Dispose of this product as hazardous waste."***

Scientific studies have shown:

- ***Fluoride is implicated in genetic disorders, cancer and low IQ levels in children.***

- *Calcium levels in the body decrease as fluoride levels rise.*

- ***People who ingest fluoride risk problems as the muscles, connective tissues and bone tissue undergo degenerative changes.***

- ***Fluoride does NOT stop tooth decay!***

And, the following comments were quoted from http://www.nofluoride.com/quotes.htm:

"Fluorides are general protoplasmic poisons, probably because of their capacity to modify the metabolism of cells by changing the permeability of cell membrane and by inhibiting certain enzyme systems." -Journal of the American Medical Association (*JAMA*), Sept 18, 1943

"Segments of the population are unusually susceptible to the toxic effects of fluoride. They include....people with deficiencies of calcium, magnesium, and/or vitamin C, and people with cardiovascular and kidney problems." -United States Public Health Service Report (NATIONAL INSTITUTES OF HEALTH-91/17, p. 112, Sec.2.7, April 1993)

"...fluoride exposure, at levels that are experienced by a significant proportion of the population whose drinking water is fluoridated, may have adverse impacts on the developing brain." -Greater Boston Physicians for Social Responsibility, May 2000

"The plain fact that fluoride is an insidious poison harmful, toxic and cumulative in its effects, even when ingested in minimal amounts, will remain unchanged no matter how many times it will be repeated in print that fluoridation of the water supply is 'safe.'" -Dr. Ludgwig Grosse, Chief of Cancer Research, U.S. Veterans Administration

***"Fluoride has been shown to adversely effect the central nervous system, causing behavioral changes, increased hip fractures** and reproduction problems."* -Natick Report Research Team (Research Microbiologist, U.S. Army, Dr. B. J. Gallo; Environmental Chemist, J. Kupperschmidt; Apollo Program Project Scientist, Dr. N. R. Mancuso; U.S. Army, Natick Research Labs, A. Murray; Molecular Biologist, Dr. Strauss)

"I am appalled at the prospect of using water as a vehicle for drugs.** Fluoride is a corrosive poison that will produce serious effects on a long range basis. **Any attempt to use water this way is deplorable." -Dr. Charles Gordon Heyd, **Past President of the American Medical Association**

They are not only using our drinking water as a vehicle for the delivery of drugs, as noted, but also **"even for a proven environmental toxin"!**

It's Not Just In The Water!

Even if you aren't drinking fluoridated water, or taking SSRI antidepressants, you could still be getting fluoride from many hidden sources, such as your soft drinks, as well as beer or wine, or even tea or fruit juices.

According to research reported in the *Journal of the American Dental Association*, after examining the fluoride concentrations of 332 soft drinks, *"The fluoride levels of the products ranged from 0.02 to 1.28 ppm, with a mean level of 0.72 ppm. Fluoride levels exceeded 0.60 ppm for 71 percent of the products"* (Vol. 130, No. 11, pp. 1593 – 1599). And in another study conducted in Mexico City, Mexico, the fluoride concentration of 283 samples of soft drinks, juices, and bottled water, available in the metropolitan market of Mexico City, were found to range from 0.07 to 1.42 ppm (*International Journal of Paediatric Dentistry*, Vol. 14, Issue 4, p. 260).

Some Possible Hidden Sources Of Fluoride To Watch Out For

Fluoridated Tap Water

"Since [the 1940s], the percent of individuals consuming fluoridated water in the US) has steadily increased. ***The increase in percentage of communities with fluoridated water has resulted in an increase in the mean content of fluoride not only in soft drinks and fruits, but in canned goods (notably soups),*** *leading to increased intake of fluoride by individuals in communities with nonfluoridated water." –Fomon SJ, Ekstrand J, Ziegler EE. (2000). Journal of Public Health Dentistry 60(3):131-9.*

"Because the main component of most beverages is water, the fluoride content of these products closely parallels the fluoride content of water used in their processing." *-Levy SM, Guha-Chowdhury N. (1999). Journal of Public Health Dentistry 59:211-23.*

Infant Formula

"Our analysis shows that ***babies who are exclusively formula fed face the highest risk; in Boston, for example, more than 60 percent of the exclusively formula fed babies exceed the safe dose of fluoride on any given day.****"*
-Environmental Working Group, March 22, 2006.

"Fluoride is now introduced at a much earlier stage of human development than ever before *and consequently alters the normal fluoride-pharmacokinetics in infants.* ***But can one dramatically increase the normal fluoride-intake to infants and get away with it?"*** *-Luke J. (1997). The Effects of Fluoride on the Physiology of the Pineal Gland. PH.D. Thesis. University of Surrey, Guildford. P. 176.*

Processed Cereals

"Cereals processed in a fluoridated area had fluoride concentrations ranging from 3.8 ppm to 6.3 ppm…" -Warren JJ, Levy SM. (2003). Dental Clinics of North America 47:225-43.

"Infants who eat large quantities of dry infant cereals reconstituted with fluoridated water could ingest substantial quantities of fluoride from this source." -Heilman JR, et al. (1997). Journal of the American Dental Association 128(7):857-63.

Tea

"Another important source of fluoride ingestion is tea... [T]he fluoride content of tea has been found to range from 0.1 to 4.2 ppm fluoride, with an average of about 3 ppm." -Levy SM, Guha-Chowdhury N. (1999). Journal of Public Health Dentistry 59:211-23.

Wine

"Researchers from California State University in Fresno conducted a 5 year study (1990-1994) on vineyards throughout the San Joaquin Valley. They found that '[m]ultiple applications of Cryolite during the growing season significantly increase fluoride in wines.' Notably they found fluoride levels between 3 – 6 ppm in Zinfandel, Chardonnay, Cabernet Sauvignon, Chenin Blanc, Thompson Seedless, Barbera, Muscat Candi, Ruby Cabernet; and levels between 6 - <9 ppm in French Colombard and Zinfandel... At 6 ppm one glass of wine (175 ml) would have delivered as much fluoride as about a liter of optimally fluoridated water!" -Connett E, Connett P. (2001). Pesticides and You 21: 18-22.

Beer

"Beers brewed in locations with high fluoride water levels may contribute significantly to the daily fluoride intake, particularly in alcohol misusing subjects and this may contribute to alcohol-associated bone disease." -Warnakulasuriya S, et al. (2002). Clinica Chimica Acta 320: 1-4.

Increase In Fluoride Exposure

"Based on this review, we conclude that fluoride intakes of infants and children have shown a rather steady increase since 1930, are likely to continue to increase." *-Fomon SJ, Ekstrand J, Ziegler EE. (2000). Journal of Public Health Dentistry 60(3):131-9* (http://fluoridealert.org/f-sources.htm).

Additional warnings about tea were published in the *American Journal of Medicine* (2005 January, pp. 78-82), claiming Lipton™ Instant (2003) tea had the highest levels of fluoride at 7.7 ppm.

One specific website (http://www.nccn.net/~wwithin/fluoride.htm), devoted to the dangers of fluoride, also notes the following:

Don't drink tea: *Tea contains between 4.4 and 12 ppm of fluoride. Just one cup can be enough for an overdose.*

Take supplements of calcium and magnesium salts to help reduce fluoride absorption from the stomach and assist in elimination.

Avoid fluoride-containing drugs: *If you are taking the following, contact your doctor for a fluoride-free alternative:* ***Prozac (fluoxetine),*** *Rohypnol* *(flunitrazepam), Diflucan (fluconazole, Flixonase or Flixotide (fluticasone), Stelazine (trifluoperazine, Fluanxol or Depixol (flupenthixol) or Floxapen (flucloxacillin), and asthma drugs that use propellants containing fluoride: Ventolin and Becotide.*

Non-stick coatings, such as Teflon, are made of fluoride. ***Scrapes and other damage can release a significant amount of fluoride into cooking.***

The scrapes in Teflon™ cookware just mentioned, brings to mind another concern. Under the Teflon™ we will find aluminum! Then if you recall, earlier when we discussed Chronic Fatigue, the fluoride (found in Prozac™ and some water systems), combined with aluminum, results in the production of Proxy Nitrite, which among other things contributes to chronic fatigue. When Teflon™ cookware becomes worn, it's as though you are cooking with fluoride and aluminum. Then, acid foods such as tomatoes are the worst for leaching aluminum from the cookware. It's best to replace any Teflon™ cookware with cast iron, glass, or possibly stainless steel.

More About Teflon™

The following article was announced on *ABC News* (February 23, 2007):

*PFOA (Fer****fluoro****octanoic Acid), also known as C8, is a key chemical used in the manufacture of Teflon and the protective coating that prevents grease stains on boxes and wrappers* [i.e. microwave popcorn, French fry boxes, candy bars].

Preliminary findings of a study at the Johns Hopkins Bloomberg School of Public Health have linked the chemical to lower birth weights among newborns.

The study sampled the blood of 300 newborns and looked at their blood levels of ***a variety of fluorinated chemicals*** *in relation to their birth weight, head circumference and other developmental markers.*

The higher the level of exposure the infants had to PFOA, the lower their birth weight and head size.

Ninety-five percent of American, including children, have PFOA in their blood. PFOA has been classified as a "likely carcinogen".
(http://blogs.abcnews.com/theblotter/2007/02/early_findings_.html)

Studies have proven that the moment a Teflon pan is heated, this toxic chemical is absorbed in your bloodstream, and the above article not only exposes the potential dangers to newborns and infants, but also verifies that Teflon is indeed a dangerous "fluorinated chemical".

Removing Aluminum and Fluoride

Although the best option is obviously to avoid both fluoride and aluminum, at times it might be too late, so the next best thing is to remove them before they do any more damage.

Removing Fluoride

It's interesting that even thousands of years ago, the Egyptians were fully aware of the dangers associated with Fluoride in their water. And the Chinese were also concerned about fluoride found in their well water in some provinces, yet we continue "adding" it to our water systems! The aluminum industry just found a convenient way to dispose of a well-known environmental toxin, and have gotten away with it for years, and at our expense.

The Egyptians discovered long ago that gold was effective in the removal of fluoride in the body, although I'm not sure exactly how they accomplished it. It's amazing that, thousands of years ago, they were fully aware that fluoride is a serious toxin, (something that many scientists today still seem to be ignoring).

There just happens to be a product containing gold that I am aware of. It's a colloidal gold liquid, containing a concentration of approximately 50 parts per million. It's a super small molecule that is rapidly absorbed. According to David Hinkson, the founder of the company *Water Oz™*, some symptoms of a gold deficiency appear to be brain dysfunction, depression, gland dysfunction, and insomnia

Interestingly, those symptoms just happen to be very similar to the side effects associated with Prozac™. And it appears that the Egyptians were right all along, although we just happen to have technology now to produce a colloidal form that readily absorbs. According to David Hinkson, **gold *"neutralizes fluoride poisoning"*** (noted in the *Water Oz Retail/Buyer's Club Catalog*, 2004, p. 10).

It's important to incorporate a molecule small enough to penetrate the blood-brain barrier, as fluoride also can. What convinced me that their products can rapidly absorb, was regarding their liquid magnesium. At times, it can resolve a headache, (especially tension headaches). With my wife, it will normally resolve a headache in less than five minutes. Their colloidal minerals can be purchased through *Water Oz™* by calling (800) 547-2294.

As we discussed, every single molecule of Prozac™ contains "3 molecules of fluoride"! And if you recall, Dr. Cade discovered that Prozac™, (and thus fluoride), not only accumulates, but also remains in the brain for years. If you consider that fluoride damages hormone receptors, suppresses enzyme action, and disrupts the iodine receptors found throughout the brain, you can see **the wisdom in "getting the fluoride out"!**

In addition to the colloidal liquid gold, another way of accomplishing the removal of fluoride involves using the supplement Iodoral™, which contains both iodine and potassium iodide (as we previously discussed). It will help kick start the thyroid gland by removing accumulated fluoride and replacing it with the proper form of iodine necessary for producing the thyroid hormone. In his book *Iodine: Why You Need It – Why You Can't Live Without It* (2004), Dr. David Brownstein discovered that ***"after one day of supplementation [referring to the Iodoral™], fluoride excretion increased 78%"*** (p. 88). However, he also goes on to note that ***"My experience has shown that in an iodine deficient state, it takes from three to six months of iodine supplementation before iodine saturation is reached"*** (p. 88).

Dr. Brownstein states that many different conditions such as thyroid disorders, chronic fatigue, fibromyalgia, and cancer of the breast and prostate are often the result of an iodine deficiency, and he goes on to note that ***"The most important facet of iodine supplementation is that it helps patients improve their health and helps them feel better"*** (p. 88).

I personally purchase Iodoral™ from the *Women's International Pharmacy*, as the owner Wally Simons, R.Ph. is a good friend whom I trust, although there are likely other sources. They can be contacted at (800) 699-8143.

It would also be helpful to take fish oil to help rebuild the hormone receptors in the brain, (which fluoride damages), and Iodoral™ (iodine/iodide), to also restore the iodine in the receptors of the thyroid and the brain, which fluoride replaces. Iodine is necessary for efficient metabolism in both the body and brain. The Iodoral™ should soon begin restoring normal balance in the brain.

Removing Aluminum

Malic acid, made from apples, helps remove aluminum, as does silicon. Malic acid comes in capsules, and a common source of silicon is horsetail, which comes in both capsules and tea.

There is also a homeopathic remedy called Silicea, which comes in tiny pills that melt in your mouth. The suggested dosage is six tablets, three times a day, for a total of 18. It normally comes in bottles of one thousand. Both Malic acid and Silicon (in various forms) are normally available at most health food stores.

Just To Summarize:

It was stated that *"fluoride kills red blood cells,"* which would reduce the oxygen delivery to the brain, increasing the risk of acquiring cancer, (cancer hates oxygen). This is just one way that Prozac™ helps promote cancer.

It was also stated that fluoride *"damages gastric mucosa, resulting in the symptoms of irritable bowel syndrome."* The problem is, **90% of serotonin is actually produced in the intestinal tract!** Thus, anything (such as the fluoride in Prozac™) that damages the intestinal mucosa, would likely impair the body's efficient production of serotonin, (the very hormone targeted by all SSRI antidepressants, including Prozac™). Although, as I noted, Prozac™ does not contain, nor can in any way produce, serotonin.

We have a potentially dangerous drug that absolutely no one (especially pregnant mothers or children) should be placed on by their doctor. Although Vioxx™ posed a proven cardiovascular risk, and was rightfully pulled from the market, in my opinion, **Prozac™ and the other SSRI antidepressants pose a "far greater risk" for creating both physical and mental damage, than Vioxx™ possibly could.** To the best of my knowledge, there are far more potential side effects associated with SSRI antidepressants such as Prozac™ and Paxil™, than any other class of drugs on the market.

And the FDA somehow decided that Prozac™ (which contains fluoride) is perfectly safe for our children? I don't know about you, but I believe it's about time for a serious unbiased FDA reevaluation, (or possibly just a complete overhaul of the FDA)! Maybe they just didn't have adequate time or resources to fully evaluate Prozac™, although I do, and already have, and I can guarantee you that Eli Lilly (the makers of Prozac™) will definitely not like the results! Although, my guess is, Eli Lilly has to be fully aware of the risks associated with Prozac™. Especially due to the many lawsuits they have quietly settled out of court over the years, and the hundreds of potential side effects listed with the FDA. Although, I believe that their greed is finally about to catch up with them. We will now discuss other dangerous ways that fluoride (and thus Prozac™) can be harmful, even before birth.

CHAPTER FOUR

Damage Caused By Prozac™ - Even Before Birth

You are about to discover why anyone who might possibly value either their, or their unborn child's physical and mental health, should avoid SSRI antidepressants such as Prozac™ and Paxil™ at all costs. Especially as there are "much better" natural drug-free options available, proven to be "more effective." As we begin delving into **the "dark side" associated with these dangerous SSRI antidepressants,** which their creators are fully aware of, (yet do everything within their power to hide), **you will soon realize that I am definitely "not exaggerating"!** The effects of these drugs are so insidious, and surprisingly broad-based, that I hope I won't somehow lose you in our discovery, so please bear with me, and I'll do my utmost to not confuse you in the process.

Just so you're aware, although I will at times be referring to some politicians, (including even our president), the primary issue is strictly non-partisan. We will just be looking at the issues, and the unbelievably powerful influence that the pharmaceutical industry can have on our politicians, (regardless of their affiliation).

Broadening The Market To Begin Including Pregnant Women! Will It Soon Be Mandated?

As part of the recently established Bush-backed mental health screening, all children's mental health will soon be assessed, along with their academic standards. The Illinois State Board of Education has been given the responsibility of developing the appropriate tests, according to legislation passed in 2003. Not only that, but **the program will soon require that <u>all pregnant women</u> and children through the age of 18, be subjected to compulsory screening for "mental defects." This may soon include the mandatory prescribing of dangerous drugs such as antidepressants for pregnant women, (something far too many doctors are already doing)!** Is there no end to the tremendous influence the pharmaceutical giants seem to have, regarding decisions made by our own government, which influence the passage of legislation designed to help promote their "very profitable drugs"?

As you are about to learn, we now have "ample proof" from epidemiological studies, that the SSRI antidepressants such as Prozac™ and Paxil™ that millions of women are being placed on, and often remain on during their entire pregnancy, are creating "serious damage" to their fetus. My objective in this book is to explain exactly how they can inflict damage to the unborn child, and the tremendous consequences they will thus be required to deal with later in their life; first as a child, then later as a teenager, and eventually as an adult.

The companies producing these potentially dangerous drugs are actually fully aware of their inherent risks, although with "billions of dollars" of profit at stake they are basically ignoring the problem and continuing to promote them, which makes "perfect **business sense**." They have ample financial resources (due to the huge profits from their sales) to hire lobbyists, and basically pay off those parents who choose to file litigation. The companies deliberately settle out of court, (without assuming any responsibility), along with a non-disclosure attached, (you basically can't disclose how much the settlement was). They basically "buy off" the parents, as reasonably as they possibly can, and deliberately avoid any potential media exposure. They want to keep the public in the dark regarding how potentially dangerous their drugs can actually be (as you will soon see).

Although the primary focus of this chapter is on the effects of SSRI antidepressants on the unborn fetus, that's just the beginning, and a very small part of the overall picture. As you will soon discover, it's often the beginning of an "entire lifetime" of both physical and mental heath issues facing the child (and parent). A lifetime of poor health, as well as a much shorter lifetime, is what many children can expect.

The following true story is just one example of the dramatic influence that SSRI antidepressants can have on the developing fetus, (although advised to do so by her obstetrician), when taken during pregnancy:

> ***To the FDA Advisory Panel on Antidepressant Safely in Children,***
>
> ***My name is Sylvia Olsen and I am the mother of eight children from Salt Lake City, Utah. I suffered for many years with clinical depression and in 1988 my psychiatrist put me on an SSRI medication. I was told I would need to take it for the rest of my life. Subsequently, when I got pregnant with my eighth child in 1991, I asked if I could keep taking the medication. My doctor said there was no evidence of negative side effects, and since I was already on it, I just kept taking it.***
>
> *My son, Taylor, was born weighing much less than any of my previous seven children and displaying an irritability I had never experienced. I soon noticed his body was tense all the time and his movements stiff. The slightest sound would startle him to the point of screaming and, often, even as he slept, his arms would be held stiff and straight up from his body.*
>
> *Although I've had no experience personally taking care of "crack babies," as they used to call them, I kept thinking how he reminded me of things I had heard about them. He would cry continually and seemed to find great comfort in being wrapped very snugly in a blanket and held very tightly.*
>
> *As Taylor grew, we also had to deal with* ***episodes of unreasonable displays of anger.*** *When he got upset about something as simple as his shoe tied wrong, it was as though he had no ability to reason.* ***He would scream, kick, and flail completely out of control.*** *We would have to put our arms around him to restrain him from hurting himself or trashing his room and sit there for as long as half an hour before he would start to gain control of himself and stop screaming and gnashing.*
>
> *Although, he seemed to be bright and aware at home,* ***in school he struggled with reading, writing, spelling and math, unlike his older brothers and sisters.*** *Even though his tantrums are almost non-existent now, (we believe through the help of nutritional supplements) and his academics have improved a lot, he has always required remedial help.*

One thing that always comes up when talking to school aids who have worked with Taylor, particularly one-on-one, is that they are puzzled by one thing in his learning process. ***He will appear to understand something perfectly, a math process for instance, and even be doing it on his own for a while, when suddenly, in the middle of the same work, it's as though a light bulb goes off and he has no knowledge of even being taught the process.*** *Then, later, he knows how to do the problem again as if he never lost it! They say it appears to be some odd kind of glitch in his brain, and I believe it is just another symptom of the developmental problems due to the SSRIs I was taking when pregnant with Taylor.*

I believe there are safe and affective ways of dealing with clinical depression in children other than the use of SSRIs and that the benefits do not outweigh the risks and unknown side effects.

Antidepressants do not actually heal the human mind. If they did, then we would see a decline in depression across our nation, but we do not.

Even John March, ***chief of child psychiatry at Duke University****, who receives grants from Lilly and research funds from Pfizer, said,* ***"These medicines are not a panacea, and will not, on average, carry kids to remission."***

After eight years on these medications, I once spent several months trying to cut back by just a few milligrams and suffered terrible bouts of depression from the withdrawal. Yet, later, through the help of a nutritionist, I was able to wean off of them completely in just a three month period. That was seven years ago and I have not suffered from depression since.

[MY OBSERVATION: If you recall, her psychiatrist said she would be required to take antidepressants the remainder of her life – obviously proven wrong.]

Sincerely, Sylvia Olsen
(http://www.drugawareness.org/Archives/Survivors/record0006.html)

As you can see, there is ample proof that the fetus is influenced dramatically by the antidepressants the mother is taking during pregnancy. It's amazing how closely their symptoms actually parallel those experienced by "crack babies", as Sylvia noted regarding her son Taylor.

The legality of a drug has very little to do with its safety, (or its influence). **Don't forget, the drug companies also produced cocaine, heroin, and LSD, which were also "approved by the FDA" as being safe for our use!** In fact, the Eli Lilly Company that created, and has aggressively promoted Prozac™ for years, actually also blessed us with LSD years ago.

Newborn Withdrawal – A Shock To The Infant

The following alert, reported in the *Sidney Morning Herald*, warned **several years ago** of the dangers taking SSRIs while pregnant, and the potential withdrawal effects on newborns, as follows:

Alert Over Taking Prozac During Pregnancy

August 4, 2003

Women who use Prozac and similar antidepressants during pregnancy and breastfeeding could expose their babies to withdrawal and toxic effects, *a federal government drugs watchdog has warned.*

The Adverse Drug Reactions Advisory Committee says it has received 26 reports of ***infants with withdrawal symptoms.***

The effects were attributable to mothers taking the selective serotonin reuptake inhibitor (SSRI) drugs Aropax **[Paxil™]*****, Zoloft, Prozac and citalopram*** **[Celexa™]*****. The babies' symptoms included agitation, poor feeding, stomach upsets, convulsions, tremors, fever and respiratory disorders.*** *They began within the first four days of birth and lasted two to three days.*

There were also 13 reports of adverse effects probably resulting from the transfer of SSRIs from breastmilk to the baby.

Many of the symptoms of toxicity were similar to those of withdrawal *but in two cases involved babies sleeping for prolonged periods.*

The watchdog's August bulletin quoted a study published in the "Archives of Paediatric Medicine" which found that ***almost one quarter (22 percent) of newborns who were exposed to Paroxetine*** **[Paxil™]** ***(marketed in Australia as Aropax) from their mother in the third trimester needed prolonged hospitalization associated with neonatal complications.***
(http://www.smh.com.au/articles/2003/08/03/1059849278453.html)

It's important to remember that the vast majority of such cases are never reported, nor are the possible causes identified. Apparently, only about 1% of adverse drug-related events are ever reported to the FDA. Although the known statistics are definitely sufficient for concern, if they were all reported, the major concern of the excessive and "totally unnecessary" drugging of pregnant women might be taken more seriously, and possibly even stopped, (as it should have been long ago). Hopefully it soon will be.

As the above article explains, once the baby is born, it is "suddenly withdrawn" from the antidepressant. That's what Dr. Tracy refers to as "crashing", when someone suddenly stops taking an antidepressant. Once the umbilical cord is severed, the child is suddenly withdrawn from "all the mother's medications". This sort of nightmare is all too common with mothers taking antidepressants during pregnancy, and the description of what these newborns would experience while withdrawing, is described in the following extract from a report published in the *Drug Therapy Topics* newsletter, released by the University of Washington Medical Center, Harborview Medical Center, (February 2002, Vol. 31), from an article titled ***"SSRI Antidepressant Withdrawal Syndrome in Newborns,"*** by Elizabeth Ruby, D.V.M., R.Ph.:

> *Case reports have appeared sporadically in the medical literature describing withdrawal symptoms in neonates whose mothers took these medications during pregnancy.*
>
> *A variety of symptoms, most commonly involving the central nervous system and the gastrointestinal system, have been observed in neonates experiencing selective serotonin reuptake inhibitor (SSRI) antidepressant withdrawal. Nordeng et al.* ***described withdrawal symptoms in five infants exposed to SSRI antidepressants prenatally. These neonates exhibited symptoms of irritability, constant crying, shivering, increased tonus, eating and sleeping difficulties, and seizures. Stiskal et al. described jitteriness, vomiting, irritability, hypoglycemia, and necrotizing enterocolitis in four infants exposed to Paroxetine*** **[Paxil™].** ***In adults, similar SSRI withdrawal symptoms have been observed. In the above*** *prenatal exposures, most of the pregnant women took the SSRI antidepressants throughout the pregnancy or started taking it in the second or third trimester and continued through term* (http://uw.prnrx.org/therapyTopics.asp).

In case you wondered, **the *"Necrotizing Enterocolitis"* experienced by four of the five infants in the study exposed to Paxil™ referred to above, is defined as: *"An acute inflammatory disease occurring in the intestines of premature infants; necrosis of intestinal tissue may follow"*** (http://www.hyperdictionary.com).

And **"Necrosis" is basically dying tissue, in this case regarding the intestine. Then if you consider that 90% of serotonin is produced in the intestine, and that adequate serotonin levels are important for avoiding depression, the child could very well be starting out depressed!** Then, under the new broader guidelines, (including infants to 3 years old), the child could soon become a candidate for some antidepressant. And if so, the damage would basically continue, and at an accelerated rate as well.

The brain reacts to any sudden change, (good or bad), and that applies to the fetus, as well as adults. By slowly withdrawing before the child is born, the mother can prevent crashing herself, as well as avoiding risking the newborn child to that unnecessary stress. Thus, the sooner she withdraws, the less damage the fetus will experience. Ideally, she should never consider taking an antidepressant in the first place.

Incidentally, the pharmaceutical companies that produce SSRI antidepressants have actually known about the fetal harm for more than a decade! The *New England Journal of Medicine* reported a study, in the **October 3, 1996 issue,** that showed higher rates of premature delivery, low birth weight, admissions to intensive care units, and poor neonatal adaptation, including respiratory and feeding difficulties, and jitteriness, in children born to women who took Prozac™ during pregnancy. The question remains, just how much more proof do we possibly need, in order to prove that the FDA approval has very little to do with a drug's safety, **or that it actually has any real benefit?**

SSRI Antidepressants and Birth Defects

Although as we now know, warnings have been reported for more than a decade regarding the adverse effects of SSRI antidepressants when taken during pregnancy, *WebMD Medical News* issued another warning in 2004, as follows:

Expert Panel Says Prozac Affects Fetus

> *April 28, 2004 –* ***Taking the popular antidepressant drug Prozac late in pregnancy may be toxic to the fetus,*** *a government report shows.*
>
> *Mothers who take Prozac during the third trimester of pregnancy risk* **premature delivery,** *the report says.* ***They also put their infants at risk of "poor neonatal adaptation," including:***
>
> - *Jitteriness*
> - *Quick, shallow breathing*
> - ***Low blood sugar***
> - ***Low body temperature***
> - ***Poor muscle tone***
> - ***Trouble breathing***
> - *Weak or absent cry*
> - *Diminished reaction to pain*
> - *Not getting enough oxygen while feeding*
> - ***Increased admission to special-care nurseries***
>
> ***Prozac taken by breastfeeding mothers, the report says, may retard infants' early growth*** (http://www.webmd.com/content/Article/86/98985.htm).

Then, in the April 2006 issue of *American Journal of Obstetrics and Gynecology*, it was reported that **taking SSRIs doubled the mother's risk of delivering a stillborn infant and increased the risk of premature delivery, underweight babies, and seizures.** And again, in July 2006, the FDA issued a warning that **infants exposed to SSRIs were six times more likely to develop the often fatal lung disorder, PPH (which we will soon discuss), than infants who were not exposed.**

Yet, in spite of all this knowledge, we find that ***"Prozac* [is] *Still Prescribed to Pregnant Women"***, as the title of this next article implies. You will learn of the major influence that Prozac™ had on Melissa, and her son Cody (beginning before he was born). Not only that, but **the problems Cody experienced at birth were just the beginning.** We'll now let Melissa tell Cody's story, in her own words, (as told to reporter Jane Mundy), as follows:

> ***"My obstetrician said that I should stay on Prozac throughout my pregnancy,"*** *says Melissa Christensen.* ***"I wish he knew in 2002 what I know today – that Prozac is toxic to the fetus in the last three months."***

"My family doctor prescribed Prozac about 18 months before my son Cody was born. As soon as I knew I was pregnant, I stopped taking it. But I was only off the drug for a few days. ***After seeing my obstetrician, he told me to stay on Prozac.***

I went into pre-term labor several times before I finally had to have a C-section. *I started getting sick and losing weight, even though this was the time I was supposed to gain weight. But my baby was gaining weight – fast. I had flu-like symptoms and knew something was wrong but my OB said it was just because the baby was getting so big and I was just feeling uncomfortable.*

By January 4th, he was so big that I had to have a C-section. ***As soon as Cody was born he was put into ICU, where he stayed for five days. He had an IV and an oxygen hood and his own nurse. At one day old, Cody had an x-ray of his lungs. He had trouble breathing then he developed jaundice and his sugar levels were plummeting.***

Cody is now three years old and he has severe asthma. *When I was looking over his records, the chest x-ray showed hyper-inflation of his lungs and through my research I found out that* ***this is one of the symptoms of PPHN*** **[Persistent Pulmonary Hypertension of the Newborn].** ***Then I went on the Internet and found out how prevalent the correlation is between birth defects and Prozac.***

I'm mad about this. And I also nursed my son. My OB doubled my dose right after Cody was born – I was taking 40 mg per day. As soon as I read the book I quit taking Prozac and made an appointment with my family doctor. She prescribed another antidepressant that is considered safer.

I know that a lot of people are trying to find out more about this birth defect issue. But ***you don't know right away; it could happen months after they are born.*** *I do know this:* ***all of Cody's problems are consistent with mothers on Prozac. When I asked my OB if Prozac was safe to take during pregnancy, he said, 'We give Prozac to children'. Obviously, I trusted him.***

Now it is proven that Prozac is toxic to the fetus and causes pre-term labor. *I believe it was because of Prozac that caused Cody to be born prematurely.*

As well, he was born with all the symptoms of a child with prenatal Prozac exposure – withdrawal from Prozac. These symptoms are jitteriness, lack of sensitivity to pain, low oxygen levels, respiratory distress, low blood sugar, and weak muscle tone. Research has proven that this happens to babies at birth but that they get over it within four days. In our case ***it seems like Cody never 'got over it'.***

Cody has a wide range of problems, none of which have any other explanation, *but the drug companies have not studied the long term effects of* *prenatal Prozac exposure. I don't think people know enough about the side affects of this drug and* ***Prozac will continue to be prescribed to pregnant women if we don't do something about it. Because the drug company isn't telling them to stop taking Prozac"*** (http://www.lawyersandsettlements.com/articles/prozac-pregnancy.html).

If there is anything that is totally inexcusable, it's when an obstetrician not only places their patient on an antidepressant such as Prozac™, but even recommends she remain on it throughout her pregnancy. Especially when their patient questions its safety, as Melissa did. If there is anyone that an expectant mother should be able to trust regarding the health of her fetus, it should be her obstetrician. The criterion any obstetrician should apply is: What effect has Prozac™ had on the development of fetuses, and infants' health in the past? The question is, why didn't her doctor just take a "few minutes", and research the issue himself, (information that is readily available to everyone), as Melissa eventually did herself? That should be his job – not hers. Can you imagine how the future health of many children is being compromised as a result? The potential birth defects are not just minor, but can even be life threatening, as many die prematurely. If the child does survive, his or her quality of life will be greatly compromised. The question is, **just how many O.B.s are continuing to destroy lives, one child at a time, just due to their negligence?**

We'll now look at some other "serious disorders" that could have, (and absolutely should have), been avoided.

Prozac™ and Lung Disorders

In studies published in the *New England Journal of Medicine*, **women who took SSRI antidepressants in the third trimester of pregnancy, gave birth to babies who were six times more likely to have Primary Pulmonary Hypertension of the Newborn (PPHN), or developing the lung disorder Primary Pulmonary Hypertension (PPH), than babies not exposed to SSRIs** (http://www.lawyersandsettlements.com/case/ssri_birth_defects).

PPH is a disorder of the lungs, which severely restricts the arteries, causing the blood pressure in the pulmonary artery of the heart to rise excessively. Blood flow is thus restricted, and oxygen levels in the blood are suppressed. The baby's organs, such as the brain, kidneys and liver quickly become stressed, due to the lack of oxygen.

PPHN is a bit different than PPH, as the ductus arteriosus stays open, allowing the blood flow to bypass the lungs, which means **the blood returns to the heart very low on oxygen. PPHN is a very serious birth defect,** and is usually diagnosed within 12 hours of delivery. **Even with treatment, a newborn with PPHN may experience shock, heart failure, brain hemorrhage, seizures, kidney failure, organ damage and even death. And even babies who do survive PPHN may have long-term breathing difficulties, seizures, developmental disorders and hearing loss.**

NOTE: In case you wondered, the "ductus arteriosus" mentioned above, normally closes upon birth. It basically bypasses the fetus's lungs until they are fully developed upon birth. In the interim, the mother's lungs provide the necessary oxygen to the fetus. The worst-case scenario is when the blood flow bypasses the lungs, as with PPHN. Then with the PPH, there is a serious restriction of blood flow (and thus reduced oxygen). The brain is especially sensitive to an oxygen deficiency, as neurons soon begin to die. That is especially a concern for a young infant.

Actually, it's basically one contributor to Alzheimer's disease in the elderly, due to reduced circulation from restriction in their arteries and capillaries.

Candice Pert, M.D. was one of the two developers of the serotonin binding processes that made all of the serotonergic medicines possible. In *TIME* magazine, October 20, 1997 issue (p. 8), Dr. Pert talks about the widespread use of these drugs, and declares: ***"I am alarmed at the monsters I have created."*** Dr. Pert went on to voice her concern about the long-term use of these medications, saying that **we should expect to see the same heart and lung problems that we saw with Fen-Phen™ and Redux™, with these serotonergic antidepressants as well.** According to Dr. Tracy, never in the history of medicine has the developer of any medication come out with such a strong negative statement about the drug in question, especially while the medications are even still on the market, and being prescribed for our children! **And as Dr. Pert warned – monsters they are!**

Interestingly, **Dr. Pert warned of the very same "heart and lung conditions" (referred to as PPHN) that fetuses, born to mothers who were taking SSRI antidepressants such as Prozac™ and Paxil™, often experience upon birth.** These newborns must then be placed on respirators, while others are often born prematurely, or stillborn. And of course, the full extent of brain damage won't likely be obvious for a while, (if ever). It could easily result in a lower IQ, or possibly even early Alzheimer's disease, yet seldom is the connection ever made regarding the true cause. **It's especially difficult (if not impossible) to determine, for instance, what a child's IQ potential might have been, although we do have proof that such drugs can contribute to brain damage and lower children's IQs.**

Fluoride's Influence On The Fetus's Bone and Joint Development

First we might begin by examining how the fluoride in Prozac™ might possibly influence the formation of the fetus's bone tissue. It was discovered by researchers of the Queensland Independent Senate Team that ***"Fluoride exposure disrupts the synthesis of collagen and leads to the breakdown of collagen in bone, tendon, muscle, skin, cartilage, lungs, kidney and trachea"*** (http://www.johnston-independent.com/). Thus, any disruption in the synthesis of collagen not only has a negative influence on the creation or maintenance of bone tissue, but also many other organs and tissues throughout the body.

This was also announced in the *American Journal of Medicine* (2005 January, pp. 78-82), stating the following:

> *While consuming high levels of fluoride has been known to boost bone density, it also* ***results in bone brittleness*** *and can lead to skeletal fluorosis, resulting in:*
>
> - ***Bone pain***
> - ***Calcified ligaments***
> - ***Bone spurs***
> - ***Fused vertebrae***
> - ***Difficulty moving joints***

Considering the above finding, and the fact that so many pregnant mothers and very young children continue to be placed on Prozac™, helps explain why, according to Dr. David G.

Williams, *"Today the norm for children is a dozen or more infections, antibiotic-induced asthma, terribly impaired immunity,* ***weak bones and joints, flaccid muscles,*** *poor digestion, and* ***even arthritis before the age of 10****"* (*Health Alert* newsletter, March 2007, Vol. 24, Issue 3, p. 5).

First, the high level of fluoride in Prozac™ not only suppresses the action of enzymes involved in all bodily functions, but it also leads to the breakdown of collagen in the majority of tissue in the body, (including the joints and bones). Then, when fluoride is combined with even a small amount of aluminum, (found in common table salt or baking soda), it can take a toll on a child's immune system. Then, children whose mothers were on Prozac™ during pregnancy experience respiratory and stomach upsets, which pretty much covers all the disorders Dr. Williams refers to in his newsletter. He then goes on to state the following:

> *But not to worry –* ***an FDA advisory panel advised that Celebrex, used for joint pain and arthritis, can be given to kids as young as 2 years old! To avoid the risk of heart disease – known to be caused by Celebrex – the panel calls for "tracking these kids' health for decades."*** *Even I have a hard time believing this one. The panel vote was 15 to 1,* ***even though the members know this drug is toxic for children.*** *They claim Celebrex is safe based on a flawed, short study with children that was designed by Pfizer, the maker of Celebrex* (pp. 5-6).

So we can likely add heart disease in the near future to Dr. William's rather extensive list, and there are even more that we will soon be discussing as well.

Could you possibly imagine placing kids as young as 2 years old, on such a potentially dangerous drug as Celebrex™, very similar to Vioxx™, which was pulled, not all that long ago, due to its heart disease risk, for a disease that was until recently only experienced by the aged? Something is "drastically wrong" with this picture! **You can rest assured that Pfizer is not about to investigate the cause of the young children's arthritis.** My guess is, they are likely fully aware, although the unbelievable FDA approval just opens up a whole new market for their very profitable drug (their primary objective). **Due to the "well known risk" associated with Celebrex™, the panel actually calls for tracking the kids' health for decades! These kids are about to become unpaid victims of a very dangerous "uncontrolled study".** Unfortunately, these children are far too young to realize the risk they are being exposed to, and that their life might very well be at risk, especially if they are also placed on other medications, which is becoming an all too common practice today. When will it all end? They are creating adult diseases, (in even very young children), and then giving them more drugs known to be potentially dangerous, for conditions other drugs originally created. And we are allowing them to create a medical nightmare for innocent children who are not even aware (children who trust in our judgment). This obvious abuse absolutely must be stopped! Many spend years in prison for far less, such as taking just one life, (and we are talking about millions of innocent lives). And they are in my opinion, fully aware of the risks they are exposing even very young children to. **They are just sacrificing lives for dollars,** which is basically what it all comes down to.

We then find that the vitamin C, necessary for creating collagen, along with six additional vitamins and minerals necessary for building bone, just happen to be depleted by Prozac™! In fact, **the deficiency of all sixteen of those nutrients depleted by Prozac™ results in an even greater concentration of fluoride in the bone, (something heavy metals are well known for).**

Not only does fluoride change the structure of bone, causing it to become more brittle, but we find that ***"Fluoride is more poisonous than lead and just slightly less poisonous than arsenic. It is a cumulative poison that accumulates in bone over the years"*** (http://www.mbschachter.com/dangers_of_fluoride_and_fluorida.htm).

Further studies show:

"...fluoride damages bone even at levels added to public drinking water"
-*American Journal of Epidemiology*, October 1999

"...significant increase in the risk of hip fracture in both men and women exposed to artificial fluoridation at 1 ppm."
-*Journal of the American Medical Association* (*JAMA*), August 1992

And possibly the worst of all is the fact that *"Since 1991, the New Jersey Department of Health found that* ***the incidence of osteosarcoma, a type of bone cancer, was far higher in young men exposed to fluoridated water as compared to those who were not,"*** (and I'm certain that applies to young women as well). A very good explanation as to why so many young children are now developing bone cancer. Especially as so many children, and expectant mothers, are currently being placed on Prozac™. Due to its high fluoride content, Prozac™ presents a serious threat to the developing fetus, from the brain to the bones, and everything in between. And don't forget that **our bones don't just form our framework, but are also an important part of our immune system, and produce our red blood cells that we couldn't survive without. So, developing healthy fluoride-free bones is especially important.**

It might be worth mentioning that **the natural form of progesterone,** such as the EssProL'eve™ from *International Health* discussed in the next chapter, (**NOT Provera™**), not only helps in the brain development of the fetus, and greatly reduces the mother's risk of developing breast cancer (as previously mentioned), but as noted by Dr. Lee, M.D., one of the foremost authorities on women's hormones, **progesterone also helps stimulate bone growth, instead of contributing to osteoporosis,** as Prozac™ is well known for. Possibly one reason that Prozac™ contributes to osteoporosis is due the increase in the stress hormone cortisol, which Prozac™ stimulates. According to Dr. Lee, **high cortisol is a primary cause of osteoporosis because it blocks the bone-building effects of progesterone.** Just one more example of the many positive "side benefits" of natural supplements and hormones, versus the many negative "side effects" of all drugs. The choice should be obvious to anyone who now knows the facts, (deliberately hidden from the public's view).

A Popular Drug That Can Weaken, Rather Than Strengthen, Bones - Some Dangers Of Treating Osteoporosis With Fosamax™

Speaking of side effects, (and healthy bones), there is a class of drugs on the market that are being promoted to help prevent osteoporosis, that every woman should in my opinion avoid, at all costs. Fosamax™ is the best known, and most advertised. They are promoting its benefits based on bone scans, which won't actually show you what your bone health might actually be, or its strength. If you want to end up with weaker calcified bones, and greatly increase your chances of experiencing a hip fracture, Fosamax™ would be an excellent choice.

There are two enzymes involved in the maintenance of bone tissue, and bone is living tissue that requires constant maintenance. Osteoclasts are cells that break down old calcified bone, and osteoblasts are responsible for building new bone. Bone cells, just like every cell in the body, must eventually be replaced. The problem is, Fosamax™ suppresses the action of the osteoclasts. It thus suppresses the breakdown of old calcified bone cells, (a natural, and very important process for maintaining "strong healthy" bones that should not be suppressed). Even though the bones will continue getting calcified and weaker, it won't show up on a bone scan, so no one will be the wiser. It's a crime that they are allowed to continue placing so many, (but women especially), on such terribly destructive drugs, such as Prozac™ and Fosamax™.

Never forget that bone is living tissue, and Our Creator obviously knew that it wouldn't be wise to build new bone on top of old calcified bone. Otherwise, the bone remodeling (or maintenance) would basically stop. Consider for a moment, what would happen if it didn't. Creating new bone on top of old bone would be like remodeling an old house without removing the dry rot. Not only that, but if you continually added new bone, without first removing the old bone, the bones would have to become larger, which obviously doesn't happen. Once we understand how drugs like Fosamax™ actually work, just plain logic should tell us that they would weaken, rather than strengthen bones. Then the obvious question comes to mind: If a mother is taking Fosamax™ during her pregnancy, what influence might it have on the development of the fetus's bones?

Stress and Elevated Cortisol's Influence On The Fetus

According to Dr. Ann Blake Tracy (one of the foremost authorities on antidepressants), in her book *Prozac: Panacea or Pandora?* (1991/1994), **just one single 30 mg dose of Prozac™ increases the level of the stress hormone cortisol by an amazing 200%!** This raises the question: What if the mother is taking Prozac™, and experiencing stress as well?

We'll begin by evaluating two possible ways that maternal stress, (or taking Prozac™), during pregnancy could affect the development of the baby:

> *One is if the mother is very anxious or stressed while she's pregnant, there's reduced blood flow to the baby through the uterine arteries, the main source of blood and nutrition for the baby, and* ***this could explain why the baby doesn't grow as well and also set up a secondary stress response in the fetus.***
>
> *Second,* ***if the mother has high levels of cortisol, the main stress hormone, so does the fetus. It seems that enough cortisol crosses the placenta from the mother to the fetus to actually affect fetal levels. So if the mother is stressed, her cortisol goes up, so does the cortisol level in the fetus. This in turn could well affect the development of the brain and the future stress responses of the baby.***
>
> ***We're realizing now that the development of the brain is sensitive to the hormones that are around it, and particularly cortisol,*** *just as it is to alcohol, smoking or other drugs. And that the cortisol level that the fetus experiences will set a number of brain receptors to cortisol and this in turn will set later responses* (http://www.schizophrenia.com/prevention/Stress.child.html).

So as you can see, cortisol does cross the placenta, from the mother to the fetus. And as we learned earlier, high cortisol is also a primary cause of osteoporosis. Then the well-known neurologists and brain specialist Dr. David Perlmutter, M.D. warns that **elevated cortisol damages the area of the brain where long-term memories are stored, and hormones are regulated.** He also notes that most Alzheimer's patients have high levels of cortisol in their brains.

Another very serious concern regarding cortisol and the fetus is explained by Dr. Shawn Talbott, Ph.D., in his book *The Cortisol Connection* (2002), as follows:

> *Most notable (and scary), perhaps, are the findings that* ***chronic stress can lead to actual physical changes in the arrangement of the neurons (nerve cells) in the brain. In other words, we're talking now about stress changing both the function and the shape of your brain.*** *No wonder it doesn't work the way it's supposed to!* (p. 65).

This is extremely important if you consider that cortisol crosses the placenta, from the mother to the fetus, thus it is possible for stress to change "both the function and the shape of the brain" of the fetus! Apparently Dr. Talbott felt that the dangers associated with cortisol caused so many serious concerns, (and not just during pregnancy), that **he wrote an entire book about it!**

Research preformed by Professor Marelyn Wintour and her team at Monash University in Melbourne, suggests that **one of the most important environmental variables during pregnancy is stress, as well as its duration,** as follows:

> *This is commonly studied using sheep, as* ***the lamb normally grows to the same size as a human baby in a relatively long pregnancy, and the development of major organs including the heart and brain is very similar in humans and sheep. To simulate stress in pregnancy, Professor Wintour's team exposed sheep early in their pregnancy to a stress hormone, cortisol, for a short duration. The offspring were later found to develop high blood pressure from four months after birth, which increased in severity as they aged. Kidney development was also impaired.*** *Dr. Julie Quinlivan, working with researchers at the University of Western Australia, found that* ***injecting sheep with stress hormones later in their pregnancies and on a number of occasions produced different effects, including the later development of insulin resistance and diabetes.*** *This suggests that the timing of stressful insults can have varying outcomes.*
>
> ***The duration of exposure to stress is also crucial.*** *Dr. Quinlivan notes, "Basically, if you have a single exposure to stress hormones, the body is very resilient. But* ***if you have repeated exposure to stress, it affects the number of brain cells in a fetus's brain, the growth of the baby, and the development of the thyroid and the immune system, so it has multiple effects".***
>
> ***In addition to physical effects such as hypertension or diabetes, abnormal concentrations of cortisol in-utero can also create psychological syndromes.*** *Studies have found that* ***infants exposed to elevated levels of***

cortisol in the womb- often because their mother was under stress or depressed herself- are at increased risk of depressive disorders throughout childhood, adolescence and adulthood. Such individuals also commonly exhibit cognitive delays and long-term behavioural dysfunction.

Recent research has suggested that cortisol appears to cross the placenta more easily in female than male fetuses, *thus placing women at greater risk of developing those conditions related to excesses of this hormone in later life* (http://www.lafamily.com/display_article.php?id=1089).

Adrenal Enlargement – Caused By Continuous Cortisol Stimulation

Dr. Tracy stresses the fact that the 200% increase of the stress hormone cortisol, caused by Prozac™, is not natural, (especially on a daily basis), and tends to place an excessive demand on the adrenals, often leading to adrenal fatigue. It also results in a hair-trigger response to any stress. Apparently, several factors come into play. The greatest concern of all is when the mother is placed on, and then remains on an SSRI antidepressant such as Prozac™ or Paxil™, for several years.

The particular antidepressant, as well as the dosage prescribed, are both important, although how long the mother has been "exposed" to the drug is especially a concern, in regards to the potential for adrenal fatigue. Another variable is how often the mother is experiencing any other kind of stress, both before and during her pregnancy. Many pregnancies are at times unexpected, and possibly even unwanted, which would place an added stress on the mother, especially if it could have an influence on her career. For instance, if the mother is on Prozac™, and thus already producing a high level of the stress hormone cortisol on a daily basis, and is also experiencing additional stress from other sources, the adrenals could quite easily become overwhelmed.

This is where the fetus comes in. Although the fetus totally relies on the mother for its oxygen and nutrients prior to birth, some time during the second trimester it can begin to reciprocate at that point in its development. Its adrenals will have developed sufficiently so that it can now come to the mother's rescue by supplementing her cortisol production. Unfortunately, it comes at a price. That demand placed on the fetus's adrenals, during their developmental stage, apparently results in their enlargement. Then if the child is, in turn, placed on an antidepressant at a fairly young age, (which is now becoming all too common), that process basically continues. The adrenals continually enlarge to meet the increased demand for cortisol.

Dr. James Balch tells us, by using a CT scan to measure a person's adrenal glands, *"researchers at Duke University found that* ***people suffering from clinical depression have larger adrenal glands than non-depressed people"*** (*Prescription for Nutritional Healing*, pp. 318-319). And then, one condition that is quite common with children born to mothers on antidepressants is low blood sugar, or hypoglycemia, which according to Dr. Balch, can also lead to depression. We are obviously setting our children up for depression at a very early age. Then, according to the new expanded guidelines, that is exactly where the psychiatric evaluation now begins, (as early as 18 months); a perfect excuse for placing them on an antidepressant. What a devious and obviously well thought out marketing plan!

Once the adrenals have become enlarged, that's an indication that you're nearing adrenal fatigue, a potentially serious condition that, (like elevated homocysteine), doctors were conveniently never trained to consider. However, both conditions can only be resolved with nutrition, (something deliberately left out of most doctors' training). The pharmaceutical companies have a tremendous influence on your doctor's training, thus disease prevention and nutrition are conveniently and deliberately excluded. And then we can't forget that the vitamins and minerals, necessary for resolving adrenal fatigue, just happen to be depleted by both Prozac™ and Paxil™, (something they'd rather you weren't aware of). **The question is, if drugs that are known to deplete critical vitamins and minerals are covered by your insurance, then why aren't the vitamins and minerals necessary for resolving the deficiency they are creating, covered as well? This is an accountability that should be addressed, although one they have deliberately chosen to ignore.**

Isn't it amazing that they can conveniently "create" 374 mental conditions, (with absolutely no scientific validation whatsoever), yet they somehow entirely overlook such a very important condition, that is not only easy to diagnose, but also resolve, (and of course, without the use of drugs). As this condition will be found on your doctor's list of "AMA-approved conditions" that would be treatable with patented drugs, don't expect the solution to be covered by your insurance! As it is being "deliberately overlooked", few are aware that the condition even exists, unless of course, they go to a natural practitioner, (whose services incidentally won't be covered by your insurance as well)! This is a well-orchestrated plan to deliberately exclude vitamins and minerals from your insurance coverage, and basically promote poor health, as that's where the profit potential is.

It's not just coincidental that most people with chronic fatigue also happen to have adrenal fatigue. It can at times become so debilitating, that people can have difficulty even functioning. And only by avoiding stress (as well as antidepressants), and getting the necessary nutrients, along with adequate rest, can the condition be resolved. Adrenal fatigue would be especially difficult to resolve, for a mother with a newborn, as getting sufficient rest is often difficult. Prevention (by avoiding antidepressants altogether) would obviously be the best solution, unless it's already too late.

Nutritional Supplements To Reduce Cortisol (and Stress)

As you can now see, the potential for damage, caused by elevated cortisol, can be very extensive, (especially regarding the brain). Both the pregnant mother, and her fetus are at risk, thus, reducing cortisol is extremely important.

In his book *The Cortisol Connection* (2002), Dr. Shawn Talbott, Ph.D. suggests the following ***"cortisol-controlling nutrients"*** **in an effort to** ***"counteract the detrimental health effects of chronic stress*** **[and thus elevated cortisol]*"*:**

Vitamin C
Thiamin (vitamin B-1)
Riboflavin (vitamin B-2)
Pantothenic acid (Vitamin B-5)
Vitamin B-6
Magnesium
Zinc
Chromium

The following Amino Acids:
- *Arginine*
- *Ornithine*
- *Leucine*
- *Isoleucine*
- *Valine*

Dr. Talbott points out that ***"Women should be aware that riboflavin needs are elevated during pregnancy and lactation,"*** and also notes that ***"High-fat diets have been shown in rodent studies to impair the body's ability to restore normal cortisol levels following stress"*** (p. 117).

Another supplement I might suggest is Relora™, which contains extracts from the two herbs Philodendron and Magnolia, and is found be very effective in increasing DHEA levels while also lowering cortisol. According to the book *DHEA – Unlocking the Secrets to the Fountain of Youth*, written by Beth M. Ley (1996), ***"stress depresses DHEA production"***, which is important when you consider ***"DHEA regulates diabetes, obesity,** carcinogenesis, tumor growth, virus and bacterial infection, **stress, pregnancy, hypertension, collagen and skin integrity, fatigue, depression, memory** and immune responses"* (p. 32).

Studies done on patients with mild to moderate stress were put on a two-week regimen of Relora™ and found that it *"caused a significant increase in salivary DHEA (227 percent) and a significant decrease in morning salivary cortisol levels (37 percent),"* (*Woman's World* magazine, June 18, 2002). Relora™ is available at most health food stores and through mail order.

Prozac™ and Paxil™ - Serious Nutritional Robbers!

If adequate nutrition were important to anyone, it would be especially important to an expectant mother. In only nine months' time, her body is going to create another complete human being, with all the complex organs that we as adults have, and just from the tiny microscopic sperm and egg. To me, that's truly amazing, and obviously a tall order that would require a great deal of nutrients in order to accomplish. Any nutritional deficiency during the child's development could have a major negative influence, not only regarding the development of the fetus's, but also the mother's, physical "and mental" health.

Considering that millions of women are being needlessly placed on, and often remain on the SSRI antidepressants such as Prozac™ and Paxil™ "throughout their pregnancy," there is a "serious concern" for a major nutritional deficiency. Although all medications on the market are known to deplete nutrients, these antidepressants are unquestionably some of the worst, with a total of **"sixteen nutrients depleted"!** Not only that, but those being depleted are some of the most critical for our mental health, and for avoiding depression, (the very last thing any pregnant mother needs). So, considering that in some double-blind studies, Prozac™ for instance was found to be slightly **"less effective than a placebo,"** does it make any sense to be subjecting both the mother, and her fetus, to such a major risk of serious nutritional deficiency? And that's just a small part of the many risks associated with these medications that the developing fetus is being subjected to.

Following you will find **the 16 important nutrients depleted by Prozac™ and Paxil™**, as well as some of the many benefits that each nutrient provides. For the sake of brevity, we will be narrowing our focus to those benefits primarily important for maintaining the mother's mental health, and those necessary for avoiding depression, as well as those important for the fetus's development:

1. **Vitamin B_1 – Reduces stress and anxiety; enhances energy and learning capacity. Deficiencies can produce fatigue, poor coordination, forgetfulness, and irritability or nervousness.**

2. **Vitamin B_2 – Enhances vision, reduces eye fatigue, and strongly influences how well the thyroid gland synthesizes its hormones. Deficiencies can produce dizziness, insomnia, slowed mental response, fatigue, and anxiety.**

3. **Vitamin B_3 – Enhances memory, prevents senility, and is helpful for schizophrenia and other mental diseases. Assists in normal functioning of the nervous system, and is essential to the good health of all glands, especially the thyroid. Deficiencies can produce depression, dementia, dizziness, fatigue, insomnia, irritability, and low blood sugar.**

4. **Vitamin B_6 – Involved in more bodily functions than almost any other single nutrient. It affects both physical and mental health, and promotes red blood cell formation. It is required by the nervous system (stress resistance) and needed for normal brain function. Deficiencies can produce anemia, headaches, depression, dizziness, fatigue, learning difficulties or memory loss. A thyroid gland deficient in vitamin B_6 has difficulty converting iodine into thyroid hormone.**

5. **Vitamin B_{12} – Assists in cell formation, prevents nerve damage, and promotes normal cell growth. It assists in memory, concentration and learning, and maintains a healthy nervous system. It prevents insomnia by enhancing sleep patterns and REM sleep. Deficiencies can produce anemia, chronic fatigue, weight gain, spinal cord degeneration, memory loss, depression, degeneration of nerves, moodiness or nervousness. Deficiency can also result in a significant reduction in the conversion of T_4 to T_3 thyroid hormones.**

6. **Folic Acid – Assists in the formation of blood cells, prevents and treats folic acid anemia, regulates homocysteine levels and tissue functions, and maintains normal patterns of growth. It is considered a brain food, is needed for energy production, and is also a natural analgesic or painkiller. It assists in treating depression and anxiety, and maintains the nervous system. Deficiencies can produce anemia, fatigue, insomnia, memory problems, paranoia, and weakness.**

7. **Vitamin C – Necessary for more than 300 metabolic functions in the body. It is an antioxidant, and when combined with toxic substances (i.e. heavy metals, pollution), vitamin C can render them harmless, allowing them to be eliminated from the body. It enhances the immune system, thus promoting the healing of wounds and burns, preventing infection, and fighting bacterial infection. It assists the body with oxygen use, aids in the prevention and treatment of cancer, and assists in the production of anti-stress hormones. Deficiencies can produce tooth loss, high blood pressure, extreme weakness, depression, fatigue, and increases susceptibility to infection (especially colds and bronchial infections). Vitamin C deficiency can also cause male infertility and increased genetic damage to sperm cells, which may lead to birth defects. Pregnancy and breastfeeding increase the need for vitamin C.**

8. **Vitamin D – Prevents muscle weakness, enhances the immune system, prevents depression, and is necessary for healthy thyroid function. Deficiencies can produce skeletal malformations, retarded growth in children, insomnia, depression, visual problems, and insulin resistance.**

9. **Calcium (an essential mineral) – Assists in neuromuscular activity and the entire nervous system. Deficiencies can produce heart palpitations, muscle cramps, insomnia, nervousness, depression, or hyperactivity.**

10. **Magnesium (an essential mineral) – More than 300 enzymes are activated by magnesium, and low magnesium levels make nearly every disease worse. It is responsible for the production and transfer of energy, thus reducing fatigue. It is necessary for healthy nerves and muscular tissues, as well as nerve transmissions and impulses. It is also a natural tranquilizer, known as the anti-stress mineral, and assists in the prevention and treatment of depression and PMS. Deficiencies can produce weakness, fatigue, insomnia, nervousness, anxiety, confusion, irritability, depression, seizures, asthma, chronic fatigue, insulin resistance, type II diabetes, chronic stress, attention deficit hyperactivity disorder (ADHD), and poor memory.**

11. **Manganese (a trace mineral) – Necessary in the syntheses of thyroxine, the principal hormone of the thyroid, relieves fatigue and nervous irritability, and improves memory. It promotes a healthy nervous system, a healthy immune system, assists with blood sugar regulation and energy production. Deficiencies can produce confusion, convulsions, eye problems, hearing problems, heart disorders, irritability, memory loss, loss of muscle coordination, muscle contractions, sprains, strains, weak ligaments, tremors, abnormalities in insulin secretion, impaired glucose metabolism and pancreatic damage. Low levels of manganese are often found in people with epilepsy, hypoglycemia, and schizophrenia.**

12. **Selenium (a trace mineral) – Protects the immune system, and is necessary for conversion of the T_4 thyroid hormone to the active form T_3 hormone. Deficiencies have been linked to cancer, heart disease, exhaustion, infections, liver impairment, and pancreatic insufficiency.**

13. **Sodium (a trace mineral) – Necessary for stomach, nerve, and muscle function, and assists in making the cell walls permeable. Deficiencies can produce confusion, depression, dizziness, fatigue, headache, poor coordination, recurrent infections, muscle weakness, poor concentration, and memory loss.**

14. **Zinc (a trace mineral) – Promotes mental awareness, and is a constituent of insulin. It is necessary for the conversion of the T_4 thyroid hormone to the active form T_3 hormone. Deficiencies can produce delayed sexual maturation, fatigue, growth impairment, night blindness, decreased immune system (susceptibility to infection, recurrent colds and flu, slow wound healing), impaired memory, and propensity to diabetes.**

15. **Glutathione (an amino acid compound) – Protects the liver from alcohol-induced damage. Deficiencies can produce decreased immune system, lack of coordination, mental disorders, tremors, and contribute to oxidative stress, which plays a key role in the worsening of many diseases including Alzheimer's disease and Parkinson's disease.**

16. **Coenzyme Q_{10} (CoQ_{10}) – Enhances the immune system, and is beneficial in treating obesity, diabetes, and anomalies of mental function (i.e. schizophrenia and Alzheimer's disease). It boosts energy levels, and plays a critical role in energy production. It is also a natural antihistamine, thus it is beneficial for those who suffer from allergies, asthma, or respiratory disease. Deficiencies can produce congestive heart failure, fatigue, and decreased immune system, and has been linked to diabetes, muscular dystrophy, and periodontal disease.**

As you can easily see, **every single nutrient depleted by Prozac™ plays an important role in preventing many undesirable physical, mental, and emotional conditions, as well as the healthy development of the fetus.** It looks more like the nutrients an expectant mother should assure she is getting an adequate supply of, rather than taking a drug that is depleting them! Armed with that knowledge, why would we possibly want to take a drug that could deplete so many nutrients that are so very critical, especially to our mental health? If there is anything that would be depressing, it would in my opinion, be knowing you are taking a drug that is basically depriving you (and your fetus) of the "many benefits" provided by the above nutrients!

Following is more proof of how important prenatal nutrition is, and the effects it can have on the fetus, as stated in an article found in an issue of the *Los Angeles Family Magazine*, titled ***"You Are What Your Mother Ate: Prenatal Causes Of Adult Diseases"***, as follows:

> [Medical scientist, David Barker] *found that* ***babies born with low birth weights had a higher incidence of a number of chronic cardiovascular conditions as adults, including heart disease, hypertension (high blood pressure), diabetes and raised cholesterol. In some societies they are also up to ten times more likely to die prematurely in young adulthood.*** *These relationships were independent of the length of the pregnancy, suggesting that such outcomes were related to growth restriction in the womb rather than premature birth. Barker proposed that* ***poor maternal nutrition during pregnancy could cause genetic changes affecting the development of fetal organs, leading to increased susceptibility to chronic diseases in years to come and ultimately a shorter life span.***
>
> ***Interestingly, fetuses that are clinically malnourished during the first trimester of development are three times more likely to be obese as adults.***
>
> *Further research has been carried out by Professor Marelyn Wintour of Monash University in Melbourne.* ***Vitamin D deficiency during pregnancy for example has been suggested to correlate with the later development of schizophrenia, while low levels of Vitamin A can impair renal (kidney)***

development. Insufficient concentrations of iron and fatty acids such as omega-3 in the maternal diet have also been linked with an increased adult risk of a variety of conditions, including forms of cancer and leukemia.

According to Professor Wintour, "The most alarming finding is that the time at which the fetus is most vulnerable- early in the pregnancy or around 5-7 weeks- is when the woman may be unaware she is actually pregnant".

*It is well established that **maternal abuse of substances** such as alcohol or nicotine can have **both immediate and long term effects on factors as diverse as the brain development,** immune system, birth weight, **attention span and social skills** of the offspring. **Similar effects may also be seen after gestational exposure to certain drugs (including cocaine) or toxins such as mercury, lead or some pesticides*** (http://www.lafamily.com/display_article.php?id=1089).

NOTE: Although fluoride wasn't one of the toxins mentioned, it can be every bit as toxic as lead and mercury!

Shouldn't We Pay For Nutritional Supplements For Pregnant Women - Rather Than Antidepressants (or Any Other Drugs)?

Unfortunately, on the website of the **American Pregnancy Association** (http://www.americanpregnancy.org/pregnancyhealth/depressionduringpregnancy.html), they actually **support and encourage** depressed pregnant women to talk to their health care provider about their ***"symptoms and struggles"*** and state that ***"your health care provider may want to prescribe medication immediately."*** Coincidentally, the American Pregnancy Association states it is a non-profit organization incorporated in the State of Texas, although we have already established that Texas is where the aggressive program to promote SSRI antidepressants all started.

Then in the following article, (originally published August 19, 2004), **we learn the unbiased truth, as follows:**

***A new warning is being issued about pregnant women taking antidepressant drugs. It turns out that taking such drugs during late pregnancy puts the health of their babies at risk and leads to birth complications that may require prolonged hospitalization, breathing support, and tube feeding. This warning applies to all SSRI drugs, or what's called Selective Serotonin Reuptake Inhibitors, which include drugs like Prozac and other popular antidepressants.** The warning comes from Health Canada, and is a latest in a serious of warnings being publicized about the dangers of taking prescription drugs.*

The untold part of all of this is the rather shocking realization that doctors are actually prescribing antidepressant drugs to pregnant women.** That's because there is no FDA warning about antidepressants and pregnant women in the United States. It's not surprising, **since the FDA is typically very slow to

issue warnings about prescription drugs, even as Canada, the UK, and other countries are quick to publicize such warnings in order to protect the health of the public.

Interestingly, one of the common defenses about this link between antidepressant drugs and birth complications is that there is also a risk to the fetus if a pregnant woman remains depressed. Some people are saying that it's worth giving depressed expectant mothers antidepressant drugs because it's a greater health danger for the pregnant mother to remain depressed. ***This is absurd, since antidepressant drugs don't actually improve the mental health of anyone in the first place. Even the clinical trials involving antidepressants have been distorted and selectively chosen to shed good light on SSRIs, but as we are now learning, these drugs actually promote violent behavior and can cause people to commit suicide.***

Are these the kinds of drugs we want to be giving pregnant women? *Wouldn't it make a lot more sense to help educate women about why they might be feeling down in the first place, due to their* ***dietary imbalances and their nutritional deficiencies****, and then help them alleviate those at the core?* ***Wouldn't it make more sense to use natural methods that actually support and enhance the health of unborn children as well as the health of their mothers?***

In the case of pregnancy, I think women need to be held to a higher standard, *and in this country we need a program of education and support to help pregnant women get better nutrition and a better understanding of what is required to raise a healthy child.*

Specifically, ***I think society should pay for nutritional supplements for pregnant women, meaning that those supplements would be available free of charge to any woman of childbearing age. Yes, it would be expensive, but it would be far cheaper than giving birth to another generation of health-compromised babies who are prone to learning disabilities, diabetes, and birth defects (among other disorders). Prevention is dirt cheap compared to the cost of treating disease, and prevention starts with the mother.***
(http://www.newstarget.com/z001892.html)

I totally agree with the author, unfortunately, as long as the pharmaceutical industry remains **"in charge of our healthcare system"**, that will likely never happen. **Even inexpensive prenatal vitamins that could help prevent unnecessary birth defects are not covered!** That basically places the poor, who are just struggling to make ends meet, and thus can't afford them, at the greatest risk of all. Although the thousands of dollars necessary to repair the resultant birth defects would of course be covered. That just shows the tremendous power that these multinational giants wield, and a major issue that obviously must be dealt with. The immense, and totally unnecessary pain and suffering these children will be forced to suffer with, throughout their entire lives, is totally inexcusable, and just because the pharmaceutical companies don't want to start a trend, and even slightly open the door for insurance coverage for inexpensive, although often critical, vitamins that could greatly reduce the risk of children being born with birth defects. **It's not just accidental that, although so many drugs are covered by your insurance, not one single supplement, (no matter how beneficial), will be covered.**

The Emotional Condition Of The Pregnant Mother - An Important Issue That Should Be Considered

Our brain is the organ most influenced by a nutritional deficiency. It's basically who we are, and how we think. All mind-altering drugs, (be they legal or illegal), can have a dramatic influence on our actions, our personality, and even our perceptions, thus we're no longer who we once were! The implications can be rather scary, as in the case of Andrea Yates, a caring mother who drowned her five children, (and felt she was doing it for their benefit), although there are "many others" as well, whose misperceptions actually seem very real to them at the time. In her book *Prozac: Panacea or Pandora?* (1991/1994), Dr. Ann Blake Tracy tells us that:

> *Inappropriate serotonin and dopamine neuronal functioning* [caused by Prozac™] *is thought to* ***render one incapable of sorting through thoughts and perceptions, producing an inability to determine which of them are real and which are imaginary.***
>
> ***Psychosis enters in when patients resolve the discrepancies between illusion and reality by adopting a new set of concepts – their delusions are then accepted as reality.***
>
> ***It takes very little to create a "new reality" for the patient whose memory is so profoundly affected in this toxic state*** (p. 256).

I don't believe that drug companies deliberately create drugs that are so dangerous; they just continue trying to do the impossible, and are unwilling to accept defeat. They just go on creating artificial chemicals in a lab, in order to suppress some symptom. Unfortunately, their drugs always create far more problems than they resolve. That's especially a concern when our mind is their target. All drugs are designed to override some natural process that should instead be assisted with adequate nutrients, rather than forcefully suppressing natural functions with some chemical that is totally unnatural to our body. It never has worked, and never will. They are basically attempting to second-guess Our Creator. You'd think they would know better by now.

Scientists who create, and companies who produce these serious "mind-altering" drugs, either don't know what they are doing, or don't really care. And pharmaceutical companies, who deliberately attempt to hide known serious side effects associated with such dangerous drugs, and even continue to promote them in spite of the concern, obviously don't really care. **Any drug that can have such a negative influence on who you become, or how you think, is potentially dangerous, and in my opinion should be illegal.**

Dr. Tracy talks of many unbelievable things that patients who were placed on these mind-altering drugs by their doctor did, that were totally out of character. She calls them "divorce pills" as they can alter our personality. She claims that it is common, for couples who were happily married for many years, to get a divorce for no apparent reason after their spouse is placed on

SSRI antidepressants. People's emotions tend to go, and they sometimes go into what Dr. Tracy refers to as a disassociative state. They basically have a numbing influence on a person's personality. Many claim that it's as though they are basically coming out of a fog, and back to the real world after withdrawing. One lady called and related how, for years, while on Prozac™, her husband never really communicated with her, (they basically didn't have much of a relationship), but that all changed once he got off his Prozac™, which I helped him do. She was so elated that she could hardly contain herself. She said *"Now we talk, and finally have a real relationship."*

Does this possibly sound like you or someone you know, who is taking antidepressants? If there's any time in a woman's life when a close bond, and communication with her spouse is especially critical, it's during her pregnancy, and shortly following delivery, when the child is still young, and requires the most care. Ideally, this should be a team effort, which means neither parent should be taking antidepressants. Of greatest concern, is the influence that SSRI antidepressants have on the developing fetus, and eventually the physical and mental health of the child. Some might show up early, as birth defects, while other conditions might possibly show up later in life, although the connection to the antidepressants is seldom made.

Mandatory Mental Screening For Postpartum Depression - The Typical, Although Inappropriate Solution (Antidepressants)

In 2006, the governor of New Jersey signed legislation, **requiring health care professionals who provide prenatal care, to educate women about postpartum depression (PPD), and see that new mothers receive treatment for the disorder.** Then in a press release, it was stated that **80% of women experience some degree of depression following childbirth.** And most recently, both Illinois and Pennsylvania are also attempting to get similar legislation passed as well. They are using the very same strategy as they did with TeenScreen, although the focus now is on expectant mothers. The obvious objective is to find a way to broaden their market every way possible. For years, it was adults (especially seniors). Once they had basically saturated that market, they began targeting our kids, (even very young preschoolers). Now, the only untapped market appears to be expectant mothers.

Worst of all is the deliberate attempt to get legislation passed, (state by state), to mandate mental health screening, first with children, and now their mothers. They would rather you had absolutely no choice in the matter, (an overt attempt to take away our freedom to make choices for ourselves and our children). They have already taken away our choice regarding healthcare, by assuring that natural therapies and supplements are not covered by insurance. Then if they have their way, all our health conditions (physical and mental) will be totally controlled by the pharmaceutical industry, and mandated by our government, both state and federal.

And of course, the "accepted" treatment for PPD just happens to be counseling and **drug therapy with antidepressants!** And they are deliberately very specific as to exactly how the program is to work, assuring that they take advantage of every opportunity to diagnose a mother with PPD, who would thus be **in need of the "appropriate medication".** For example, **an excerpt from Senate Bill 15, in Illinois, reads:**

> *Physicians and other licensed health care workers providing **prenatal and postnatal care** to women **shall assess new mothers for postpartum mood disorder symptoms** at a prenatal check-up visit in the third trimester of*

pregnancy, prior to discharge from the hospital or other healthcare facility, and at the initial postnatal check-up visit and at each postnatal check-up visit thereafter until the infant's first birthday.

Physicians and other licensed health care ***workers providing pediatric care to an infant shall assess the infant's mother for postpartum mood disorder symptoms at any well-baby check-up at which the mother is present prior to the infant's first birthday*** *in order to ensure that the health and well-being of the infant are not compromised by an undiagnosed postpartum mood disorder in the mother* (http://tinyurl.com/35zkec).

And then we find that a hospital in Illinois is going overboard, when they make it appear that when a mother is even thinking about getting pregnant she should be tested for depression!

The Advocate ***Good Samaritan Hospital*** *in Downers Grove, Illinois continues to recommend that SSRIs be used to treat pregnant women even despite recent warnings concerning birth defects and other life-threatening disorders in children born to mothers who took antidepressants during pregnancy.* ***"Any woman," the Hospital warns, "who is thinking about becoming pregnant, is pregnant, or had a baby within the past year can be affected by depression or other mood disorders"*** (http://www.sierratimes.com/07/04/04/75_8_37_98_67891.htm).

Most doctors who come up with conclusions that ridiculous, are normally influenced financially by the industry producing and promoting antidepressants. (I personally think they should consider re-naming the hospital!)

Although it appears as a concern, just like TeenScreen, it's just another marketing strategy by drug companies, (an obvious attempt to get everyone possible on their highly profitable medications). Unfortunately, far too many women have been placed on, (and often remain on), antidepressants throughout their pregnancy, which just increases the potential for experiencing PPD following delivery. As we discussed, the highly elevated stress hormone cortisol, stimulated by antidepressants such as Prozac™ on a daily basis, is the best way I know of to deplete the mother's adrenals, which are responsible for producing several critical hormones.

Most importantly, **mental evaluations never have been, and never will be, based on science.** Thus, the evaluation would be based on nothing but someone's personal opinion, as would be the solution. **And, as the promotion of the program is always funded, (either directly or indirectly), by the pharmaceutical industry, the "proper solution" would obviously be influenced as well.**

According to psychiatrist, Dr. Grace Jackson, author of *Rethinking Psychiatric Drugs: A Guide for Informed Consent*, ***"Prescribing SSRIs as a preventative measure during pregnancy is a terrible idea"*** (http://www.sierratimes.com/07/04/04/75_8_37_98_67891.htm). In fact, regarding the overall scheme of screening all women before, during and after pregnancy and putting them on SSRIs, Dr. Jackson has stated ***"In sum, there could not be a more foolhardy public health practice than this one."***

As you will soon discover, **there is a very good explanation for PPD, (based on science – not conjecture).** Then as usual, there are effective drug-free solutions available.

Suddenly Going From An Unbelievable High, To An Unexplainable Low (No – It's Not The Bipolar Disorder, Or Coming Off Cocaine) Instead, A Surprisingly Common Phenomenon (PPD)

In his March 2007 *Alternatives* newsletter, Dr. David G. Williams does an excellent job of explaining exactly how PPD develops, as follows:

> ***PPD is a very real problem, but it definitely doesn't stem from a drug deficiency.*** *The added nutritional and hormonal stress of pregnancy often leaves the mother's body chemistry totally out of balance following childbirth.* ***One of the most common problems seems to stem from depletion of the adrenal (or stress) glands.***
>
> *Physical or mental stress, poor diet (excess sugar or carbohydrates), skipping meals, alcohol, and smoking are some of the primary causes of weakened adrenals. During and immediately before pregnancy a poor diet, particularly consuming too much sugar or high-carbohydrate meals, will quickly weaken the adrenals.* [NOTE: Coffee is also a stimulant known to deplete the adrenals, as is the NutraSweet™ found in diet beverages.]
>
> *During the first three months of pregnancy many women experience a great deal of fatigue and a total lack of energy.* ***Beginning sometime during the second trimester they oftentimes get a huge burst of energy and heightened sense of well-being. These women will say things like, "This is the best I've ever felt in my life." And this newfound energy remains with them until they give birth, when all of the sudden it feels like the whole world collapses around them (PPD).***
>
> ***During the second trimester the child's adrenal glands begin to develop, along with the thyroid, pituitary, and other glands. And since the mother and child share a circulatory system she begins to benefit from the baby's hormones. In effect, she begins to "feed off" the baby. She begins to experience more energy and that overall sense of well-being. It couldn't get any better. Her body has discovered a fresh new source of everything she's been missing.***
>
> ***But when the baby is born, the mother is abruptly cut off from her newfound lifeline. Within a day or two of giving birth, the mother can go from the highest high to the lowest low and never know what hit her. No one offers her an explanation.*** *If anything, she might be told it's normal to experience the depression and fatigue and it's something she just needs to work through – and* ***maybe some antidepressants might help*** (p. 167-168).

Recommended Drug-Free Solution For Postpartum Depression

✓ Dr. Williams continues:

> *The underlying problem, however, needs to be corrected.* ***The adrenal glands (and often the thyroid and pituitary glands) must be given nutritional support.*** *Sugar has to be eliminated. Additional minerals, B vitamins, and essential fatty acids (predominantly omega-3s) must be added to the diet.* ***I've seen dramatic changes in just a matter of days through proper nutritional support, particularly using glandular supplements for the adrenal, thyroid, and pituitary glands. The problem isn't correctable with drugs*** (*Alternatives*, 2007 March, p. 168).

✓ **It just so happens that *Standard Process*™ is a company that has a dietary glandular formula for women called Symplex F**, which contains all three glandulars (adrenal, pituitary, and thyroid extracts), which Dr. Williams recommends, along with ovary extract. They also have another formula called Drenamin™, with several plant-based nutrients specifically formulated for helping rebuild weakened adrenals. Their products are only available through doctors (including chiropractors).

✓ **The adrenals (especially when depleted) need adequate salt.** The only salt I would recommend is Celtic sea salt, sold through the *Grain & Salt Society*. It comes in coarse crystals and fine ground. As the "coarse" is cheaper, I would recommend swallowing one teaspoon daily with water. Or you can use the "fine" for everyday seasoning. That's the only salt I have used the past 18 years, and unlike the common table salt, it's actually healthy, (as it contains over 80 trace minerals). Celtic sea salt is available at most health food stores, or directly through the *Grain & Salt Society* by calling (800) TOP-SALT, or by visiting http://www.celtic-seasalt.com/ .

✓ **Avoid stimulants and stressors.** As Dr. Williams recommended, **avoid coffee, sugar, and NutraSweet™**, as they all stress the adrenals. And most importantly, **avoid physical or mental stress as much as possible. I would also recommend avoiding drugs such as Prozac™, which greatly increase the level of the stress hormone cortisol.** If you happen to experience unavoidable stress for some reason, just take a couple capsules of the very calming herb, valerian root. It will safely help you relax, and appears to do so without causing drowsiness.

✓ **Stay hydrated!** Don't forget to **drink at least ten 8-ounce glasses of water daily,** which is especially important during pregnancy. The nausea many women experience during pregnancy is often the result of inadequate water intake.

✓ It's also important to **take a potent vitamin B-complex such as B-100, as well as a good multi-mineral containing at least calcium, magnesium, and zinc.**

✓ **Essential fatty acids such as flax and fish oils also play an important part in our mental health.** I would recommend a minimum of two large soft gels of Flax seed oil, and two of fish oil, daily.

Applying all of the above recommendations throughout pregnancy, would greatly reduce the risk of experiencing PPD. Just remember that the typical approach of ***"drugs for everything, and nothing but drugs for anything"*** is a dangerous and self-destructive approach that never has, and never will, truly resolve any health issue, (physical or mental). In the next chapter, we will be discussing some ways to create an optimum environment for the fetus. Our objective will be to assure that your child is born healthy, and to avoid unnecessary birth defects, or premature birth.

CHAPTER FIVE

Creating An Optimum Environment For Fetus Development

This particular subject might very well deserve a separate book, (which I might eventually write), although it's such a critical issue to all mothers (and fathers), that I will at least discuss a few concerns of greatest importance here. You will find that several things I will be discussing should increase your child's IQ, rather than lowering it, (as drugs such as Prozac™ and Paxil™ can easily do). Not only that, but two issues we will be discussing, should also greatly reduce the mother's breast cancer risk in the process. Rather than creating "tremendous damage" to the fetus (and mother), which these antidepressants are well know for, our natural solutions will instead provide "many benefits" to both the mother, and the fetus, (all positives, and absolutely no negatives).

We will now evaluate what might be the optimum environment for creating the healthiest child possible, and then explain how you can provide it. As it's the mother's body that's responsible for creating the child from its very inception, (obviously a major project), it's up to her to assume that responsibility. The mother's diet, and whether she takes nutrients, or instead chooses to rely on drugs, plays a major role in the fetus's development. By far the greatest problem we are currently experiencing, is the bad advice women are continually receiving from their doctor, such as recommending that they continue taking an antidepressant during their pregnancy – something that even many obstetricians, (who should know better), continue recommending.

We will be applying a little basic logic that should make perfect sense to anyone familiar with even the basics of nutrition, (and if you're not, then hopefully you soon will be). As we learned, SSRI antidepressants such as Prozac™ and Paxil™ are known to contribute to serious birth defects, lower children's IQ, and often lead to premature birth as well. Worst of all, is the damage that takes place during the fetal development stage, which will influence their physical and mental health throughout their entire life. We will now evaluate some things we all require to maintain healthy cells, and an adequate level of energy.

✓ **Nutrients.** Maintaining the mother's health, while also creating another complete human being in only nine months, is obviously a tremendous challenge to any mother's body. Rather than taking a drug such as Prozac™, **"known to deplete a total of 16 critical nutrients"**, the mother should instead be taking extra vitamins and minerals. Then, as we discuss later in this book, in the chapter on "Contributors To Depression", **microwave cooking will destroy sixty to ninety percent of the critical nutrients in food.** Not only that, but when foods in plastic containers are heated, the **toxic xenoestrogens (estrogen mimics)** in plastic are released into the food. The xenoestrogens have a similar influence on the woman's body, (and the fetus), as the estrogen made by the mother's ovaries, except **xenoestrogens are considerably more potent,** (thus, a little goes a long way). This contributes to estrogen dominance, which can be a major concern for both the mother and the fetus.

Nutrition should be a mandatory part of every doctor's training, (but especially obstetricians), although unfortunately it's not. The mother's nutrition is by far the most critical during pregnancy. **All pregnant women should take a high-potency vitamin B complex (B-100), a quality multi-mineral (containing calcium, magnesium, and zinc), and at least 4,000 mg of ester-C with bioflavonoids, in divided doses, daily.**

✓ **Healthy Fats.** We should consider how we can assure that the fetus's cells and cell receptors are healthy, (an important issue for the mother as well). For example, trans fats, or hydrogenated fats, found in most fast foods and processed foods, (as well as margarine and most cooking oils on the market shelves), build unhealthy cell walls and receptors in both the body and brain, and even block the absorption of good fats! This will have a tremendous influence on your child's future health, as building healthy receptors will assure the efficient utilization of all hormones, from insulin in the body, to serotonin and dopamine in the brain. You should avoid any food or oil that lists hydrogenated or partially hydrogenated fat or oil, and be sure to cook with extra virgin cold pressed olive oil.

You should also take a minimum of one tablespoon of flax seed oil, and a tablespoon of fish liver oil daily, (referred to as essential fatty acids or EFAs). How efficient the process of getting nutrients into the cell, and toxins out for their removal, depends on the health and permeability of each cell's wall, in addition to the health of the hormone receptors, (another benefit of EFAs such as fish and flax oil). Instead, according to Dr. Sherry Rogers, M.D., **the fluoride in Prozac™ actually damages hormone receptors.**

It has also been found that Cod liver oil (which naturally contains EFAs and vitamin D), taken during pregnancy, may reduce the risk for Type I diabetes. According to a study conducted in Norway, **when mothers took cod liver oil during pregnancy, their offspring had a lower risk of developing Type I diabetes** (*Diabetologia*, 2000, pp. 1093-1098). And it would be so easy to do, and the mother would benefit as well. Avoiding Type I diabetes is such a major issue, as it's a terribly destructive disease, and requires daily injections of insulin.

✓ **Celtic Sea Salt.** And while we're on the subject of transporting nutrients into the cell and removing toxins, (regardless of what your doctor might have told you), **"you do need salt"! You just need a complete salt,** such as Celtic sea salt through the *Grain & Salt Society*, which not only contains over 80 trace minerals in an ionic (easily absorbable form), but also both "sodium and potassium", (the primary issue). Common table salt is not only missing the many trace minerals, but also the critical cofactor, potassium. Not only that, but it also contains **"aluminum",** added as a non-caking agent, **for your convenience**! Then, they even bleach the salt, so it will be more pleasing to the eye, (how thoughtful of them). Celtic sea salt is available at most health food stores, or directly through the *Grain & Salt Society* by calling (800) TOP-SALT, or by visiting http://www.celtic-seasalt.com/ .

Now back to the subject as to why you need the complete unadulterated salt, as created by nature. Every single cell in our body contains a sodium/potassium pump that requires "both minerals", not just the sodium found in common table salt. The pump's function is transporting nutrients into each cell, as well as the removal of toxins. So, having both healthy cell walls, (via healthy fats), and adequate sodium and potassium, (via the complete salt), is important for maintaining healthy cells, and efficient cell function, which is the basis of every organ, (including the brain). Sodium without potassium, (as found in common table salt), causes edema (fluid retention).

And the aluminum, added to common table salt, is especially a concern for anyone also taking Prozac™. As we discuss under Chronic Fatigue, the fluoride in Prozac™ poses an even greater threat when aluminum is also present. The fluoride/aluminum combination begins depleting the energy molecule ATP, while also suppressing two of the most critical antioxidants in the body, and greatly reduces the immune function as well. Not only that, but fluoride can very efficiently transport aluminum through the blood brain barrier, into the brain, greatly increasing the risk for developing Alzheimer's disease, (and what about the fetus's brain?). My guess is, the majority of women on Prozac™ are also consuming common table salt containing aluminum, (a bad combination).

There are many sources of aluminum, other than common table salt. Baking powder, antacids, antiperspirants, and aluminum containers that soft drinks and beer are sold in, for instance, are just a few examples. I once saw an analysis of the minerals found in broccoli, and would you believe that one was a trace amount of aluminum! The highest concentration would likely be when vegetables are grown in areas where there is more pollution and thus acid rain, which leaches aluminum from the soil. Then we not only absorb aluminum from antiperspirants, but the perspiration being suppressed is our body's attempt to remove the environmental toxins that the liver is lacking enzymes to detoxify, (basically double trouble).

I should also mention that an adequate level of both sodium and potassium, (found in the complete salt), is critical for efficient nerve transmission in the brain, and according to Dr. F. Batmanghelidj, M.D., **when combined with water, sea salt is actually an excellent source of energy for the brain!** This would be especially important for someone on a reduced carbohydrate diet in an effort to lose weight, and do so without creating hypoglycemia, (the lack of energy to the brain). Incidentally, **the amino acid L-glutamine just happens to be another alternate source of energy for the brain. We don't actually need as much glucose as you might think.**

✓ **Sufficient Water.** Dr. Batmanghelidj also stresses the importance of drinking eight to ten 8-ounce glasses of water daily, for many reasons. That is especially important for an expectant mother. Water is a solvent, important for efficient toxin removal. Not only is the mother's body producing toxins, (as we all do), but the fetus does as well, especially during the third trimester when it's more fully developed. At that point, the fetus is larger, and thus there are more cells producing toxins. While we're on the subject, another problem associated with Prozac™ is that it's highly protein binding, and thus very difficult for the liver to metabolize. As a result, it greatly reduces the liver's ability to efficiently metabolize and remove toxins. Then the fluoride in Prozac™, combined with even a small amount of aluminum, can make a bad problem even worse. As a result, the amniotic fluid, (or the fetus's environment), can become even more toxic.

According to Dr. Batmanghelidj, author of *Your Body's Many Cries For Water,* the morning sickness that some women experience is often a sign of dehydration. Also, any deficiency of water would contribute to a more toxic environment, with more toxins, and less water in the amniotic fluid. This means the mother's blood would become more toxic as well, (actually very similar to the uncomfortable symptoms some experience during detoxification). This problem can become even worse if the mother has the candida yeast infection, often caused by antibiotics or birth control pills, and worsened by simple sugars often found in soft drinks, and fruit juices – an issue we will now address.

Why Is The Mother More Prone To Develop Candidiasis During Pregnancy? And What Influence Can The Candida Yeast Infection Have On The Child?

Donna Gates, nutritional consultant and author of *The Body Ecology Diet*, brought up some interesting issues regarding the fetus's development, in an article published in *A Grain of Salt* newsletter (Winter 2007 issue). In her article titled *"What Every Girl & Woman Needs To Know If They Ever Want To Have A Baby"*, she stresses the importance of establishing a healthy inner-ecosystem prior to pregnancy if possible, and notes that *"Studies show that* ***as many as 85% of women have a vaginal infection"*** **that they pass on to their newborn**

babies instead of the beneficial bacteria, which also compromises the young child's immune system. She also stresses that, (referring to the mother), ***"Your immune system is weakened so that your own antibodies do not see your developing baby as an enemy. This makes it more difficult for your immune system to stave off bacterial, viral and fungal infections."*** Incidentally, the fungal infections referred to is the candida yeast infection.

She then explains that:

> ***Babies who lack an abundance of beneficial bacteria start life with gastrointestinal pain like colic reflux and even infant constipation.***
>
> ***When a woman has a systemic fungal infection (candidiasis) she can infect her baby, and neither of them may have any visible symptoms!***
>
> *Babies born with yeast in their gut (inherited from mothers with candidiasis) lack the normal healthy bacteria that establish a thriving immune system.* ***A baby's blood-brain barrier isn't formed until six weeks after birth. Before the blood-brain barrier is formed, there is potential for fungal, bacterial and viral infections to enter your baby's brain*** (p. 6).

In order to fully understand Candidiasis (the candida yeast infection), and how to treat it, be sure to read the chapter on Candida, later in this book, which I cover this condition in considerable detail.

How Prozac™ Compromises The Liver's Detoxification Function - Exposing The Fetus's Brain To Excessive Toxins, Especially When Combined With Alcohol (Possibly Produced By Candida)

Although consuming alcohol while taking antidepressants is contraindicated, (not recommended), it's a concern that far too many, (including doctors), tend to ignore. According to Dr. Tracy, SSRI antidepressants cause terrible cravings for addictive substances, (especially alcohol)! Not only that, but SSRI antidepressants (such as Prozac™) also greatly potentiate the effect of alcohol. It's the very same P450 enzyme in the liver that attempts to metabolize Prozac™ that is also attempting to metabolize and remove "another toxin", alcohol. We then learn from Dr. Tracy that **Prozac™ actually potentiates alcohol by "ten times", although with the more potent Paxil™ it's even worse at "forty times"!** That would help explain why women on Paxil™ during pregnancy often experience the worst birth defects.

That is especially a concern for a mother with the candida yeast infection, who may also consume too much sugar. Incidentally, the yeast infection actually causes cravings for sugar, (its favorite food), just compounding the problem. Then as the liver is basically "tied up" for so long, attempting to metabolize the antidepressants, your brain (and that of the fetus) is basically exposed to the toxic alcohol much longer than it would normally be, (especially with Paxil™).

One thing alcohol is known for, is temporary destabilizing of the blood-brain barrier, which would normally prevent toxins from gaining access to the brain, (a concern for the mother). As Donna Gates just indicated, the problem with the fetus is, it's not until the child is approximately six weeks old that its blood-brain barrier is finally formed. If that weren't true, it would obviously be rather difficult to get all the nutrients through the blood-brain barrier to accommodate the rapidly developing brain of the fetus, yet toxins can easily gain access to the fetus's brain!

Then, as the detoxification process in the liver is being compromised by the Prozac™ or Paxil™, more toxins will not only remain in the bloodstream, but can now gain access to the brain as well. That brings up one more concern; the metabolizing of alcohol actually involves two passes through the liver, (referred to as phase I and phase II detoxification). During the first phase, an enzyme called alcohol dehydrogenase converts alcohol to an even more toxic substance called acetaldehyde (a molecule very similar to formaldehyde). Then finally in the last phase, acetaldehyde is finally converted to acetic acid (basically vinegar) and water. The problem is, when the liver is overloaded with drugs such as Prozac™ or Paxil™, which are so difficult to metabolize, the detoxification process can take considerably longer than it normally would.

A serious concern is that the candida yeast basically turns the body into a brewery. As a matter of fact, people who never drank alcohol in their entire life have been arrested for having a high blood level of alcohol, just because they had candida, and had consumed sugar, **(the higher the sugar intake, the higher their alcohol level will be).** This has been confirmed in tests. Then, anyone with candida who is also taking an SSRI antidepressant, (such as Prozac™ or Paxil™), should expect the very same potentiation (10 to 40 times) of the alcohol produced by the candida in their body. Under the right (or should I say wrong) set of circumstances, the body can quite easily become a very efficient brewery. **Alcohol is still alcohol, no matter what the source might be.** We actually cover this issue in considerable detail in the Candida chapter, later in this book.

Most mothers are actually warned by their doctor to avoid alcohol, due to the danger to the fetus, of developing the fetal alcohol syndrome, although seldom (if ever) are they warned of the candida/alcohol connection, or the part that sugar can play if they do have the yeast infection, (which as we learned, is surprisingly common). By far, the greatest concern is when a woman is also taking Prozac™ (or even worse Paxil™), which "greatly increases the risk of brain damage, due to excessive alcohol". That is especially a concern for the fetus, whose brain is rapidly developing.

Following is an article regarding research published in the June 2007 issue of *Alcoholism: Clinical & Experimental Research*, which helps explain the dangers of alcohol during pregnancy, whether by ingestion or produced by Candidiasis.

Alcohol Use During Pregnancy Leads To Greater Risk Of Extreme Preterm Delivery

Preterm delivery, and particularly "extreme prematurity" – defined as less than 32 weeks of gestation – are major contributors to perinatal sickness and death worldwide. A new study has found that maternal alcohol use during pregnancy can contribute to a substantial increase in risk for extreme preterm delivery.

Robert J. Sokol, distinguished professor of obstetrics and gynecology and Director of the C.S. Mott Center for Human Growth and Development at Wayne State University, and his colleagues, collected data on exposure to alcohol , cocaine and cigarettes, as well as corresponding outcomes, from 3,130 pregnancy women and their infants. Of the newborns, 66 were extremely preterm, 462 were mildly preterm, and 2,602 were term deliveries.

Findings indicated that alcohol and cocaine, but not cigarette, use were associated with an increased risk of extreme preterm delivery; alcohol accounted for the lion's share of the risk. Furthermore, the effects were greater in pregnancies among women older than 30 years of age.

Researchers have seen what appears to be a greater susceptibility to neurobehavioral effects and anatomic congenital anomalies in pregnancies among older women. "This is an important finding," he said, "because a woman could have been drinking during pregnancy when she was younger and had no effects, but could be more susceptible later."

Given that the patient population was 92 percent African American, added Sokol, the results will need to be confirmed elsewhere, using similar methodology. "The baseline risk for preterm delivery is higher among African Americans than whites in the United states," he said. "There are known ethnicity effects for prenatal alcohol exposure, so studying pregnancies among whites would be sensible, yet if I had to guess, I think we would see changes in the same direction."
(http://www.sciencedaily.com/releases/2007/05/070524164514.htm).

Although Sokol mentioned the known ethnicity influence regarding alcohol exposure, one thing he didn't address is the fact that both Oriental and Native American women are at the greatest risk. Their P450 enzyme in the liver that metabolizes alcohol is less effective than other nationalities. As a result, the acetaldehyde, which as you just learned, is a metabolite of alcohol produced in the first stage of the breakdown of alcohol, is not removed nearly as rapidly. And, as acetaldehyde is similar to formaldehyde, and even more toxic to the brain than alcohol, Oriental and Native American women should be at a much greater risk than others would be.

We must not forget that any time there are toxins such as fluoride or alcohol, (or even acetaldehyde), in a pregnant mother's blood stream, the fetus will also be exposed. This is especially a serious concern during the first trimester, (the first three months), as that's when the fetus's brain is rapidly developing, and its brain would be especially vulnerable to such serious toxins at that time. And as we learned, its blood brain barrier is not even developed yet.

All cells in our body produce toxins as a byproduct of normal metabolism, (which applies to the fetus as well). Thus, the mother's liver is faced with an even greater demand of eliminating an increasing level of toxins as the fetus continues to grow. Then, if the mother is taking antidepressants, (or possibly any other medications, as well), we can easily see an obvious problem, (a potential for toxic overload)!

Other Influencing Factors Regarding Premature Births

One thing I should mention is that, when a child is born prematurely, in my opinion, it's because the environment that the fetus is being exposed to, is extremely unhealthy, and not conducive to its further development inside the mother, (exactly the environment that SSRI antidepressants such as Prozac™ and Paxil™ are known to contribute to). Then other factors such as the mother's diet, (including her water consumption), her thyroid function, whether she has the candida yeast infection, and her pH (acid/alkaline level), are just a few factors that could influence the environment of the developing fetus.

Both adequate thyroid function, and a sufficient oxygen level, also plays a critical role in the fetus's development. **The very first thing every mother should do is to check her thyroid function.** In the chapter on Hypothyroidism, I show you how you can easily check it yourself, and how to effectively resolve it if it's too low. Women are ten times as likely as men to experience the condition, and it's often related to elevated estrogen, or stress (including the stress hormone cortisol produced by Prozac™).

The pH (acid/alkaline) level plays an important part on how much oxygen the fetus will be getting. When your pH is low (too acidic), you will be depleting critical oxygen. Although oxygen can increase the pH, making your body more alkaline, your oxygen will be depleted in the process, (obviously not desirable). Also, the more toxic your body is, the more acidic it becomes. All drugs are very acidic, as is sugar, coffee, and alcohol. Interestingly, although common table salt is acidic, Celtic sea salt is instead alkaline! Most processed foods are acidic, while fresh fruits and vegetables are normally alkaline. As water helps remove toxins, it also helps alkalinize the body. Even your thyroid hormones play an important part in detoxification, and thus efficient oxygen utilization. An adequate level of both the thyroid hormone and oxygen is necessary for optimum energy production, and a healthy environment for the fetus.

Prozac™ not only contributes to an acidic condition, and thus the depletion of oxygen, but according to Dr. Tracy, Prozac also constricts the arteries. Thus, reducing the oxygen delivery to the fetus as well, (obviously a very bad combination, and "totally unnecessary").

Although the mother's body should be a much healthier environment for the fetus's development than the outside world, at times it's not, or nature wouldn't be forcing it out prematurely. Premature birth is not just accidental, and it's not just a coincidence that by far the greatest number of women experiencing both birth defects and premature births, just happen to be taking drugs such as Prozac™ and Paxil™. The more we learn about their potential damage to the fetus, the more apparent that will become.

Avoid Smoking During Pregnancy!

Something else to consider, regarding potential damage to the fetus, as well as a risk for premature delivery, is smoking. As noted by Robert Sokol (the professor of obstetrics and gynecology and Director of the C.S. Mott Center for Human Growth and Development at Wayne State University, mentioned in an earlier article), *"Although we found smoking to be associated with mild preterm, but not extreme preterm, delivery, **smoking remains a recognized risk for preterm delivery** and should still be considered a problem from the fetal perspective."*

Not only that, but following is an article, *"adapted from a news release issued by Elsevier"*, announcing that ***"Smoking during pregnancy can increase*** **[the]** ***risk of ADHD in*** **[the]** ***child".***

> *Women smokers who become pregnant have long been encouraged to reduce or eliminate their nicotine intake. A new study being published in the June 15th issue of Biological Psychiatry provides further reason to do so, as it presents new evidence that **in utero exposure to smoking is associated with attention deficit/hyperactivity disorder (ADHD) problems in genetically susceptible children.***

Rosalind Neuman, Ph.D., one of the study's authors, explains the findings: "When genetic factors are combined with prenatal cigarette smoke exposure, the ADHD risk rises very significantly. When the child has either or both of two specific forms of dopamine pathway genes (DAT and DRD4), and was exposed to cigarette smoking in utero, the risk for having combined type ADHD (many inattention and hyperactive/impulsive symptoms) increased 3 to 9 fold."

These data highlight ***a new risk of maternal smoking, increasing the risk for ADHD in their children. ADHD, in turn, increases the risk for substance abuse.*** *Thus, it appears that in utero exposure to nicotine may help to perpetuate a cycle across generations that* ***links addiction and behavioral problems.****"*

This article appears in Biological Psychiatry, Volume 61, Issue 12 (June 15, 2007), published by Elsevier (http://www.sciencedaily.com/releases/2006/02/060206171449.htm).

The Dangers Of Chlorine

Although sufficient water is extremely important during pregnancy, "good" water is even more important. As we learned in the previous chapter, fluoridated water causes a host of health issues for both the mother and the baby, but as you are about to learn, chlorinated water also causes health risks, (especially regarding thyroid function), and even potential miscarriages!

As noted in his book *Essential Oils Desk Reference, second edition*, (June 2002), Dr. D. Gary Young, N.D., points out that ***"Chlorine is one of the most reactive and toxic elements known to man"*** and goes on to warn that *"When put in the public water supply as a disinfectant, it creates disinfection byproducts (DBP) that* ***can cause cancer, birth defects, and spontaneous abortions"*** (p. 419). Dr. Young goes on to warn:

Once ingested or inhaled, chlorinated chemicals leach into the fat cells and become trapped. THMs (trihalomethanes) are very volatile – this means they can be inhaled during bathing as well as consumed in potable water. Showering, washing dishes, and flushing a toilet can also contaminate the air with trihalomethanes.

Once trapped inside the body, the chemically bind with and damage DNA.

Several studies have been done on pregnant women to determine the effects of THMs in drinking water. Following are just a few:

A California Department of Health study surveyed 5,144 pregnant women and fount that pregnant women who consumed more than 5 glasses of water a day containing more than 75 ppb (parts per billion) had double the risk of spontaneous abortion. Researchers at the University of North Carolina at Chapel Hill also examined the link between THMs and miscarriages in populations living throughout central North Carolina. They found that ***women who suffered the highest exposure to THM in the drinking water had almost triple the risk of miscarriage.***

Another study conducted by the U.S. Department of Health and Human Services examined the effect of THMs in the water supply of 75 towns throughout the state of New Jersey. When scientists compared levels of THMs to the frequency of birth defects, they found that ***women who consumed water exceeding 80 ppb THMs had triple the risk of giving birth to infants with neural tube defects.*** *The authors suggested that one of the reasons for this may be due to the fact that vitamin B12 may be disrupted in the body due to chloroform, a common THM.*

An even larger epidemiological study by the National Institute of Public Health in Norway surveyed the effects of chlorinated water on 141,077 infants born in Norway between 1993 and 1995. Researchers found that ***the higher the chlorine content of the water and the higher the organic matter in the water, the higher the risk for birth defects including cardiac defects, respiratory tract defects, and urinary tract defects.***

Murray S. Malcolm, M.D., a public health physician in New Zealand, [Wellington School of Medicine], *spearheaded a countrywide study that examined the role of THMs in triggering birth defects and cancer. He concluded,* ***"A quarter of all bladder, colon, rectal cancers, and birth defects may be preventable by reducing disinfection byproducts (i.e. THMs) exposure"*** (*Essential Oils Desk Reference, second edition*, DG Young, June 2002, p. 419).

Some Telling Statistics That Should Be Taken More Seriously (Your Child's IQ Could Depend On It)

In a recent survey, it was discovered that a greater percentage of children, in both Japan and China, were prepared academically to attend college, than the students in the United States. Why, might we ask, could that possibly be true? First, far more expectant mothers, and school age children in the U.S., are taking iodine-depleting, brain-damaging, I.Q.-lowering drugs. Second, the average child in Japan gets far more iodine from their diet (found in sea foods), than children in this country. Then, China appears to be the country that has taken the iodine deficiency potential the most seriously, and they have thus aggressively addressed the issue.

Back in 1993, China identified the connection between the level of fluoride in drinking water, and children's IQ, as follows:

It has been reported that ***fluoride can penetrate the fetal blood-brain barrier and accumulate in cerebral tissue before birth, thereby apparently affecting the children's intelligence.*** *In the present study, conducted in April 1993, this hypothesis was further investigated by comparing the performance on IQ tests administered to 320 randomly selected children, age 7 to 14, residing in central Shanxi Province, China, in two suburban villages with significantly different fluoride content in drinking water.*

The results of this study indicated that ***intake of high-fluoride drinking water from before birth has a significant deleterious influence on children's IQ*** *in*

one of two similar villages. No real differences were found for gender. ***In the high-fluoride village of Sima the number of children with IQ of 69 or below was six times that in the healthier low-fluoride village of Xinghua.***
(http://www.fluoridation.com/brain.htm)

If you noticed, all the children were still drinking water containing fluoride. One village just had higher concentrations of fluoride in their drinking water than the other. The question is, although "six times" as many children with a low IQ is phenomenal, if the second group were to drink water with "no fluoride", wouldn't you normally expect an even greater difference? The Chinese actually took the results of this study very seriously, and thus proceeded to address the problem. They were also aware that fluoride is an iodine suppressant, thus avoiding an iodine deficiency (whatever the cause) became their primary focus. The obvious solution should be two-pronged. First would be eliminating all iodine suppressing chemicals (such as fluoride). And second, add iodine to salt or foods that people consume daily. Insufficient iodine translates to low thyroid function, which then leads to many different undesirable conditions, including lower IQ, depression, fatigue, (and obviously poor grades).

As pointed out by Dr. Sherry Rogers, M.D., (*Detoxify or Die*, 2002), in a one-year study of 39,000 children in the United States, comparing those drinking fluorinated versus non-fluorinated water, it was discovered that instead of building strong healthy teeth, **fluoride actually damaged brain enzymes and lowered IQs!** She also found that **fluoride had been linked to behavioral disorders, and birth defects**, (which was just discussed in detail in the previous chapter, regarding the fetus). Another key issue she discusses regarding the brain is that, **once in the cell membrane, fluoride causes damage to hormone receptors, leading to their malfunction!** This is obviously a major concern, as brain cells have receptors for several hormones that influence our moods, our memory, and our energy level, as noted in the following study:

> ***Fluoride studies in rats can be indicative of a potential for motor disruption, intelligence deficits and learning disabilities in humans.*** *Humans are exposed to plasma levels of fluoride as high as those in rat studies.* ***Fluoride involves interruption of normal brain development. Fluoride affects the hippocampus in the brain, which integrates inputs from the environment, memory, and motivational stimuli, to produce behavioral decisions and modify memory.*** *Experience with other developmental neurotoxicants prompts expectations that changes in behavioral functions will be comparable across species, especially human and rats* (*Neurotoxicology and Teratology*, Vol. 17, No. 2, p. 176, **"Neurotoxicity of Sodium Fluoride",** Muellenix, Denbesten, Schunior, Kernan, 1995).

Just to put things in perspective, **although only about one part per million of fluoride is normally found in artificially fluoridated water, we find that every single molecule of Prozac™ actually consists of three molecules of fluoride,** as we previously mentioned. Therefore, if just drinking fluoridated water with a fairly low concentration of fluoride was found to create behavioral disorders and lowered IQs, then Prozac™ should be expected to have an even greater effect on children. Then keep in mind that some children taking Prozac™ are also drinking fluoridated water, which often contains another thyroid suppressant (chlorine) as well!

One Underlying Contributor To A Child's Lower IQ: Prozac's Fluoride Is Causing Iodine Deficiency Disorder (IDD)

Some developing countries, although China in particular, appear to be very concerned about a serious health problem that is associated with a deficiency of iodine in the diet. **One of the greatest contributors to an iodine deficiency in the United States is fluoride!** If you consider that **Prozac™ contains high levels of fluoride**, and that fluoride is a toxic thyroid suppressant, as well as a known iodine agonist, and that a low level of iodine retards brain development, and contributes to mental retardation, you can easily see why Prozac™ is such a serious threat. Then, `as fluoride also reduces the action of enzymes, and damages hormone receptors in the brain, you can now understand how broad its influence can be.

The International Council for Control of Iodine Deficiency Disorders' website, (http://indorgs.virginia.edu/iccidd), devoted to research on the iodine deficiencies in several countries, stresses that the problem is very serious, as follows:

> ***IDD [Iodine Deficiency Disorder] is the single most widespread cause of mental retardation in children. In the early stages of life, it retards brain development by preventing the fetal brain from establishing sufficiently dense cell networks. Later it can manifest itself as low academic test scores or mental retardation.***

The children at the greatest risk for an iodine deficiency are those exposed to fluoride, (especially a concern regarding Prozac™), before they are even born. Many adults are also iodine deficient, as the majority of our dietary iodine comes from iodized salt, and most doctors still recommend avoiding salt, which incidentally is poor advice, (and not just due to its iodine content)! Then on the grocery shelves, you will find both iodized and non-iodized salt, (for no apparent reason). Many aren't even aware of the importance of adequate iodine in the diet. Then, most processed foods list salt (not iodized salt) as an ingredient. Unfortunately, years ago the decision was made to replace iodine (important to the thyroid) with bromine (a thyroid suppressant), as a dough conditioner! This was a poor decision with absolutely no justification. As a result, most baked goods on the store shelves now contain bromine, also contributing to poor thyroid function. This is also a major contributor to obesity in both children and adults.

In some developing countries, due to the poverty, poor education, and remoteness of some villages, it's difficult to assure that everyone gets iodized salt, although in several countries they are actually very aware of the concern, and are thus taking steps to try to eliminate the problem. China appears to be the country taking the lead in attempting to find the best way to resolve this major issue. Unfortunately, it's an issue that doesn't appear to be taken nearly as seriously in this country, although we could quite easily resolve if we so chose, yet it's an issue we appear to be continuing to ignore. Not only are we adding the known iodine agonist, "fluoride", to the drinking water in many cities, but we are also giving it to pregnant mothers in the form of SSRI antidepressant drugs. We couldn't do much more to assure that many in the nation will be iodine deficient, (suffering with IDD), without totally banning iodine altogether. A major contributor to poor health, especially regarding the fetus, is a low thyroid condition, from inadequate iodine intake, or from iodine depletion by the bromine added to baking goods, and fluoride added to our drinking water and widely prescribed drugs, (although these are all things that you can easily avoid, if you so choose).

Unfortunately, in the U.S. we're continually looking for ways to improve children's academics in school, while damaging their brains, and lowering their IQs, often even before they are born. And then we somehow justify placing as many children as possible on mind-altering drugs, sometimes even before they start school. If we're truly searching for a way to improve children's grades, the answer should be obvious: Get them, (and their mothers), off these dangerous IQ-lowering drugs. Their entire future, (and thus our nation's), depends on whether we start taking action, or just continue ignoring the obvious problem, as we have in the past. If it wasn't obvious before, hopefully it is by now.

China is fully aware, (as we should be), that their nation's future lies in the potential of the upcoming generation. The U.S. is currently falling behind in that regard. The only way we can expect to stop the current trend, is to "just say no" to all mind-altering I.Q.-lowering drugs, beginning with expectant mothers, and ending with the elderly, who would prefer to avoid unnecessarily retiring in an Alzheimer's ward.

What Else Can You Do To Influence Your Child's IQ? Actually, Far More Than You Might Think!

It's not just accidental that the parents' IQ doesn't always determine what their child's IQ might be. It's likely that the parents' education and vocabulary might at least have some influence on their children's IQ, although it often begins very early with the environment provided by the mother during the fetus's brain development.

✓ As previously mentioned, **EFAs are extremely important to both the developing brain, as well as all though life.** Research has shown that infants of mothers who supplemented with EFAs had higher IQs, psychomotor development and eye-hand coordination at 4 years of age (*Indian Journal of Pediatrics*, 2005, pp. 239-242). **And, although this pertains to raising your child's IQ, after it is born, more research has found that *"infants receiving formulas not supplemented with fatty acids score significantly lower on tests assessing IQ-related skills than do infants receiving supplemented formulas"*** (*Psychiatric Times*, 1998, December, Vol. XI, Issue 12). And then, ***"intake of EFAs during preschool years may also have a beneficial role in the prevention of ADHD, while enhancing learning capability and academic performance"*** (*Indian Journal of Pediatrics*, 2005, pp. 239-242).

✓ As we likely learned by now, antidepressants such as Prozac™ and Paxil™ create the worst possible environment for the development of the fetus's brain, (or body in general). So avoiding them must become our top priority. Remember, these SSRI antidepressants not only produce excessive stress hormones, but they also contribute to nutrient depletion (for mother and baby), which may very well affect birth weight. And studies have shown that, while ***"babies born with low birth weights had a higher incidence of a number of chronic cardiovascular conditions as adults, including heart disease, hypertension (high blood pressure), diabetes and raised cholesterol,"*** we find that ***"A recent collaborative study between scientists in Britain and Queensland found that high birth weight is linked in later life to an elevated IQ"*** (http://www.lafamily.com/display_article.php?id=1089).

✓ Another concern worth mentioning is the statin (cholesterol lowering) drugs that many are being unnecessarily placed on by their doctor. This is such a widespread practice that I believe it deserves mentioning. Other than antidepressants, they are one of the worst drugs on the market, and in my opinion "totally unnecessary"! They can weaken your heart, damage your kidneys, zap your energy, and even make you wonder where your memory went. Not only that, but they are suppressing the liver's ability to produce cholesterol, and the greatest demand for cholesterol just happens to be the brain and nerves, as well as producing hormones critical for the fetus, (such as progesterone).

Elevated cholesterol is not, and never has been the risk that it was made out to be. The true risk factor is elevated homocysteine, which few doctors discuss with their patients, (unless they are a natural practitioner). **Not only does elevated homocysteine contribute to damage to the arteries, but the neurons in the brain as well. And the folic acid, along with vitamins B_6 and B_{12}, necessary for controlling homocysteine, just happen to be depleted by Prozac™!** As you can see, Prozac™ appears to be multi-talented when it comes to destroying your physical and mental health, (as well as that of your fetus).

✓ If your cholesterol level is excessive, (other than providing an increased demand for the developing fetus), you likely have a low thyroid condition, which incidentally can have a substantial influence on your child's IQ, (and yours). I cover the condition in considerable detail under the chapter on Hypothyroidism. As I mentioned, far more women experience the problem than men, and it's one of the greatest contributors to both fatigue and depression, (and the very reason so many women are "unnecessarily" placed on antidepressants). This is another travesty in medicine today, and women are by far the most abused in that regard.

Another example was the excessive prescribing of the hormone replacement therapy (HRT), using the "artificial hormones", (Premarin™ for estrogen, and Provera™ for progesterone), which not only contributed to fluid retention, and weight gain, but also increased the risk for breast cancer. These unnatural hormones are unhealthy, and have many troubling side effects, and in my opinion, do not belong in any woman's body. Not only that, but most menopausal women already have enough estrogen, (and more often than not – too much). Even if she no longer has ovaries, a woman's fat tissue, and even her adrenals, are capable of producing estrogen, (and we can't forget the xenoestrogens). Worst of all, elevated estrogen suppress the thyroid, (a major contributor to depression)!

✓ British physician Katherina Dalton, a pioneer in progesterone research who spent decades **treating pregnant women with progesterone**, **observed that women she treated *"had children with higher IQs and calmer dispositions",*** (*What Your Doctor May Not Tell You About Breast Cancer*, Dr. John Lee, M.D., 2002, p. 102). Just the opposite is true of children whose mothers are instead placed on antidepressants. They would likely tend to have lower IQs, and more inclined to experience ADHD, not to mention an increased risk for developing diabetes and cancer!

When supplementing with progesterone cream, it is important to use **natural progesterone**, and not the synthetic progestins in tablet form usually prescribed by medical doctors for hormone replacement therapy, as they are the altered synthetic form of the hormone that are responsible for many negative side effects. **You do not need a prescription for natural progesterone cream.** Both pregnenolone tablets and progesterone cream are available from many health food stores, mail order, and even some pharmacies. *International Health* sells a natural progesterone cream called EssProL'eve™, which comes in a 3-ounce dispenser that automatically dispenses the proper amount. It is applied topically for transdermal delivery (absorption through the skin). To order EssProL'eve™, contact *International Health* by calling (800) 481-9987, or visit http://internationalhealth.net/defalut.asp.

Reducing The Mother's Breast Cancer Risk

Another important issue for the mother is, both the Iodoral™ and natural progesterone (in cream form, applied topically), greatly reduce the risk of the mother acquiring breast cancer.

According to the National Cancer Institute, ***"A woman who has her first child after the age of 35 has approximately twice the risk of developing breast cancer as a woman who has a child before age 20"*** (http://www.cancer.gov/cancertopics/factsheet/Risk/pregnancy).

It is also advised that *"After pregnancy, breastfeeding for a long period of time (for example, a year or longer) further reduces breast cancer risk by a small amount,"* which would benefit both mother and child, unless the mother was taking a drug such as Prozac™ or Paxil™. In that case, the child would be unnecessarily exposed to the toxic fluoride, and elevated cortisol, even longer.

Other than the thyroid, the highest concentration of iodine is found in women's breast tissue. When the level of iodine is low, the risk of acquiring breast cancer is greater, and as we're aware, the fluoride found in Prozac™ disrupts the iodine, reducing the iodine level. Also, women who acquire breast cancer normally have elevated estrogen and a low level of progesterone in their breast tissue as well. The natural progesterone keeps the estrogen levels in check, basically preventing the problem. And if you really want to prevent the problem, you should definitely avoid Paxil™! According to Dr. Tracy, ***"the possibility for breast cancer is 700% greater after Paxil use. I suspect similar results to come in with the other SSRIs"*** (*Help! I Can't Get Off My Antidepressants!*, audiotape, 1999). As you can see, Paxil™ (and likely other SSRIs, which would include Prozac™) greatly increases the risk for acquiring breast cancer.

Something else to consider is regarding statin (cholesterol lowering) drugs, and the importance of cholesterol. An article by Sally Fallon and Mary G. Enig, Ph.D., originally posted on The Weston A Price Website (http://www.westonaprice.org/moderndiseases/statin.html), titled *"The Dangers Of Statin Drugs – What You Haven't Been Told About Cholesterol Lowering Medications"* pointed out that "***Hypercholesterolemia* [high cholesterol] *is the health issue of the 21st century. It is actually an invented disease, a 'problem' that emerged when health professionals learned how to measure cholesterol levels in the blood."*** With that in mind, the article went on to note that ***"In one trial, the CARE trial, breast cancer rates of those taking a statin went up 1500 percent."*** That's a significant increase, yet doctors continue placing women on cholesterol lowering medications, (if they only knew – and now you know).

Any study with that kind of results, showing how the drugs that many women are taking are increasing their risk of acquiring breast cancer by an amazing 1500%, should have made front page news, yet very few are even aware! Worst of all, it's a drug for a non-disease, which absolutely no one needs!

A Cancer Cure – Deliberately Suppressed Decades Ago – Would Have Destroyed The Huge Profit Potential Of The Cancer Industry

Interestingly, about 65 years ago, a man named Harry Hoxsey, from Texas, was successful in curing tens of thousands of those with cancer, whose doctors had basically given up on them, as they were considered as incurable, (referred to as Stage IV cancer). Hoxsey named his formula "The Hoxsey Formula", and other than a few herbs, it contained potassium iodide, sometimes just referred to as iodide, (**one of the two ingredients in Iodoral™**).

You might wonder why doctors are still resorting to the use of the very toxic chemo and radiation therapy, and have been for decades. The answer: That's where the money is! Both the AMA and the American Cancer Society took Hoxsey to court, over and over, and eventually put him out of business. Combined, they have tremendous financial resources, which we are unfortunately supporting, (whether we like it or not). In my book *A Drug-Free Approach To Healthcare,* (which is now available in a new *Revised Edition*), I discuss several natural options to choose from, if you or a loved one acquires cancer. It's best to avoid cancer in the first place, if you can, thus I also discuss the causes of cancer, so you can avoid them. True medicine should be based on disease prevention, not symptom suppression. Although diseases considered as incurable are often curable using natural therapies, it's best to prevent them, as the damage they inflict must be repaired.

As you have learned, just by getting off Prozac™, Paxil™, or any other SSRI antidepressant, and adding Iodoral™ and natural progesterone cream, you can increase your child's intelligence, (and his or her chance for a more successful future), while helping yourself avoid the dreaded breast cancer as well; A tremendous benefit for two people, (mother and fetus), and definitely well worth the effort. All the things you do to avoid cancer, will help the fetus as well, thus you will both benefit. Although drugs can be very unpredictable, and rather frustrating, natural supplements are instead very refreshing. Your body will be ever so grateful for caring.

Doesn't the natural drug-free approach make a lot more sense, especially if you want to maintain your health, while also assuring that your fetus will be exposed to a healthy environment during its development as well?

Avoid The Dangerous Anti-Seizure Drug, Valproic Acid (Depakote™)

Another prescription drug to avoid is the anticonvulsant/antiseizure drug Depakote™ (generic name: valproate or Valproic Acid)! According to a report published by the American Academy of Neurology, ***"24 percent of the children of mothers who took valproate showed an IQ in the mental retardation range"*** (*New York Times*, May, 4 2007).

This is especially a concern when you take into consideration the domino effect, and the fact that **45 of the top 200 most prescribed drugs (nearly one-fourth!) list "seizures" as a potential side effect.** Thus, you can easily see how you could end up being prescribed an antiseizure medication. Following are the 45 prescription drugs (most commonly prescribed – although there are likely hundreds more), found to potentially cause seizures, along with their generic names, and what they are most commonly prescribed for:

1. **Advair Diskus™ (generic name: fluticasone & salmeterol)-** Prescribed to treat asthma.
2. **Proventil™ (generic name: Albuterol)**- Used to treat bronchospasms, associated with asthma.
3. **Xanax™ (generic name: Alprazolam)**- Benzodiazepine, used to treat anxiety disorders.
4. **Elavil™ (generic name: Amitriptyline)**- Tricyclic antidepressant.
5. **Amoxil™ (generic name: Amoxicillin)**- A Penicillin antibiotic.
6. **Aricept™ (generic name: donepezil)**- Used to treat Alzheimer's disease.

7. **Avelox™ (generic name: moxifloxacin)**- A fluoroquinolone antibiotic.
8. **Soma™ (generic name: Carisoprodol)**- Muscle relaxant.
9. **Celexa™ (generic name: citalopram)**- SSRI antidepressant
10. **Keflex™ or Keftab™ (generic name: Cephalexin)**- A cephalosporin antibiotic.
11. **Cipro™ (generic name: ciprofloxacin)**- A fluoroquinolone antibiotic.
12. **Klonopin™ (generic name: Clonazepam)**- Benzodiazepine, used to treat seizures and panic (anxiety) disorders.
13. **Ritalin™ or Concerta™ (generic name: methylphenidate)**- Central nerous system stimulant used to treat ADD and ADHD.
14. **Valium™ or Diastat™ (generic name: Diazepam)**- benzodiazepines used to relieve anxiety.
15. **Diovan HCT™ (generic name: valsartan & hydrochlorothizide)**- An ACE inhibitor plus a thiazide diuretic, used to lower blood pressure and decrease edema (swelling).
16. **Effexor XR™ (generic name: vanlafaxine hydrochloride)**- Serotonin / norepinephrine reuptake inhibitor prescribed as an antidepressant, and to treat anxiety.
17. **Prozac™ or Sarafem™ (generic name: fluoxetine)**- SSRI antidepressant
18. **Humalog™ (generic name: Insulin Lispro)**- Man-made insulin, used in the treatment of diabetes to lower high blood sugar levels.
19. **Humulin 70/30™ (generic name: Insulin Isophane & Insulin Regular)**- Man-made insulin, used in the treatemtn of diabetes to lower high blood sugar levels.
20. **Humulin N™ (generic name: Insulin Isophane)**- Man-made insulin used in the treatment of diabetes to lower high blood sugar levels.
21. **Vicodin™ (generic name: hydrocodone & acetaminophen)**- Narcotic pain reliever.
22. **Imitrex™ (generic name: Sumatriptan)**- Serotonin 5-HT_{1D} Receptor Agonist, used to treat vascular headaches such as migraine and cluster headaches.
23. **Imdur™ (generic name: Isosorbide Mononitrate)**- A member of the nitrate family, prescribed to dilate blood vessels and prevent chest pain.
24. **Lantus™ (generic name: Insulin Glargine)**- Man-made insulin used in the treatment of type 1 diabetes.
25. **Lescol XL™ (generic name: fluvastatin)**- Statin cholesterol-lowering drug that blocks the production of cholesterol in the body.
26. **Lavaquin™ (generic name: levofloxacin)**- A fluoroquinolone antibiotic.
27. **Levothroid™ or Synthroid™ (generic name: levothyroxin)**- used to treat hypothyroidism.
28. **Lexapro™ (generic name: escitalopram oxalate)**- SSRI antidepressant
29. **Ativan™ (generic name: lorazepam)**- Benzodiazepine, prescribed to treat anxiety and seizures.
30. **Omnicef™ (generic name: cefdinir)**- Antibiotic.
31. **OxyContin™ (generic name: Oxycodone)**- Narcotic analgesic.
32. **Paxil™ (generic name: Paroxetine)**- SSRI antidepressant.
33. **Paxil CR™ (generic name: Paroxetine)**- SSRI antidepressant.
34. **Phenergan™ (generic name: promethazine)**- Antihistamine, also used as a sedative.
35. **Promethazine & Codeine** – Antihistamine and narcotic analgesic combination, commonly used in the form of a syrup cough suppressant.
36. **Remeron™ (generic name: mirtazapine)**- antidepressant.

37. **Risperdal™ (generic name: risperidone)**- Antipsychotic medication used for the treatment of schizophrenia and mania associated with bipolar disorder.
38. **Seroquel™ (generic name: quetiapine)**- Antipsychotic medication used for the treatment of schizophrenia and mania associated with bipolar disorder.
39. **Singulair™ (generic name: montelukast)**- a Leukotriene inhibitor, used to prevent asthma.
40. **Skelaxin™ (generic name: metaxalone)**- Muscle relaxant.
41. **Restoril™ (generic name: temazepam)**- Benzodiazepine used to reduce anxiety and epilepsy.
42. **Ultracet™ (generic name: acetaminophen & tramadol)**- pain reliever combination.
43. **Wellbutrin SR™ (generic name: bupropion)**- Antidepressant. Also used to treat bipolar depression and ADD.
44. **Zoloft™ (generic name: sertraline)**- SSRI antidepressant.
45. **Zyprexa™ (generic name: olanzapine)**- Antipsychotic, used to treat symptoms of schizophrenia and bipolar disorder.

It's scary, to say the least, that so many medications can contribute to something as serious as seizures! That tells us they are obviously having a major influence on the brain. Then, on the above list of medications, a surprising number are those many pregnant women are likely currently taking. I can see several major concerns that could dramatically influence the fetus.

First is the potential danger to the fetus, if the mother begins experiencing seizures. And possibly even worse is, if the mother is placed on the drug Depakote™, which many doctors prescribe for the seizures, as there is about one chance in four that their child could wind up with mental retardation!

Possibly most important of all is, seldom (if ever) does a woman need any of the medications that can contribute to seizures in the first place. And this is just one of many examples. As you likely know by now, all drugs (legal or illegal) are inherently dangerous, (and some can be outright scary), especially during pregnancy!

Promising New Research, Currently In Progress - New Baby Formula Will Fight Fat

Following is a portion of a story adapted from a news release issued by *Society of Chemical Industry* (http://www.sciencedaily.com/releases/2007/04/070423080517.htm):

> ***Infant formula and other baby foods that provide permanent protection from obesity and diabetes into adulthood could be on shop shelves soon,*** *reports Lisa Melton in Chemistry & Industry, the magazine of the SCI.*
> *The foods, under development at the Clore Laboratory at the University of Buckingham, will be supplemented with leptin, the hunger hormone. Those who take the foods early in life should remain permanently slim.*
>
> [Mike] *Cawthorne's group has already demonstrated that* ***supplementing infant rats' diets with leptin means that they never get fat or develop diabetes*** *(AM J Physiol Regul Integr Comp Physiol, doi: 10.1152/ajpregu.00676.2006). Even animals fed a high-fat diet remained slim.* [Sounds a lot like some people I know.]

Providing leptin [early] *enough effectively hard-wires the body's energy balance. In fact, whether one is fat or thin may be determined before birth. Feeding the hormone to pregnant rats has been found to have a lifelong impact on their offspring's predisposition to obesity.* ***Animals born of leptin-treated mothers remain lean even when fed a fat-laden diet, while those from untreated dams gained weight and developed diabetes.***

The difference boils down to energy expenditure. The offspring of leptin-treated mothers burn up more energy.

Edinburgh researcher Jonathan Seckl says. "We need to know whether leptin is acting pre- and post-natally, figure out how it works, and dissect the possible side-effects before this becomes a potential approach for humans. Nonetheless, this is good science," he says.

Promoting An Easier Delivery, And A More Rapid Recovery

Dr. John Christopher's son, David, now produces many herbal formulas developed by his father. They have one formula in particular, which a mother can begin taking about six weeks prior to the expected delivery date. It strengthens the female organs, and should help make the delivery much easier. It's an herbal formula called Prenatal™. One of David Christopher's employees indicated that she had taken the Prenatal™ formula prior to having her first child. She claims she was in labor only 30 minutes, and had an easy delivery, with absolutely no complications. A long difficult delivery can place stress on both the mother and the fetus. It also increases the risk of trauma to the fetus, potentially resulting in brain damage.

Although, if you do have a cesarean section, (which is becoming all too common now days), there are a couple supplements I would recommend. One is to take eight 1,000 mg tablets of ester C, in divided doses, throughout the day, to help increase the collagen necessary for rebuilding tissue, (just remember that Prozac™ has just the opposite effect). Then begin taking three capsules of the protolytic (protein digesting) enzyme Vitalzyme™, twice daily. It helps in the healing process by reducing inflammation, as well as digesting and removing necrotic (dead) tissue in the bloodstream, (resulting from surgery), which helps thin the blood and improve the circulation, and thus promotes healing. And according to Dr. William Wong, N.D., Vitalzyme™ greatly reduces the amount of scarring following surgery.

Both the Prenatal™ formula, and Vitalzyme™, are commonly sold through health food stores, however, Prenatal™ can be purchased by calling *Dr. Christopher's* at (800) 453-1406, to find a store that handles it. And to purchase Vitalzyme™, call *World Nutrition* at (800) 548-2710 or visit http://worldnutrition.info.

Now that we know how you can avoid unnecessary risks, and help insure that you will have a better chance of carrying the fetus to full term, have an easy delivery, as well as a healthy baby, we need to look at another potential risk (the unnecessary drugging of young kids). As it quite often starts with Ritalin™, or one of its close cousins, that's where we will now start.

CHAPTER SIX

"ADHD" – A Contrived Condition With Absolutely No Validation!

The Diagnosis, The Medications, and Real Causes of the Symptoms

Something to consider is: If there is absolutely no "valid diagnostic test" for ADHD, then how can they possibly justify prescribing a potentially dangerous stimulant like Ritalin™ to kids, for an non-diagnosable condition? The truth is, they just go on doing it, without any justification! The question is: Who is going to stop them, (so far no one)!

Following is an extract from an on-line article titled ***"Ritalin – The Hidden Effects,"*** (http://www.healthliesexposed.com/articles/article_2006_05_26_2415.shtml), by Jon Rappaport, an independent investigative reporter who has published numerous articles on medical issues in both the US and Europe:

> ***On November 16-18, 1998, the National Institute of Mental Health held the prestigious "NIH Consensus Development Conference on Diagnosis and Treatment of Attention Deficit Hyperactivity Disorder [ADHD]." The conference was explicitly aimed at ending all debate about the diagnoses of ADD, ADHD, and about the prescription of Ritalin.*** *It was hoped that at the highest levels of medical research and bureaucracy, a clear position would be taken: this is what ADHD is, this is where it comes from, and these are the drugs it should be treated with. That didn't happen, amazingly. Instead, the official panel responsible for drawing conclusions from the conference threw cold water on the whole attempt to reach a comfortable consensus.*
>
> *Panel member Mark Vonnegut, a Massachusetts pediatrician, said,* ***"The diagnosis [of ADHD] is a mess."***
>
> *The quite conventional and orthodox panel essentially said it was not sure ADHD was even a valid diagnosis. In other words,* ***it virtually admitted that ADD and ADHD might be nothing more than attempts to categorize certain children's behaviors---with no organic cause, no clear-cut biological basis, no provable reason for even using the ADD or ADHD labels.***
>
> ***The panel found "no data to indicate that ADHD is due to a brain malfunction*** *[which malfunction had been the whole psychiatric assumption]."*
>
> ***The panel found that Ritalin has not been shown to have long-term benefits. In fact, the panel stated that Ritalin has resulted in "little improvement on academic achievement or social skills."***
>
> *Panel chairman, David Kupfer, professor of psychiatry at the University of Pittsburgh, said,* ***"There is no current validated diagnostic test [for ADHD]."***

Yet at every level of public education in America, there remains what can only be called a voracious desire to give children Ritalin (or other similar drugs) for so-called ADD or ADHD.

Beverly Eakman, author and president of the 2001 National Education Consortium, pointed out that ***"Children are being diagnosed with a list of behaviors that in 1987 was literally voted into existence by the American Psychiatric Association and inserted in the DSM-IV, Diagnostic and Statistical Manual of Mental Disorders****. Within one year 500,000 children in the U.S. were diagnosed with the disorder"* (http://www.ritalindeath.com/ADHD-Controversy.htm).

Even the U.N.-sponsored International Narcotics Control Board, back in March 2000, blasted the United States for over prescribing stimulants such as Ritalin™, pointing out that ***"America consumes more than 90 percent of all the methylphenidate* [Ritalin™] *taken worldwide"*** (http://www.salon.com/news/feature/2000/03/21/prozac).

And, although the following might appear extreme, it is far from an isolated example. According to an on-line article by Arianna Huffington, titled "P is for Preschoolers... And Prozac," the father of one fourth-grader at an elementary school in Millbrook, New York, commented that ***"Half of the students in his son's school were on Ritalin, and the school nurse had to go along on field trips to administer the kids' medicine"*** (http://ariannaonline.huffingtonpost.com/columns/column.php?id=240).

And it's no wonder, if you consider that child neurologist Fred Baughman, author of *The ADHD Fraud: How Psychiatry Makes "Patients" of Normal Children*, reports that ***"10 million of the 50 million school children in the nation are on one or more psychiatric drug"*** (http://www.sierratimes.com/07/02/27/75_7_243_126_94769.htm).

The following article is alarmingly accurate in its portrayal of what is happening to our children:

Schoolchildren Are Increasingly Dosed With Both Ritalin and Anti-Psychotic Drugs, Says New Research

Researchers from the Children's Hospital at Vanderbilt have found that ***anti-psychotic medications are being prescribed at an alarming rate for Tennessee children with Attention Deficit Hyperactivity Disorder, or ADHD. The use of anti-psychotic drugs has more than doubled since 1996,*** *and today children are not only being dosed with Ritalin -- a powerful narcotic drug -- but now anti-psychotic drugs to mask other symptoms related to behavioral disorders.*

Dosing our children with powerful narcotics in order to alter their brain chemistry rather than teaching them how to avoid the foods that cause these behavioral disorders in the first place.

We turn our children into literal druggies by forcing them onto extremely dangerous narcotic and anti-psychotic drugs.

ADHD is not a behavioral disorder, nor is it some sort of mysterious chemical imbalance in the brain. *It is simply the natural effect of pursuing a diet that is very high in refined carbohydrates and very low in optimum nutrition.*

They load up on high-sugar breakfast cereals, soft drinks, candy bars, sweets, cookies, and desserts, and then, just in case they don't have enough sugar in their system already, when they go to school they get rewarded with more candy and desserts, and they even have the opportunity to purchase soft drinks and candy bars from vending machines that are actually supported and promoted by the school bureaucrats.

We have a fast-expanding collection of mental health professionals who are increasingly putting children on powerful narcotic drugs in order to mask the symptoms caused by the widespread consumption of sugars and processed foods.

The victims in all of this are, of course, the children themselves, who end up going through the public school system with increased risk for obesity, diabetes and other diseases promoted by the consumption of food ingredients like white flour or refined white sugar.

And people wonder why we have such high rates of obesity, diabetes, and drug dependency in our adult population. *It's not mystery – just look at the children we're raising in this country.* ***We're raising yet another generation of drug-addicted, chronically diseased, overweight, brain-numbed zombies – and proudly declaring it "public education"*** (http://www.newstarget.com/001622.html).

According to the U.S. Centers For Disease Control and Prevention, **as of May 2006, an estimated 3.3 million Americans, ages 19 and younger, *"are treated with addictive, dangerous, and potentially deadly drugs without demonstration of abnormality of disease"*** (http://www.ritalindeath.com/ADHD-Controversy.htm).

Why Are They Unnecessarily Drugging Our Children? And Why Are Parents Being Threatened For Refusing To Do So?

Regardless of the total lack of legitimacy of an "ADHD" diagnosis, the standard treatment by medical doctors remains to be the dangerous Ritalin-type stimulants. And **many parents have discovered that their children may only be allowed to continue school on the condition that they take Ritalin™.** There have even been accounts of **social agencies saying the parents were unfit, and threatening to take children away, unless they allow their children to be prescribed Ritalin™.**

The previously mentioned on-line article by Arianna Huffington also relates one of the patients Dr. Peter Breggin discusses in his book, ***Reclaiming Our Children***, as follows:

> *One of Breggin's patients is Michael Weathers, a fourth-grader at the Alden Place Elementary School in Millbrook, N.Y., who* ***was given a succession of psychiatric drugs, including Ritalin and Paxil, starting in the second grade. When his parents, disturbed by the manic side effects, took him off the drugs, the school reported them to Child Protective Services, charging them with, among other things, medical neglect****.*
>
> (http://ariannaonline.huffingtonpost.com/columns/column.php?id=240)

And this didn't just start happening, but has **become a widespread problem of taking away parents' rights.** As seen in this report published in the *USA Today*, **August 8, 2000**, this obviously has been going on for many years:

> ***Some public schools are accusing parents of child abuse when they balk at giving their kids drugs such as Ritalin, and as judges begin to agree, some parents are medicating their children for fear of having them hauled away.***
>
> *It's an emerging twist in the growing debate about diagnosing and medicating children with attention deficit disorder (ADD) and attention deficit and hyperactivity disorder (ADHD):* ***An Albany, NY, couple put their 7-year-old son back on Ritalin after a family court ruled that they must continue medicating him for ADD.***
>
> *Child protective services visited another New York couple to check out anonymous allegations of "medical neglect" after they took their son off Ritalin and other drugs because of side effects, the couple said.*
>
> *"This is relatively new, but it's happening," says Maryland psychiatrist Peter Breggin, who is aware of similar cases in Boston. Often, he says,* ***divorced parents disagree on medicating kids, and judges recently have ruled in favor of the parent who wants to medicate. The Albany case is the first pitting educators against parents that progressed to a judge's ruling.***
>
> *"This is going to be happening more and more," says psychologist Peter Jensen, who is on the board of Children and Adults With Attention Deficit Disorder a parents group that advocates combining drug and behavior treatments.*
>
> ***As many as 3.8 million schoolchildren are diagnosed with ADD/ADHD, according to the American Academy of Pediatrics.***
>
> *At least 2 million take Ritalin, a stimulant, for symptoms such as inattentiveness, impulsivity and sometimes hyperactivity. Many others are treated with different drugs.*

But should parents be forced to put their children on drugs?

The long-term effects of children taking stimulants have not been studied. *And psychology professor William Frankenberger, who has studied ADD/ADHD at the University of Wisconsin-EAU Claire for more than 20 years, says it's* ***"disturbing to take a decision like that out of parent's hands"*** (http://www.resultsproject.net/USA_Today.html).

In an accompanying article, several parents described their personal stories. One couple had a police officer come to their door. Only the fact that they had gotten a second opinion, in writing, that their son did not need to take any medication, saved them from possibly having him taken into protective custody. The parents had decided to take him off of the medications that he was on (Ritalin™, Dexedrine™, and Paxil™) due to the serious side effects they were causing. That is **"a very dangerous combination of drugs"** that absolutely no child should ever be placed on! **There are likely hundreds of similar horror stories like these, and this kind of abuse should not be allowed to happen! Especially when you consider that the very existence of the "disease" that Ritalin™ is prescribed for, is unproven, as well as Ritalin's unproven "benefits."**

In her book, *No More ADHD* (2001), Dr. Mary Ann Block states:

Let me clear this up right now. ADHD is not like diabetes and [the stimulant used for it] is not like insulin. Diabetes is a real medical condition that can be objectively diagnosed. ***ADHD is an invented label with no objective, valid means of identification.*** *Insulin is a natural hormone produced by the body and it is essential for life. [This stimulant] is a chemically derived amphetamine-like drug that is not necessary for life. Diabetes is an insulin deficiency.* ***Attention and behavioral problems are not a [stimulant] deficiency.***

The following is summarized from *Talking Back to Ritalin* (1998), by Peter R. Breggin, M.D. (http://www.antipsychiatry.org/ritalin.htm):

- *Several million children are being treated with Ritalin and other stimulants on the grounds that they have attention deficit-hyperactivity disorder (ADHD) and suffer from inattention, hyperactivity, or impulsivity. The stimulants include: Ritalin (methylphenidate), Dexedrine and DextroStat (dextroamphetamine or d-amphetamine), Adderall (d-amphetamine and amphetamine mixture), Desoxyn and Gradumet (methamphetamine), and Cylert (pemoline). Except for Cylert, all of these drugs have nearly identical effects and side effects. Ritalin and the amphetamines can for most purposes be considered one type of drug.*

- ***The number of children being drugged has escalated several-fold in the last few years.***

- ***Ritalin and amphetamine have almost identical adverse effects on the brain, mind and behavior,* including the production of drug-induced behavioral disorders, psychosis, mania, drug abuse, and addiction.**

- ***Ritalin and amphetamine frequently cause the very same problems they are supposed to treat--inattention, hyperactivity, and impulsivity.***

- ***A large percentage of children become robotic, lethargic, depressed, or withdrawn on stimulants.***

- ***Ritalin can cause permanent neurological tics* including Tourette's syndrome.**

- ***Ritalin can retard growth in children*** *by disrupting the cycles of growth hormone released by the pituitary gland.*

- ***The recent finding that Ritalin can cause cancer in some animals was not taken seriously enough by the drug company or the FDA.***

- ***Ritalin routinely causes gross malfunctions in the brain of the child. There is research evidence from a few controlled scientific studies that Ritalin can cause shrinkage (atrophy) or other permanent physical abnormalities in the brain.***

- ***Withdrawal from Ritalin can cause emotional suffering, including depression, exhaustion, and suicide.*** *This can make children seem psychiatrically disturbed and lead mistakenly to increased doses of medication.*

[MY NOTE: Proper nutritional supplementation during withdrawal can help prevent the withdrawal reactions noted. That is important for both Ritalin™ and antidepressants. If handled properly, withdrawal should be relatively trouble-free.]

- *ADHD and Ritalin are American and Canadian medical fads.* ***The U.S. uses 90% of the world's Ritalin.*** *CibaGeneva Pharmaceuticals (also known as Ciba-Geigy Corporation), a division of Novartis, is the manufacturer of Ritalin. It is trying to expand the Ritalin market to Europe and the rest of the world.*

- ***Ritalin "works" by producing malfunctions in the brain rather than by improving brain function.*** *This is the only way it works.*

- *Short-term, Ritalin suppresses creative, spontaneous and autonomous activity in children, making them more docile and obedient, and more willing to comply with rote, boring tasks, such as classroom school work and homework.*

- *Short-term,* ***Ritalin has no positive effect on a child's psychology or on academic performance and achievement. This is confirmed by innumerable studies and by many professional reviews of the literature.***

- *Longer-term, beyond several weeks,* ***Ritalin has no positive effects on any aspect of a child's life.***

- ***Labeling children with ADHD and treating them with Ritalin can*** *keep them out of the armed services,* ***limit their future career choices,*** *and* ***stigmatize them for life.*** *It can* ***ruin their own self-image,*** *subtly* ***demoralize them, and discourage them from reaching their full potential.***

- ***There is no solid evidence that ADHD is a genuine disorder or disease of any kind.***

- ***There is a great deal of research to confirm that environmental problems cause ADHD-like symptoms.***

- *A very small number of children may suffer ADHD-like symptoms because of physical disorders, such as lead poisoning, drug intoxication, exhaustion, and head injury. Physical causes may be more common among poor communities in the United States.*

- ***There is no proof of any physical abnormalities in the brains or bodies of children who are routinely labeled ADHD.*** *They do not have known biochemical imbalances or "crossed wires."*

- ***ADHD is a controversial diagnosis with little or no scientific or medical basis. A parent, teacher, or doctor can feel in good company when utterly dismissing the diagnosis and refusing to apply it to children.***

- *Ciba* [pharmaceutical company] *spends millions of dollars to sell parent groups and doctors on the idea of using Ritalin. Ciba helps to support the parent group, C.H.A.D.D., and organized psychiatry.*

- ***The U.S. Department of Education and the National Institute of Mental Health (NIMH) push Ritalin as vigorously as the manufacturer of the drug, often in even more glowing terms than the drug company could get away with legally.***

- ***Ritalin is addictive and can become a gateway drug to other addictions. It is a common drug of abuse among children and adults.***

According to a survey released May 16, 2006 in Washington, D.C., by the Partnership for a Drug-Free America, ***"Four and a half million teenagers (19 percent) report abusing prescription medications to get high. This includes amphetamines like Ritalin and Adderall."*** This is likely due to the fact that the same survey, of more than 7,300 teenagers in grades 7-12, shows that ***"40 percent of teens think that prescription drugs are 'much safer' than illegal drugs."***

Are Prescription Drugs Any Safer Than Illegal Drugs?

Lucas A. Catton, President of the Foundation for Social Improvement and director of the International Drug-Free Alliance notes, regarding the study:

> ***People are being fooled every day into thinking that prescription drugs are generally safe.***
>
> ***Maybe the fact that these drugs are ruining the lives of so many teenagers will help adults wake up to see what is happening around them, but it shouldn't have had to come to this point.***
>
> ***...the recent additional findings about the dangers of antidepressants as well as the link between psychiatrist authors of the Diagnostic and Statistics Manual (DSM-IV) and pharmaceutical companies are more indicators that a corrupt system must be changed.***
> (http://www.emediawire.com/releases/2006/5/emw388413.htm)

Something to consider: The very same companies produced LSD, heroin, and cocaine, (once considered as legal, and aggressively promoted), that are now producing very similar "legal drugs", such as Ritalin™, Prozac™, and Paxil™. Not only that, but they were all approved by the FDA as "perfectly safe" for our use! They are all basically stimulants that target the very same hormones.

The following information, found in the *Life Extension's Disease Prevention and Treatment, expanded fourth edition*, (1991/2004, pp. 143-147), might help explain:

Ritalin Abuse

> ***The DEA classifies methylphenidate*** **[Ritalin™]** ***and amphetamine as Schedule II drugs (<u>those with the very highest potential for addiction and abuse</u>), a category that also includes methamphetamine, cocaine, and the most potent opiates and barbiturates. <u>Methylphenidate is derived from the same family as cocaine and gives a similar, brief 4-hour high, making it an increasingly popular recreational drug.</u>***
>
> *Ritalin tablets are often taken crushed and snorted like cocaine for a quick burst of energy.* ***<u>Emergency room admissions due to Ritalin abuse have also climbed rapidly,</u> and <u>severe side effects</u> such as hyperthermia, hypertension, <u>strokes,</u> <u>seizures,</u> and <u>death</u> are often observed.***

These drugs tend to create a dependency, and an imbalance in brain chemicals, often leading to the manic-depressive, or bipolar disorder, (discussed in a later chapter). Nothing would make a child more difficult for his or her teacher to deal with! Not only that, but when they go from the manic to the depressive state, they are much more prone to commit suicide. The higher the high, the lower the following low will be.

So what do we expect, when we are prescribing these potent drugs, with "the very highest potential for addiction and abuse" to our children, at such an alarming rate? Furthermore, another study from Massachusetts General Hospital (MGH), appearing in the April 2006 issue of the *Journal of the American Academy of Child and Adolescent Psychiatry*, reported the following:

> *The results showed that participants* [in the study] *with ADHD were more likely than those without ADHD to report* ***misusing their medication, with 11 percent admitting selling their drugs, 22 percent reporting they took too much, 10 percent getting high and 31 percent admitting they had taken their medication along with alcohol or other drugs.***
> (http://www.sciencedaily.com/releases/2006/03/060330162120.htm)

Possibly this is why recent research discovered that **adult** ADHD-drug use is increasing more than ever. The following news release from Medco Health Solutions, Inc., by chief medical officer Dr. Robert Epstein, M.D., M.S., was posted September 16, 2005, at *WebMD Medical News,* as follows:

> ***ADHD Drugs: Adult Use Doubled in 4 Years***
>
> *ADHD drug use grew more among adults than among kids and teens from 2000 to 2004, states a Medco news release.*
>
> *The growth in adult ADHD drug use outpaced increases in pediatric use by nearly 44%, notes Medco. Pediatric use was defined as use by patients aged 19 or younger.*
>
> ***The greatest growth in ADHD drug use was among adults aged 20-44.***
>
> *Medco's survey tracks prescription drug use,* ***not medical diagnoses*** *of ADHD.*
> (http://www.webmd.com/content/Article/112/110271.htm)

Not surprisingly, **research shows that over the past five years Ritalin™ has become the number one injected substitute for heroin in the United States** (http://www.uhuh.com/education/ritpsych.htm#c.%20Hazardous%20Heart%20Attacks%20Caused%20by%20Ritalin). And along with the legal use of Ritalin™, comes a large market for illegal use of the drug on the streets. And it's no wonder, as reported in the *Wall Street Journal* by Marilyn Chase (May 17, 1999), *"Nadine Lambert, a professor of education, followed almost 500 children for 26 years. She argues that* ***exposure to Ritalin makes the brain more susceptible to the addictive power of cocaine and doubles the risk of abuse."*** Doesn't it make more sense to stop the exposure altogether, and make these drugs illegal, just as heroin and cocaine now are? Anything that can increase the risk of a child becoming addicted to a drug such as cocaine in the future should be avoided at all costs! Cocaine or heroin addiction can totally destroy a person's life, so why increase that risk with our children?

Jeffrey's Story – A Little Boy Improperly Diagnosed With ADHD On Ritalin™ At Four – Graduates To Zoloft™ At Six Not Really ADHD – Just A Food Allergy!

We absolutely must take the time necessary to identify and then resolve the underlying problem. Often, something as simple as a minor dietary change or the elimination of an allergic food is adequate. Even eliminating sugar is often sufficient, and can make a major difference in both a child's behavior and his or her grades.

A prime example is my assistant's son named Jeffrey, who was diagnosed with ADHD at the age of three. Almost daily he would completely terrorize his preschool classroom, often biting and hitting other children and the teachers, to the point that his teachers strongly suggested medication. Just after turning four, Jeffrey was placed on Ritalin™, three times a day, under the direction of his pediatrician. When that didn't succeed in calming his outbursts, his dosage was increased, to the point that his pediatrician indicated it was standard protocol to try a stronger drug, as Jeffrey was already taking the highest dosage of Ritalin™ allowed. Thus, time-release Dexedrine™ was prescribed, which then resulted in many serious side effects. He had difficulty staying awake, appeared more like a zombie when he was awake, and complained of terrible headaches. Not only was the Dexedrine™ unsuccessful in calming Jeffrey, but within one week of changing his medication, Jeffrey was kicked out of preschool due to his continued uncontrollable behavioral problems. After observing the many severe and varied side effects Jeffrey was experiencing, his mom decided to stop giving him the Dexedrine™.

By May of his first grade year (age 6), the County Mental Health counselor announced, after just **one** visit, that Jeffrey's problems were actually "emotional" and that a new drug Zoloft™ was especially beneficial for that sort of problem. Jeffrey began taking Zoloft™, and did so through the summer, until November of that year, (a total of 6 months). During this time, he continued to complain of terrible headaches on a daily basis, began to experience difficulty in remembering things, and also wet the bed nightly.

After my assistant went to work for me, we were discussing Jeffrey's behavior and problems with bed-wetting, as well as his difficulty remembering. A milk allergy is often the underlying cause of bed-wetting, as well as headaches, and after discovering he was also on Zoloft™, that would likely explain his difficulty remembering. Together we decided to wean Jeffrey off Zoloft™, eliminate both milk and excess sugar from his diet, and give him a calming herb called Valerian Root, twice daily. Although calming, Valerian will not (and did not) cause drowsiness, but instead helps in staying focused, which is important to a child with ADHD.

Jeffrey also began taking flax seed oil soft gels, calcium, magnesium, zinc, vitamin C, and a good vitamin B-100 complex. By third grade, Jeffrey was doing fourth grade math and fifth grade reading, and his memory is just fine. He is now 12 years old, goes months with only an occasional short-lived *"fit"*, and is no longer troubled with any headaches or bed-wetting, which is much more relief than any prescription drug ever provided. Incidentally, just this past year Jeffrey was able to stop taking his Valerian on a daily basis, as he seems to no longer need it.

Although Jeffrey is just one prime example, there are many other children in the nation needlessly placed, and often left on these potentially dangerous drugs for years. A food allergy is quite often the underlying problem, and sugar, milk, wheat, eggs, and sometimes chocolate are the most common allergens. If necessary, an ALCAT (allergy blood test) can be performed in a lab, which can identify up to 150 different allergens. As you can see, although the natural solution is often very simple, it is seldom considered, and as usual with our broken healthcare system, the child is instead placed on dangerous drugs, and often left on them for years.

With Proper Diagnosing Psychiatric Drugs Can Be Avoided – Our Children Are Worth The Effort!

Following are just three examples of modern medicine's willingness to turn to dangerous medications, instead of searching for the true underlying cause of the problem (found at http://www.fightforkids.org/a_call_to_moms.htm):

#1: "Allergies and School Failure"

At 15, Betsy was depressed and suicidal each year in the late summer when ragweed pollen was in the air in northern Michigan. During her first visit to Dr. Doris Rapp's clinic she appeared normal until she was tested for an allergy to ragweed. Then she crawled into the office bathtub and refused to come out. She screamed, was untouchable, and complained of so much abdominal pain that she pulled her knees to her chest and held her stomach. After she was given a neutralizing allergy treatment, she felt entirely normal within a few minutes. Betsy was a persistent school failure until her allergies were recognized and treated, and her academic work and demeanor in school improved dramatically.

#2: "Sugar Junkie"

Carl was a darling 3-year-old youngster with a charming personality—until he ate sugar. His mother noticed that when Karl ate party food or candy, his total personality quickly and dramatically changed. He was videotaped as he gleefully devoured eight cubes of sugar. Just as the mother had predicted, within less than an hour he switched from Dr. Jekyll to a Mr. Hyde. At first he stopped playing quietly and began to whine. Then he became more irritable, stomped his feet, wiggled in his chair, tossed his toys over his head, and threw pieces of a puzzle at his mother. When he was given the correct allergy treatment, within a few minutes he was transformed back into his adorable self. His mother was in tears. She realized she was not a bad mother and he was not a bad kid.

#3: "Color Blind Not 'Disordered'"

Warren was diagnosed as hyperactive. He was impulsive, restless and inattentive. He also had breathing problems, episodes of partial hearing loss during ear infections and a heart murmur. Originally at school, he had good report cards and was never in trouble with the teachers. Then he started getting into squabbles and scrapes with kids who used to be his good friends. He was prescribed a psychotropic drug for his "hyperactivity." A proper medical evaluation discovered Warren was color-blind, his EEG showed abnormal but non specific brain wave patterns and a carbon monoxide assay revealed a blood saturation of this deadly gas at the dangerous 20% level. Carbon monoxide was displacing the oxygen in Warren's bloodstream, drastically reducing the supply of oxygen to his brain. His fidgeting, falling academic performance and purposeless hyper behavior were all symptoms of low-level carbon monoxide poisoning. Warren's parents immediately called the gas company and had their heating system overhauled. Within 3 weeks, his carbon monoxide level had dropped to 3%. Within 6 months, his EEG was normal and his color-blindness was resolved. He improved at school.

Incidentally, had they known, one way they could have eliminated the carbon monoxide poisoning would have been to give Warren high doses of vitamin C daily. It rapidly converts deadly carbon monoxide into carbon dioxide, which is easily eliminated in the lungs. This allows the red blood cells to again absorb oxygen, and deliver it to the brain as nature intended. For serious carbon monoxide poisoning, giving vitamin C intravenously is recommended.

We must seriously ask ourselves why years ago, no one ever heard of giving children drugs to control their behavior, or for depression. Back then, we somehow did just fine without them. Just a slight diet modification, or identifying some allergen, is normally all that is necessary to resolve the same problems that children are being placed on potentially dangerous drugs for every day. As most doctors were never trained in nutrition, that is something they seldom consider, although that should always be the very first consideration.

Some Potential Causes of "ADHD" Symptoms

✓ **Hypoglycemia.** In his book, *Nutrition and Mental Illness* (1987), Dr. Carl C. Pfeiffer, Ph.D., M.D. explains that ***"glucose deficiency drastically alters the function of the brain,"*** and that *"the physical and emotional disturbances in the hypoglycemic disorders vary according to the severity of the disorder and the affected individual."* It is important to note that **just a few of those "emotional" symptoms include: depression, irritability, fatigue, nervousness, insomnia, mental confusion or forgetfulness, <u>inability to concentrate</u>, <u>disruptive outbursts</u>, anti-social behavior, and even suicidal tendencies.** There is more detailed information on this condition in the Hypoglycemia chapter.

✓ **Food Allergies**. According to research done by Cornell Medical Center, and published in the *Annals of Allergy* (1976), ***"73% of children with attention deficit hyperactive disorder (ADHD) responded favorably to a diet that eliminated reactive foods and food additives. They concluded that dietary factors play a significant role in a majority of children with ADHD"*** (pp. 149-160). As you now know, there can be very serious effects associated with common food allergies, which we just discussed in Jeffrey's Story.

Dr. Carl C. Pfeiffer, Ph.D., M.D., in his book, *Nutrition and Mental Illness* (1987), explains the part that allergies play, and the related symptoms, as follows:

> ***The allergic child may suffer from the so-called allergic-tension-fatigue syndrome described by Dr. Frederic Speer in 1954, which results in irritability, hyperactivity, and impaired concentration, thus adversely affecting school performance.*** *Food dyes or additives may cause the symptoms. The most commonly implicated types of food are milk, wheat, egg, beef, corn, cane sugar, and chocolate. Allergy runs in families.*
>
> *Food intolerance, lack of absorption of food, and relief with fasting are three key pointers to the food-allergic patient. These patients usually have a low blood histamine, a fast pulse, and food idiosyncrasies which may be expressed as strong likes and dislikes.* **Favorite foods are often the offending foods, so the patient is like an addict, eating the offending food to obtain a psychological high** (pp. 48, 50).

Incidentally, the symptoms that Dr. Speer labeled as allergic-tension-fatigue syndrome, way back in 1954, would be called "ADHD" today. In this case, the contributing factor was either food or additives that contributed to the condition, although that is an even greater concern today, as more and more additives are now being added to processed food.

✓ **Milk.** Dr. Robert Cade, M.D., and his colleagues at the University of Florida, have identified a milk protein, casomorphine, as ***"the probable cause of attention deficit disorder and autism"*** (*AUTISM*, 1999, p. 3). Incidentally, it has been found that eighty percent of cow's milk protein is casein, which breaks down in the stomach to produce a peptide casomorphine (http://orisis.sunderland.ac.uk/autism/).

✓ **Malnutrition.** As reported in the November 2004 issue of the *American Journal of Psychiatry* (161:A62), ***"malnutrition at age 3 predisposes children to outward-directed behavioral problems, e.g., hyperactivity and aggression, at ages 8, 11, and 17. Malnutrition may therefore affect later behavior by impairing brain development."*** More specifically, a study conducted at the University of California in 2004 found that *"**a lack of zinc, iron, vitamin B, and protein in the first three years of a child's life** was linked to negative behavior later on. Children who were fed poorly were found to be more likely to fight, take drugs, and bully others"* (http://www.associatedcontent.com/article/207888/artificial_food_additives_linked_to.html).

Studies reported in the September 1997 issue of *Pediatrics*, found that a large percentage of US children are not obtaining even the Recommended Daily Allowance (RDA) of nutrition through their meals. Results from the 3307 children studied, are as follows:

> [The studies] *found that* ***only 1% met all the recommendations. Furthermore,, 64% of children studied failed to meet the minimum RDA requirements for vegetable intake and of the 36% that actually met these requirements, ¼ of all the vegetables they consumed were in the form of French fries!*** (http://www.naturaladd.com/resources/articles/nutrition_adhd.html)

Although this is an issue we discussed in the previous chapter, under the development of the fetus, it might be worth noting here also, that **malnutrition begins at inception, or nine months before the child is born.** The child's nutritional status reflects that of the mother. If you recall, **of greatest concern is when the mother has been placed on an SSRI antidepressant (such as Prozac™ or Paxil™). Not only is the developing fetus exposed to high doses of two substances known to create brain damage (cortisol and fluoride), but also the depletion of 16 critical nutrients is creating a major nutritional deficiency as well.** Under those circumstances, you should expect the child's brain development to be "seriously compromised" at birth.

Then, due to the behavioral problems associated with malnutrition, as noted, modern medicine's next step would often be to place the child on the very same drugs that created the condition initially. This would basically add insult to injury, and greatly compromise the child's future potential, and seldom does the child have any say in the matter, although it's his future that is at stake. It's our responsibility to make sure that the decisions we make are in the child's best interest, and not just for our convenience, (or their teacher's)!

✓ **Essential Fatty Acid (EFA) Deficiency.** EFAs are necessary for the proper development and functioning of the brain and the entire nervous system. There have been numerous studies and research done that link EFA deficiencies to ADHD symptoms, resulting in a misdiagnosis of the "disease". One study found that **patients with low EFA levels had more temper tantrums, as well as problems with learning, health and sleep,** than those with high levels of the EFAs (*American Journal of Clinical Nutrition*, 2000, Burgess, J.R., Stevens, L., Zhang, W., Peck, L., 71, pp. 327S-330S).

Another study, performed and reported by the University of South Australia, gave more than 130 children with ADHD a combination of fish oil and evening primrose oil for up to seven months. At the end of the trial, almost half of the children showed a reduction in their symptoms, and according the head scientist, Natalie Sinn, ***"the results suggest that an inadequate diet could cause ADHD"*** (http://www.abc.net.au/news/newsitems/200606/s1668130.htm).

And, yet another study confirms the following:

Recent research is showing that boys with ADD have EFA deficiencies.

Omega-3 EFAs are concentrated in a few tissues including the brain. More specifically, a substance termed "Docosahexaenoic acid" (DHA), converted from Omega-3 EFAs, is the most abundant Omega-3 EFA in the brain.

EFAs cannot be produced by the body. They have to come from the food we eat.

*Thus, **in spite of an adequate diet, some individuals are not able to convert EFAs into essential components (for example, DHA and EPA from Alpha-linolenic acid) and this may lead to behavioral, learning and health problems.** To complicate matters further, it seems that consumption of foods with high levels of transfatty acids (as found in cooking oils, margarine, etc) blocks the production of DHA and EPA from the original food source.*

*Modern eating means that many children (and adults) are eating too much of some fats – the omega-6 fats and hydrogenated and trans fats - in manufactured and fried foods. **This can severely damage brain development and functioning*** (http://www.causeof.org/efa_d.htm).

Something else to consider is, the majority of foods now served in school cafeterias contain mostly hydrogenated Omega-6 fats, which block the absorption of the beneficial Omega-3 essential fatty acids. Anything that can potentially damage brain development (and function) in children should not be part of their diet. That, along with the excessive consumption of sugar and starches, are major contributors to behavioral disorders, and less than optimal brain development.

✓ **Zinc Deficiency**. Studies have confirmed **a definite link between zinc deficiency and hyperactivity** (*Biological Psychology*, 1996, pp. 1308-1310). Other studies have proven that *"clinical manifestations in **severe cases of zinc deficiency include emotional disorder**,"* as well as *"A moderate deficiency of zinc is characterized by **mental lethargy**"* (*Journal of Clinical Endocrinology and Metabolism*, 1985 August, pp. 567-589).

Researchers have also identified a possible link between these zinc deficiencies and EFA deficiencies, noting that they recognized that ***"a zinc deficiency could cause a fatty acid deficiency"*** (*Biological Psychology*, 1989, pp. 222-228).

✓ **Vitamin B deficiency.** The B vitamins are necessary for the production of neurotransmitters, as well as normal functioning of the entire nervous system. Many experts believe that ***"one of the main causes for inattention, hyperactivity, impulsivity, temper tantrums, sleep disorders, forgetfulness, and aggression are caused by faulty neurotransmissions in the brain"*** (http://incrediblehorizons.com/mimic-adhd.htm).

✓ **Sugar.** Although there are skeptics, as well as those who choose to ignore the facts, it has been proven that **sugar most definitely alters moods, and causes hyperactivity.** The following information was found in *Life Extension's Disease Prevention and Treatment, expanded fourth edition*, (1991/2004, pp. 143-147):

> ***Sugar is certainly the single most damaging food linked to ADHD and a variety of other disorders.***
>
> ***The sudden release of insulin and drop in blood glucose caused by refined sugar intake (reactive hypoglycemia) rapidly raises adrenaline, causing a fight or flight response and the aggressive behavior, hyperactivity, and attention problems found in ADHD.*** *Upon sugar feeding, people with ADHD release only half the catecholamines (adrenal hormones such as norepinephrine and epinephrine that counterbalance a rapid drop in glucose due to high insulin) as controls.*
>
> ***In addition, many of the children with ADHD became more hyperactive following the glucose intake*** *in an effort to trigger their adrenal glands to produce more catecholamines. The most recent studies show that ADHD is linked to catecholamine dysfunction and energy disorders in brain neurons because it is improved by medications that enhance catecholamine function.* ***The results of this and other studies on sugar and ADHD emphasize the importance of well-balanced meals rich in protein and complex carbohydrates, which raise catecholamine levels and control fluctuations in glucose.***

In case you wondered, **the "catecholamines" they referred to, are a class of neurotransmitters, which includes norepinephrine,** (also known as noradrenaline), epinephrine, (also known as adrenaline), and dopamine. **Norepinephrine mediates (or promotes) learning ability, mental activity, attention span, and mood,** and is basically associated with the reward system. **A deficiency of these neurotransmitters is often implicated in depression, yet an elevated level can evoke paranoia, aggression, and anger, and can be induced by sugar, as well as amphetamines, (such as Ritalin™), which can at times over stimulate norepinephrine or dopamine. As usual, a delicate balance of all neurotransmitters is extremely critical, thus more is not always better,** (something only our body can effectively regulate). If you noticed, although an adequate level of neurotransmitter such as norepinephrine and dopamine are important for avoiding depression, for instance, an elevated level actually contributes to some very undesirable conditions, such as paranoia, aggression, and angers, thus maintaining that delicate balance is critical.

NOTE: Stimulant drugs such as Ritalin™ (and Prozac™) "do not" produce neurotransmitters. They basically over stimulate their use, by suppressing the normal reuptake of any "excess in the synapses", eventually depleting their availability for other intended uses. By doing so, they also reduce the sensitivity of their respective receptors, thus disturbing the normal delicate balance between the calming and stimulating neurotransmitters. A whole cascade of mental disorders can then potentially result, with the bipolar disorder being the most common. Excessive highs, followed by depressive lows, are typical of any stimulant, and quite similar to someone on cocaine. This issue is discussed in considerable detail later, in the chapter on Bipolar Disorder.

✓ **Lead Poisoning / The Fluoride Connection.** The U.S. Centers for Disease Control states that **lead poisoning can cause learning disabilities, behavioral problems and at high levels, seizures and even death, and is a highly significant risk factor in predicting higher rates of ADD, ADHD, and learning disabilities.** In fact, *"research shows that children with even mildly elevated lead levels can suffer from reduced IQs, attention deficits, and poor school performance"* (http://incrediblehorizons.com/mimic-adhd.thm).

And, according to research published in the *International Journal of Environmental Studies* (September 1999), **average blood lead levels are significantly higher in children living in communities where water is treated with silicofluorides (the cheaper form of fluoride),** most commonly used to fluoridate America's drinking water. **Silicofluorides are used by over 90% of U.S. fluoridated towns and cities.** Thus, **the majority of fluoridated drinking water actually contains two toxins that are very damaging to the brain (fluoride and lead).**

✓ **Bromine,** a liquid heavy metal, is another concern. It is often used as a dough conditioner in baked goods, as well as a clouding agent in many popular drinks. **Toxicity of bromine has been reported from ingestion of some carbonated drinks (i.e. Mountain Dew™, AMP™ Energy Drink, some Gatorade™ products), which contain brominated vegetable oils** (*Clinical Toxicology*, 1997, pp. 315-320). Bromine **is still used today in many prescription medications** (i.e. asthma treatment). Dr. David Brownstein, M.D. notes the following:

> **Bromine intoxication** *(i.e. bromism) has been shown to cause delirium, psychomotor retardation,* ***schizophrenia,*** *and hallucination.* ***Subjects who ingest enough bromide feel dull and apathetic and have difficulty concentrating. Bromide can also cause severe depression, headache, and irritability.***
>
> ***Recent research has demonstrated that some symptoms of bromide toxicity can be present with low levels of bromide in the diet*** (*Iodine: Why You Need – Why You Can't Live Without It*, 2004, p. 78).

✓ **Mineral imbalance and mineral deficiencies caused by excess phosphate intake.** According to research by Hertha Hafer, pharmacist and author of ***The Hidden Drug – Dietary Phosphate (Cause of Behaviour Problems, Learning Difficulties and Juvenile Delinquency)***, **phosphates in particular trigger ADD symptoms in children that were not recognized in earlier studies.** Hertha Hafer has been studying the dietary connection to ADD and ADHD for more than 20 years, which led her to discover **phosphorus as the common component in the foods that affect ADD children**, as published in her book. Although Feingold suggests elimination diets that do often work, Hafer claims that **a reduced phosphate diet provides consistent results**, and reports studies of thousands of families in Germany, Switzerland and elsewhere in Europe to substantiate her claims.

> ***Phosphate is a very common ingredient in our modern diet of processed foods. It is a highly versatile food-additive, which is of great interest to food manufacturers. It is used in the preservatives, emulsifiers, stabilizers, thickeners, it is added to the flour aerators in self-raising flours, it is put into soda and cola drinks in the form of phosphoric acid, and so on.***
>
> ***There are some people who have sensitivities to the high intake of phosphate minerals. The result is an upset in the delicate mineral balance, leading to other mineral deficiencies affecting the nervous system and resulting in all the symptoms, which are typical of the problem behaviour of the ADD child. Other people do not have this sensitivity and can consume relatively high amounts of phosphate in their diet without observable adverse effects. The tendency to the sensitivity is hereditary.***
>
> ***In some ways a comparison with diabetes is an apt one. A diabetic has a condition which is irreversible and which requires dietary modification for life. The management of phosphate sensitivity requires a parallel approach.***
>
> ***ADD is not a condition with a long history, unlike a wide range of other health problems which have been recorded regularly for hundreds or thousands of years. It is not reported today in countries where people continue to eat a traditional diet of unprocessed foods. But in countries in which there has been progressively a big shift to processed and convenience foods during the last century and in which natural foods high***

in phosphate have become available throughout the year, ADD has become a major problem.

These two developments have proceeded a parallel: the greater the intake of processed, convenience phosphate-rich food, the higher the incidence of ADD.

It is very probably that there is a link between phosphate sensitivity and a range of other afflictions of modern society. These include: alcoholism and more serious drug addictions, depression, juvenile delinquency, adult criminality and accidental deaths (i.e. the high incidence of deaths of young males in road accidents) and the epidemic of teenage and young adult suicides (http://phosadd.com/diet/diet.htm).

Of all the minerals, phosphate has the most influence on the pH of our bodies. If excess phosphate is the underlying cause of ADD, your saliva pH will have a reading of 7.5 or above. The saliva of a non-medicated ADHD child will be distinctly alkaline; pH readings in the range 7.5 to 8.5 are common. Although most people tend to be too acidic, rather than alkaline, either too high or too low pH can be a concern. Medications (including Ritalin™) are normally acidic, which in this case might bring their pH closer to the normal range, although that won't solve the underlying problem, (and should not even be considered as the proper solution). Reducing phosphates in the diet should be the natural (and sensible) approach.

Additional information regarding Hertha Hafer's low-phosphate diet and recipe suggestions, as well as links to more than 15 published research reports of evidence supporting its connection to ADD and ADHD symptoms, is available by visiting the website http://phosadd.com/mainpage/main33.htm. Laboratory tests are available for mineral deficiencies.

✓ **Magnesium Deficiency**. The mineral magnesium has a profound influence on the regulation of the central nervous system. Studies have found that **chronic (long-term) magnesium deficiency can result in hyperactivity, impaired reaction to external stimuli, irritability, fatigue, and poor mental concentration**, all of which could easily produce a misdiagnosis of ADHD, resulting in a prescription for dangerous drugs. According to an assessment of magnesium levels in children with Attention Deficit Hyperactivity Disorder (ADHD), researchers ***"examined 116 children with ADHD and found that 95% of those examined were deficient in magnesium"*** (*Magnesium Research*, 1997, Tadeusz Kozielec & Barbara Starobrat-Hermelin, Vol. 10, No. 2, pp. 143-148).

✓ **Calcium Deficiency**. In his August 2006 newsletter, *Health Alert* (Vol. 23, issue 8), Dr. Bruce West points out that ***"children who are deficient in calcium will often also be hyperactive, unable to concentrate in class, highly ticklish, jumpy, fidgety, and very difficult to calm"*** (p. 7). Interestingly, **calcium is depleted by Ritalin™ and other stimulants!** Calcium helps buffer the pH when the body is too acidic (low pH). It is also calming to the brain, and should be taken in combination with magnesium.

✓ **Artificial fluorescent lighting**. Pioneer light researcher, Dr. John Ott, coined the term "malillumination" to describe sun deficiency and the negative, harmful effects of artificial pink or cool-white fluorescent lighting on behavior, learning, health, hardiness and longevity. **Research has proven that *"cool-white florescent bulbs, (which are used in virtually all [school] classrooms) cause: bodily stress, hyper-activity, attention problems and other distress leading to poor learning performance."*** In 1973, Dr. Ott researched four 1st-grade classes in Florida, and found that some students in the classes with cool-white **fluorescent lighting demonstrated hyperactivity, fatigue, irritability, and attention deficits.** However, **students in the classrooms with full-spectrum lighting showed improved behavior and classroom performance, as well as overall academic achievement, within one month of the new lights being installed.** Not only that, but ***"Several learning-disabled children with extreme hyperactivity problems miraculously calmed down and seemed to overcome some of their learning and reading problems while in the classrooms with full-spectrum lighting"*** (http://www.fullspectrumsolutions.com/lighting_for_schools.shtml).

Further studies (by Hollwich, 1980), discovered that **cool-white florescent lighting actually produced increased levels of stress producing hormones**!

Dr. Jacob Liberman, author of the book ***Light: Medicine of the Future*** (1991), puts it in perspective, as follows:

> ***For years we have been labeling and re-labeling children who appear to have difficulties we do not understand.*** *We test and tutor them continually, only to find out that they are usually very bright but that for some reason outside of our understanding they do not achieve in the expected manner within the traditional learning environment. Although the labels for these children have changed from dumb, stupid and lazy to dyslexic, minimally brain dysfunctioned, and learning disabled* [and ADD], ***the labels nonetheless scar them for life...***
> (http://www.fullspectrumsolutions.com/lighting_for_schools.shtml)

✓ **Inorganic Growth Hormones.** Another interesting suggestion is the ingestion of growth hormones, sited by Dr. John Douillard, D.C., Ph.D., as follows:

> *Growth hormones are stimulants injected into animals to increase growth rates, and there have not been any long-term studies on the effects and use of these hormones. However, in vegetarian societies such as India, ADHD is relatively unknown. In America, on the other hand, where the diet includes large amounts of red meats, poultry, and milk, ADHD has become prevalent. The consumption of hormone-free meats, eggs, and milk, or a vegetarian diet, should be examined as potential treatment and prevention.*
> (http://www.healingpeople.com/index.php?option=com_content&task=view&id=25&Itemid=146)

✓ **Food Additives.** Pediatric allergist Dr. Ben F. Feingold, first proposed that synthetic flavors and colors in the diet were related to hyperactivity in 1973. Numerous studies since then have proven that **certain synthetic food additives can produce such symptoms as: Learning and behavioral problems, hyperactivity, irritability, bedwetting, compulsive aggression, self-mutilation, difficulty in reasoning,** and even physical illnesses such as chronic ear infections, asthma and migraine headaches. In fact, Dr. Feingold claims that **almost 50% of hyperactive children are sensitive to artificial flavors, colors and preservatives.** Unfortunately, a study reported by the National Academy of Science in 1989 found that **73% of all food additives have never been tested for neurobehavioral effects in humans** (*"Toxicity Testing: Strategies to Determine Needs and Priorities"*, NAS Press, DC).

The following success story was obtained at http://www.feingold.org/article-pg.html:

> ***A school in Worcestershire, England, has banned all additives from its meals to stop children behaving badly.***
>
> *Barnabas first and middle school in Drakes Broghton banned 27 additives – including the yellow coloring in custard – during a two-week trial.*
>
> ***Staff started the trial after discovering a study suggested one in four children have tantrums as a result of eating too many additives.***
>
> ***After two weeks staff say they noticed a market improvement in pupils' behavior.***
>
> *Head teacher Charlie Lupton said* ***children's concentration levels had also improved since the trial started.***
>
> *"More than 30% of parents noticed their children were better behaved during the trial and 18% said their children were sleeping better."*
>
> *He said* ***pupils had also commented on how much better their school meals tasted.***

According to The Feingold Program, founded by Dr. Feingold, it is important to avoid artificial (synthetic) coloring, as ***"Those colors that make the 'fruit punch' red, the gelatin green and the oatmeal blue are made from petroleum (crude oil)*** *which is also the source for gasoline"*, and artificial (synthetic) flavoring. Especially ingredient labels listed with a number that begins with "D&C", as it means that *"this coloring is considered safe for medicine (drugs) and cosmetics, but not for food"* (http://www.feingold.org/grocery.html). The question that comes to mind is, if a coloring is not considered as safe for food, then why should it be considered as safe for medications? They are normally more rapidly absorbed, and normally have a more direct access to the brain, thus they could pose an even greater risk.

Other examples of additives that The Feingold Program suggests to avoid are: Aspartame (NutraSweet™, artificial sweeteners), MSG, Sodium benzoate, Nitrites, Sulfites, as well as aspirin and other foods containing salicylate, noting *"Salicylate is a group of chemicals related to aspirin. There are several kinds of salicylate, which plants make as a natural pesticide to protect themselves."*

As you can see, children misdiagnosed with ADHD could easily be suffering from food allergies or hidden food sensitivities, or possibly from food preservatives or dyes. You can find a local allergist, associated with the *National Alliance against Mandated Mental Health Screening & Psychiatric Drugging of Children*, by visiting their website at http://www.ritalindeath.com/Allergists.htm.

✓ **Psychological Trauma.** Be sure to rule out the possibility that a child may actually be reacting to an abusive or traumatic situation or event.

Some Of The "Inactive" Ingredients in Ritalin™ May Actually Contribute to "ADHD" Symptoms

As pointed out by Dr. Feingold, synthetic dyes can cause serious reactions in some sensitive children (as well as adults), and as you are about to learn, these dangerous dyes are not only in foods, but in many medications as well. And Ritalin™ is just one!

Following is a list of "inactive ingredients" in Ritalin™, as posted on http://www.rxlist.com/cgi/generic/methphen.htm, as well as the dangers of each:

- **Polyethylene glycol (PEG) -** *"May contain ¼-dioxane which is a* ***possible carcinogen, estrogen mimic*** *and endocrine* **[hormone]** ***disruptor.*** *Moderately toxic, and possible carcinogen* [cancer causing]. *Many glycols produce* ***severe acidosis, central nervous system damage*** *and congestion.* ***Can cause convulsions****,* ***mutations,*** *and surface EEG changes"* (http://www.purezing.com/living/living_toxins_commondyes.html).
- **Lactose** - Milk sugar!
- **Sucrose** - Table sugar!
- **Zein** - Protein from corn gluten meal (used as coating).

As you can see, the last three ingredients, although they might seem "inactive", are actually three of the most common food allergens, and contributors to "ADHD" symptoms.

And, it's not just Ritalin™!

Other medications often prescribed for "ADHD" symptoms, or in combination with ADHD medications, also contain very active "inactive" ingredients that can at times contribute to the very symptoms they are prescribed for.

Prozac™ (an SSRI antidepressant) also contains Polyethylene glycol (PEG), mentioned above in Ritalin's "inactive" ingredients. And, according to the *Physicians Desk Reference, 55th edition*, (2001, p. 1127), another one of the "inactive" ingredients listed in Prozac™ is F D & C Yellow No. 6, which ***"may cause allergies, hyperactivity, and chromosomal damage"*** (http://www.purezing.com/living/living_toxins_commondyes.html).

Zoloft™ (an SSRI antidepressant) 25 mg tablets contain F D & C Red No. 40 (http://www.rxlist.com/cgi/generic/sertral.htm), which is ***"linked to allergic reactions, skin rashes, hyperactivity, and asthma, so it may be a good idea to avoid them"*** (http://www.vegetarian-restaurants.net/Additives/Artificial-Colors.htm).

Paxil™ (an SSRI antidepressant) contains F D & C Yellow No. 6 (http://www.rxlist.com/cgi/generic/parox.htm), which is ***"suspected of causing tumors in adrenal glands and kidneys. May cause allergies, hyperactivity, and chromosomal damage"*** (http://www.purezing.com/living/living_toxins_commondyes.html).

Even most doctors are totally unaware that they might be subjecting their patients to additional risks associated with the "inactive ingredients" in their medications, which can actually be "very active" as you can easily see from the above.

CHAPTER SEVEN

Problems That Can Stem From A Candidiasis Yeast Infection (An Infection Caused By The Candida Fungus)

Thousands of children are being placed on dangerous drugs such as Ritalin™ or Prozac™, when they could just be experiencing symptoms associated with the candida yeast infection, named candidiasis. Yet, something as simple as eliminating sugar from their diet would go a long way toward resolving the physical and mental conditions often associated with candidiasis.

We all have both good and bad strains of bacteria, which reside primarily in our intestinal tract. The good strains of yeast and bacteria basically control the bad ones, preventing them from overwhelming the body. The bad yeast (candida) only becomes a problem when the immune system has been compromised, or after using an antibiotic medication (something that is often over-prescribed). Then, in combination with excessive sugar or carbohydrate consumption, the candida has a perfect environment to multiply. Excessive sugar consumption is a major contributor to candidiasis, as well as cancer. They both thrive on, and ferment sugar, especially in an anaerobic (oxygen deficient) environment.

Studies show that just **one teaspoon** of sugar is sufficient to impair the immune system by **50 percent,** for several hours after consumption. Therefore, **if you continually consume even a small amount of sugar at a time throughout the entire day, your immune system will be impaired by 50 percent ALL DAY LONG!** Sugar not only weakens the immune system, but the combination of sugar (the candida's food of choice), along with a weakened immune system, (caused by eating sugar), feeds the Candida allowing it to discreetly thrive.

Note: The yeast population can actually double every 20 minutes, if fed the proper diet. When the immune system is compromised by the sugar, it is less effective in controlling candidiasis as well.

Many of the symptoms of candidiasis, as listed in the book *A Holistic Protocol for the Immune System, 6th Edition* (1989), by Scott J Gregory, are as follows:

> ***Some candidiasis sufferers feel "spacey"*** **[or inattentive].**
>
> ***Some symptoms in children that may stem from a yeast overgrowth are hyperactivity, behavioral and neurological problems****, ear and respiratory tract infection (Dr. Michael Schmidt, Childhood Ear Infections).* ***Children's consumption of sugar should be severely limited or eliminated.***
>
> ***Others experience chronic fatigue and various physical, psychological and emotional problems, even suicidal tendencies.***
>
> ***One study in a mental institution showed that 163 out of 169 persons there suffered from candidiasis.***
>
> ***Food allergies and environmental sensitivity can initiate and imitate symptoms like those of candidiasis*** (pp. 85-86).

Just the fact that, according to the previous study, **a total of 163 of 169 (all except six) patients in the mental institution actually suffered from candidiasis,** should obviously be a clue to anyone as to why they likely developed their "mental problems," especially if you consider the typical mental conditions above, which are associated with candidiasis. Although it obviously makes much more **"financial sense"** to **not attempt to resolve the problem,** and send them home. You could imagine what influence it might have on their vacancy factor! However, it would obviously make much more "health sense" to resolve the underlying problem, rather than unnecessarily placing them in an institution and subjecting them to years of dangerous psychotic drugs. These institutions are not only very depressing, but they are also where you will often find the greatest degree of "legal" drug abuse. Keep in mind that "legal drugs" can be every bit as dangerous as most illegal drugs, which were once considered legal. Often the patients themselves, or family members, have very little say regarding what medications they are placed on, and often left on for years. Their doctor normally makes that determination. As with children, they often sedate them, making them easier to manage. The medications they are placed on are often more for the convenience of the caregiver, than the welfare of the patient.

Candidiasis is also a major contributing factor to weight gain, which may be at least one contributing factor to the obesity and diabetes in children today, (considering the common diet of many children today). **The majority of the bad yeast, known as candida, thrives on sugar and carbohydrates, resulting in intense cravings, which feeds the candida, allowing it to grow. It also increases the production of insulin, which takes the sugar from the bloodstream and deposits it, as fat,** into the fat cells. And, according to the authors of *Recovery From Addiction* (John Finnegan and Daphne Gray, 1990) ***"Yeast disorders are often a main causative factor in addictions, especially alcoholism, sugar addictions, and eating disorders."*** And once the immune system is suppressed, the body is no longer able to control the bad yeast.

Other common symptoms associated with candidiasis (for which more drugs are often prescribed) are: **depression**, **mood swings**, **hypothyroidism, asthma**, chronic fatigue, and muscular or nervous system systems. Ironically, excessive drug use (prescription and over-the-counter) suppresses the immune system, promoting candida growth even further. Some of the worst are antibiotics, estrogen and oral contraceptives, cortisone and corticosteroids (such as Prednisone), **SSRI antidepressants (such as Prozac™),** and chemotherapy agents.

How Candidiasis Contributes To Brain Damage

All yeasts convert sugar and digestible carbohydrates to acetaldehyde under anaerobic (oxygen-deficient) conditions, and the intestinal environment is sufficiently anaerobic for this process to occur. Acetaldehyde is the first and most toxic poison created by alcohol metabolism in the liver. It is a carcinogen also found in cigarette smoke, car exhaust, and even embalming fluid. Scientists consider acetaldehyde to be much more toxic to the body than the alcohol itself.

The potentially harmful acetaldehyde is transported to the liver, along with digested food. In the liver, it is oxidized to harmless acetate (basically vinegar) and water, by a zinc-containing enzyme called aldehyde dehydrogenase. Unfortunately, due to a genetic difference, the aldehyde dehydrogenase enzyme appears to be less efficient in the metabolizing of acetaldehyde in the liver of many Orientals and Native Americans, causing it to circulate throughout the body and brain much longer, (something these nationalities should be aware of).

Acetaldehyde binds strongly to proteins (just like the SSRI antidepressants do), and, like the closely related substance formaldehyde, it has significant potential for damaging organs. Even during moderate production, **acetaldehyde can bind to the cells of the brain**, as well as the intestine, liver, and blood vessels. And during excessive acetaldehyde production, the bonding is cumulative and can at times become irreversible when exposure to the acetaldehyde is prolonged.

At least part of the acetaldehyde is found within the brain, and there is research to confirm that, in two autopsies of FM (fibromyalgia) patients, **Candida was still found in the brain and its fluid. Then, once the acetaldehyde enters the brain, it hinders the production of acetylcholine, a key neurotransmitter.** Any disturbance in the availability of the neurotransmitter, acetylcholine, will destabilize the natural functions of the autonomic nervous system, (which controls cardiovascular, respiratory, and digestive functions, and many other involuntary activities). This can potentially result in **erratic thinking and deranged behavior, as well as defective short-term memory, which is why these mental disturbances are quite common in people with Candidiasis.** Actually, many neurotransmitters can be bound to acetaldehyde, which results in the formation of **"false neurotransmitters"** that are thought to **contribute to conditions such as depression, anxiety,** the vague uneasiness sometimes associated with stress, **schizophrenic-like symptoms, difficulties with concentration, and possibly even complete lapses in memory.**

Then, if you also combine other medications such as cholesterol lowering and antihypertensive drugs, which are responsible for severe nutrient depletion, and reduced circulation to the brain, you are basically compounding the problem. The SSRI antidepressants such as Prozac™, Paxil™, Celexa™, and Zoloft™, are also notorious for nutrient depletion, (actually, a total of sixteen, **including vitamin B_6**). According to Dr. Sherry Rogers, M.D., **just a deficiency in vitamin B_6 alone, actually causes the released acetaldehyde from Candida to be even more damaging to the brain, increasing the potential for permanent brain damage**. Thus, the risk of developing either dementia, or Alzheimer's disease, in the future would be much greater. So, we are not just looking at depression and behavioral problems, but also the potential for serious irreversible brain damage!

And, as these SSRI antidepressants are also very difficult for the liver to metabolize, thus they contribute to elevated acetaldehyde as well. Not only that, but as both Prozac™ and Paxil™ are known to greatly potentiate (increase the level) of alcohol, and as acetaldehyde is a metabolite of alcohol, they will also increase the level of acetaldehyde that the brain will be exposed to, causing even more brain damage!

How To Tell If It's Candidiasis

It is best to determine if you have candidiasis by performing some sort of test, which incidentally you can likely do yourself. As Dr. Bruce West, D.C. has suggested, you can test for candidiasis by spitting into a glass of water. If saliva floats, there is not a candida problem.

You can also take this quick quiz. If you answer yes to more than half of the following questions, more than likely your symptoms are yeast-connected.

1. Have you taken repeated "cycles" of antibiotic drugs?
2. Have you ever taken birth control pills?
3. Do you suffer from recurrent digestive problems?

4. Do you suffer from hives, psoriasis, or other chronic skin conditions?
5. Do you suffer from headaches or earaches?
6. Do you suffer from unexplained pain or swelling in your muscles or joints?
7. Do symptoms seem to occur after exposure to tobacco, perfume and other chemicals?
8. Do you crave sugar, breads or alcoholic beverages?
9. Do symptoms seem to worsen after consumption of sugar, breads or alcoholic beverages?
10. Do you suffer from rectal itching or itching of the genitalia?
11. Do you feel bad all over but no one can seem to find the cause?

Natural Solutions For Treating Candidiasis

NOTE: Several issues should be addressed, <u>simultaneously</u>, in order to effectively eliminate the Candida yeast. Serious measures are sometimes necessary to overcome this very aggressive fungus infection. Following are several options to consider.

<u>#1 Avoid or Eliminate the Known Contributors</u>

As noted earlier, the likelihood of developing candidiasis greatly depends on the number of contributors the body is exposed to, thus **eliminating or avoiding as many factors as possible** should obviously be your very first step, as well as watching what you eat. These factors include:

- Stress (physical and emotional) – **Prozac™ produces stress hormones**
- Lack of sleep – **both Ritalin™ and Prozac™ can cause insomnia**
- Allergies (such as food and additives)
- Alcohol **(cravings caused by Prozac™)**
- Caffeine
- Smoking or nicotine
- Environmental Toxins
- Excessive Drug Use (over-the-counter, legal or illegal) – especially antibiotics
- Insufficient stomach acid – especially those with type "A" blood or the use of antacids
- Chlorinated Water (in some water systems, and most commercial swimming pools)
- Fluoride (found in some water systems and Prozac™)

<u>#2 Remove the Primary Food Source</u>

Remember, when you are feeding yourself, you may also be feeding the candida as well, thus **it is important to avoid:**

✓ **Sugar and Simple Carbohydrates** (Candida's primary source of food). This includes honey and syrups. And remember, alcohol is sugar!

✓ **Avoid all fruits** (they are full of sugar!)

✓ **Acidic foods** (Candida thrives on an acidic environment. Some examples of acidic foods are: tomatoes, limes, pickles, and vinegar.

✓ **Yeast and all fermented foods**. Any form of bread. Avoid foods labeled "enriched" and all grains containing gluten (wheat, oats, rye, and barley). Remember, alcohol is also a yeast!

✓ **Molds**, such as:
- o Any leftover foods that have not been frozen, as mold grows quickly on any food that isn't eaten as soon as it is prepared.
- o Fruit juices. Not only are they full of sugar, but most fruits used for making juice often contain mold.
- o Aged Cheese.
- o Mushrooms.
- o Dried fruits.
- o Potatoes.
- o Sprouts.
- o Also avoid moldy places, such as basements.

#3 Rebuild the Weakened Immune System To Its Full Potential

Aside from decreasing stress and increasing rest, you will likely be required to change your diet (and definitely avoid sugar). Increasing your nutritional supplementation and eliminating any nutrient depleting medications is also helpful. Just keep in mind that the recommended daily allowance (RDA) of all supplements is normally the average suggested dosage. The most beneficial dosage for a particular individual can sometimes vary considerably between individuals.

✓ **Garlic.** Just one of the suggested supplements listed by the School of Natural Healing, as it **assists in enhancing the immune system.** It has been said that the builders of the pyramids ate garlic daily for endurance and strength, considering it to be one of the most valuable foods on this planet. **Garlic is known as a potent immune system stimulant** and even touted as being a **natural antibiotic**. Additionally, **garlic is also effective against fungal infections, as it aids in removing parasites, and has proven effective in fighting both candida and yeast vaginitis**.

✓ **Vitamin C**. Supplementing with vitamin C not only enhances the immune system, but it can increase iron absorption by as much as 30 percent. It is important to remember that vitamin C can easily be depleted by many things, such as:

- **Alcohol**
- **Antibiotics**
- **Caffeine**
- **Estrogen and oral contraceptives**
- **Histamine H_2 blockers (i.e. Tagamet™, Pepcid™, Zantac™)**
- **NSAIDs (i.e. ibuprofen)**
- **Steroids and corticosteroids**
- **Physical and Emotional Stress (and Prozac™)**

They not only deplete vitamin C, but are detrimental to your overall health as well, so they should be avoided whenever possible.

Be sure to take the **esterfied form of vitamin C**, as it is not acidic and is metabolized by the body easier. In fact, esterfied vitamin C enters the bloodstream and tissues **four times faster** than standard forms of vitamin C. It is buffered with calcium, which helps maintain a more alkaline pH, and avoids the removal of calcium from the bones, which could contribute to osteoporosis. It moves into the blood cells more efficiently and also stays in the body tissues longer. I would recommend 2,000 mg to 4,000 mg of Ester-C with bioflavonoids daily, in divided doses.

✓ **Iron** is required for a healthy immune system, as well as energy production. Incidentally, iron deficiency is also more prevalent in people with candidiasis. In my opinion, the best form of organic iron is blackstrap molasses, as it is a natural form that won't accumulate at toxic levels as some forms of iron can. One or two tablespoon daily is normally adequate.

✓ **Castor oil** has been found to improve the function of the thymus gland and other parts of the immune system, as well as treating liver disease. Cold-pressed castor oil should be available at your local health food store. Just be aware that castor oil is also a laxative.

✓ **Zinc.** Just as a zinc deficiency can cause deterioration of the liver and the immune system, as well as a propensity to diabetes, zinc supplementation enhances the immune system and the healing process. I would recommend 50 mg daily.

✓ **Ginger** is naturally rich in zinc, and can be made into tea or added to meals. It can also be taken in capsule form, and is readily available as well as inexpensive.

✓ **Lower histamine levels.** Since elevated histamine levels add to allergic conditions and further weaken the immune system, it is important to reduce histamine levels if elevated. Furthermore, Dr. Carl C. Pfeiffer, Ph.D., M.D. claims that **those with high histamine levels actually tend to unconsciously crave sugar to relieve the pressure caused by a histamine imbalance, which would just feed the candida.** For more detailed information, you can refer to the "Histamine" section in the chapter on Bipolar Disorder.

#4 Correct Any Nutritional Deficiencies Caused by the Candida

✓ **Calcium and Magnesium.** Not only does candidiasis deplete calcium and magnesium, but it has been documented that **patients low in magnesium are more prone to develop chronic (long-term) candidiasis** (*Depression – Cured at Last!*, Dr. Sherry Rogers, 1997). Incidentally, Prozac™ depletes both calcium, and magnesium as well.

Although many formulas contain 2 to 1 calcium to magnesium ratios, I recommend the opposite, as do some other doctors. While the normal recommendation might be the adequate for building bone, magnesium is actually used for many different functions throughout the body. When in our youth, our magnesium to calcium ratio is normally 3 to 1, in favor of magnesium. I personally take 1,000 mg of calcium and 2,000 mg of magnesium daily.

It would also be helpful to take 1,000 IU of vitamin D_3 to enhance the calcium absorption, (something I do, as well). During the winter months, or when you are not exposed to direct sunlight, is the time when you're more inclined to be deficient in vitamin D.

✓ **Vitamin K** is produced by the good bacteria in the intestines, thus when the good bacteria is missing, vitamin K is normally deficient. Not only does a deficiency interfere with insulin release, and glucose regulation in ways similar to diabetes, but a deficiency of vitamin K can also produce abnormal bleeding disorders. Vitamin K helps escort calcium to the bones, helping prevent osteoporosis. Incidentally, vitamin K also assists in converting glucose to glycogen for storage in the liver, thus promoting healthy liver function. I personally use one soft gel daily of SuperK™ with K_2, by Life Extension™, which contains 9 mg of vitamin K_1 and 1 mg of vitamin K_2. One daily should be adequate.

✓ **Vitamin B_1** is commonly depleted by candida infections, and yet can easily go completely unnoticed. Vitamin B_1 (thiamine) assists in the production of hydrochloric acid, which is necessary for proper digestion and a healthy digestive tract (preventing candidiasis), as well as reducing stress, and enhancing energy and circulation. One vitamin B-100 complex (which includes 100 mg of B_1, along with the other B vitamins) daily should normally be adequate, unless you drink alcohol, which is notorious for B_1 depletion, then an additional 100 mg of B_1 might be necessary. Best of all, just don't drink alcohol, as it just contributes to candidiasis!

#5 Repair your liver

The authors of *Recovery From Addiction* (Finnegan & Gray, 1990) tell us that **the link between candidiasis and liver damage is so strong that it can often cause severe liver damage,** requiring months or even years to correct. They point out that *"Specific nutrients feed and regenerate the liver and glands, so that as people recover they can slowly introduce more good quality complex carbohydrates into their diets and be able to metabolize them"* (p. 41). Following are just a few supplements, which have proven to be beneficial for liver detoxification and repair.

✓ **Alpha Lipoic Acid (ALA), Selenium, and Milk Thistle,** is a combination used by Dr. Burt Berkson at the Integrative Center of New Mexico, New Mexico State University to successfully treat patients suffering from cirrhosis of the liver, as noted in the March 2002 issue of Dr. David G. Williams' *Alternatives* newsletter (Vol. 9, No. 9, p. 70).

Dr. Berkson published a report detailing a treatment program, as follows:

> *Each patient was given 600 milligrams of alpha lipoic acid, 400 micrograms of selenium, and 900 milligrams of Silymarin (milk thistle extract) daily in three divided doses. He reports that* ***all responded positively to the treatment within a short period of time and none required transplant surgery****. All feel fine and returned to work without any problems.*

This is obviously a much better solution than resorting to a liver transplant, and the accompanying dependence on a lifetime of anti-rejection medication.

✓ **Golden Seal** is extremely effective for cleansing the liver, as well as proving **beneficial for those with liver damage and yeast disorders.** According to the late legendary herbalist Dr. John Christopher, M.H., N.D., 3 to 6 capsules a day for 1 to 3 months has proven to be effective.

✓ **Chamomile tea** has powerful anti-fungal capabilities, known to **effectively battle candidiasis, as well reduce stress.** Chamomile is also one of a few plants that have been **established to have properties that rebuild the liver.** In fact, researchers found two compounds of chamomile (azulene and guaiazulene) that are able to **initiate new growth of liver tissue** in rats that had portions of their liver surgically removed.

✓ **Lecithin** is a type of lipid (fat) that is needed by every living cell in the body. It not only **helps repair liver damage, but it also enhances the immune system,** and enables fats, such as cholesterol and other lipids, to be dispersed in water and removed from the body. Lecithin granules are the least expensive and can easily be sprinkled on cereals or soups, salads, or juice. I would recommend two to four tablespoons of granules daily. I just swallow the lecithin granules with water, as it has very little flavor.

✓ **Dandelion root** is a multi-talented herb, and **extremely beneficial for candidiasis sufferers,** in many ways. **It improves liver function,** as well as increasing the flow of bile and improving digestion. Available as a supplement in capsules. Two capsules, twice daily, should normally be adequate.

✓ **Potassium supplementation** can **promote strong liver function,** just as a potassium deficiency can result in weak liver function. Normally, 100 mg daily should be sufficient.

#6 Do The Liver Flush

Once we have healed the liver, removing stones lodged throughout the bile ducts in the liver should prove beneficial. Most adults actually have dozens of stones in their liver or gallbladder, (or both). The process is quite easy, takes only three days, and is painless. The stones are softened, and then removed by working their way through the intestinal tract. They are quite easy to identify, as they float. They normally vary in size, from large grains of sand to the size of marbles, and normally range in color from green to yellow.

As the bile helps digest fats and remove toxins, eliminating any restrictions to its efficient flow would definitely be beneficial. The only thing you need to order is *Super Phos 30™*. One 4-ounce bottle is normally sufficient for about 8 flushes, and costs approximately $30. It is available through *NMS Publishing*, by calling (718) 871-1363, or by writing to:

Paul Oberdorf
NMS Publishing, Dept. JF
5711 14th Avenue
Brooklyn, NY 11219

You will also need 3 quarts of apple juice (no sugar added), one cup of pure extra-virgin olive oil, one 12-ounce can of Classic Coke™ (something I wouldn't "normally" recommend), and the juice of one fresh-squeezed lemon, and then **follow the instructions that come with the *Super Phos 30™*.**

Considering the potential benefits, I believe it's well worth the little effort involved. I personally did two flushes myself, about one month apart, and got nearly twice as many stones the first time as I did the second time. Most people are quite amazed at how many stones were eliminated. Remember, they have been accumulating for a lifetime. For some of us, it's much longer than others, as in my case (1933 was a long time ago)! Life was so much simpler back then, when most of these drugs had yet to be created, although we somehow seemed to manage without them. That was also a long time before we "somehow" developed 374 different mental conditions! It was only after discovering that we had so many different mental conditions, which we weren't even aware of years ago, that the need for mind-altering drugs suddenly became a major concern, (apparently due to a void that we somehow needed to fill, or possibly a rapidly developing industry that needed financing)!

#7 Kill the candida and prevent it from coming back

✓ **Colloidal Silver.** Super Silver™, available through *International Health LCC*, is 10ppm purified colloidal silver, and purified water. It contains no artificial ingredients, preservatives, or additives, and when taken in the doses specified, is completely safe for human consumption, or can be applied to the skin or eyes. It's perfectly safe for young children as well.

As noted in the *ASAP™ Silver Solution* [now referred to as Super Silver™] *Information & Usage Guide* (*International Health*, 2003), research performed by microbiologist Jason Henrie, at the University of California at Davis, tested the ability of the ASAP™ Silver Solution to inhibit the growth of yeast. The following observations were reported:

> ***ASAP Silver Solution definitely inhibits the growth of yeast and the difference between treatments is statistically significant.*** *The maximum growth rate and the final population are the same, so inhibition is due to a delay in the onset of growth. It is important to note that ASAP was applied in only one dose and that in a real-world situation it will be applied multiple times. It is evident that a single 10ppm application could prevent the further growth of a small population of yeast for 24 hours, allowing ones immune system time to respond. Even more, multiple 10ppm applications could conceivably prevent the growth of yeast indefinitely* (pp. 27-28).

Super Silver™ is made by a special patented process, and proven in laboratory tests to be more effective than other colloidal silver products, and at a much lower concentration. Super Silver™ can be purchased by calling *International Health* at (800) 481-9987, or on their website http://internationalhealth.net/default.asp.

✓ **Coenzyme Q_{10}** (CoQ_{10}) has proven beneficial in treating candidiasis. It is also extremely effective in stimulating the immune system, protecting the stomach lining against ulcers (and maintaining healthy intestinal flora), and is a natural antihistamine (thus assisting in fighting allergies as well). Unless you have been taking medications that deplete CoQ_{10}, 100 mg daily should be sufficient. Statin (cholesterol lowering) medications are some of the worst drugs for CoQ_{10} depletion, in which case I would recommend 200 mg daily, (and **get off the statin**)! In my book *A Drug-Free Approach To Healthcare*, (which is now available in a new 2007 *Revised Edition*), I explain in detail the damage they create, and why in my opinion they are totally unnecessary. Everyone I know, who took my advice and got off them, felt much better once they did!

✓ **Folic Acid and PABA (Para-Amino benzoic Acid)** are both water-soluble cofactors of the B-vitamin family, and necessary for the maintenance of healthy intestinal bacteria, thus **preventing candidiasis.** They also promote a healthy digestive/intestinal tract and **assist in depression.** They are both depleted by alcohol, estrogen, and oral contraceptives. Both are normally found in a good vitamin B-complex, (I suggest B-100).

✓ **Vitamin E.** In a report in the *Journal of the American College of Nutrition* (1983), Robert S. London, M.D. of Baltimore tells of controlled research studies using **vitamin E**, resulting in **significant improvement regarding candidiasis symptoms such as: mood swings**,

headache, craving for sweets, increased appetite, fatigue, depression and insomnia. Doses ranging from 150 to 600 IU of vitamin E were used, with **300 IU per day appearing to be optimal** (*The Yeast Connection – A Medical Breakthrough*, William Crook, 1983/1986). Keep in mind that vitamin E can be easily depleted by alcohol, antibiotics, aspirin, laxatives, estrogen and oral contraceptives, NSAIDS (i.e. ibuprofen), and **all cholesterol-lowering drugs.** Always take the natural vitamin E. Avoid the one with an "L" following the "D". Just think of the "L" as standing for "built in a **L**ab".

✓ **Essential Fatty Acids (EFAs)** are beneficial for treating and preventing candida, as well as **preventing the fungus from destroying cells.** They also super enhance the immune system. Either flax seed oil or fish oil should work. I would recommend four 1,000 mg soft gels of either, or two of both, daily. Incidentally, **EFAs have also proven beneficial with ADHD, depression and bipolar disorder.** As with all supplements, they have many "benefits". The difference with drugs is, the drugs have many "side effects"!

✓ **The mineral Copper**. According to Dr. Sherry Rogers, research has found that animals given copper have more resistance to bad yeast. Three mg daily should be sufficient. Be aware that excessive levels of copper can be toxic, (so in this case, more is not always better).

✓ **Aloe vera juice.** The aloe vera plant is well known for its healing effect of stomach and colon disorders. Its juice **kills bacteria, parasites, and candida in the digestive tract.** It also normalizes stomach acid production, aids in digestion thus preventing deficiencies, and has been found to benefit food allergy sufferers. One tablespoon of aloe vera juice, twice daily, **improves blood sugar levels, and reduces sugar cravings (for those attempting to give up sugar).**

✓ **Probiotics – The most common are: *Lactobacillus acidophilus* and *Bifidobacterium bifidum*,** which provide many beneficial functions in the intestinal tract. Taking a probiotic supplement (such as *lactobacillus acidophilus* or *Bifidobacterium bifidum*) not only helps return the intestinal flora to its healthy balance, and inhibits the growth of current and future candida in the digestive tract and vagina, but it also enhances the absorption of nutrients from food. There are many probiotic formulas, containing various beneficial bacteria, and in various concentrations of each. One alternative to probiotic supplements is to eat plain unsweetened yogurt that contains live yogurt cultures.

✓ **Valerian Root.** Known for its relaxing effects, this calming herb also supports healthy bacteria levels in the body, as well as reducing stress (an immune suppressant, and another contributor to candidiasis).

✓ **L-Glutamine** is an amino acid that not only helps prevent candidiasis, but also protects the intestines and the liver, as well as maintaining a healthy digestive tract, and promoting proper pH balance. As an added benefit, glutamine also provides an alternate source of energy for the brain, reducing cravings for carbohydrates.

#8 Make sure the candida has been completely eliminated

In her book *Depression Cured at Last!* (1997), Dr. Rogers describes the following scenario to avoid:

> *A common mistake is someone who got better on a program to eradicate yeast.* ***But they did not go far enough to discover why they were vulnerable enough to get it in the first place. So they never totally get rid of it. It begins to drive persistent cravings.*** *But since they feel worse eating sugars (it causes the growth of further yeasts), they suck down more anti-fungals.* ***This is a great way to foster the growth of Candida species that are highly resistant to anti-fungals.*** *And* ***taking anti-fungals while you are on antibiotics will foster resistant fungi even faster.*** *Always be suspicious if you have "chronic* [long-term] *yeast" or "chronic" anything. For what it really means is that the* ***total load has not been addressed*** (pp. 172-173).

#9 Be persistent!

Don't give up until you have totally eradicated your yeast infection, (it will be well worth your effort)! Then avoid the things we just discussed that will lead to the onset of another episode. In order to be successful in your endeavor, you absolutely must be more persistent than the yeast! As usual, I am basically providing you with different options to choose from, and you don't necessarily have to incorporate them all, unless you choose to, (although the more the better).

As I often stress, due to our bio-individuality, we won't all experience the same results from the very same therapy. Some serious systemic cases of candida infection that has migrated from the intestinal tract, throughout the body, often respond the best to oxygen therapy. This is a therapy that some natural practitioners incorporate in their practice.

Incidentally, according to Dr. William Wong, N.D., Ph.D., **150 mcg of molybdenum daily *"acts to keep yeast* [candida] *from making alcohol out of your carbohydrates"*** (*10 Natural Treatments You Haven't Heard Of Until Now*, Wong, 2000, p. 129). Thus, it might be wise to take molybdenum to prevent the candida from producing alcohol, which is metabolized into the even more toxic acetaldehyde, until you have eliminated the candida.

NOTE: If all else fails, some natural practitioners use I.V. hydrogen peroxide therapy to resolve systemic candidiasis (difficult cases that have migrated from the intestine to other areas of the body).

CHAPTER EIGHT

Solutions For Treating "ADHD" – Modern Medicine's Attempt Vs. The Drug-Free Approach

Ritalin™ - Yet Another One Of Modern Medicine's Solutions

If you recall, **under "Jeffrey's Story", he was placed on Ritalin™ at the age of "four", yet it was warned that Ritalin™ should not be used with children under six years of age!** A surprising number of doctors tend to totally ignore, (or possibly just don't take the time to read), such warnings. It appears that no one seems to hold them accountable. An M.D. can pretty much, at his or her own discretion, prescribe any drug, for nearly anything he or she might choose, and do so with absolutely no justification. There is something drastically wrong with the way medicine is being practiced in the nation today. If the doctors are not willing to read, and then follow manufacturer's warnings, they should at least make sure the patient has the opportunity to do so. It should also be spelled out in simple terms that absolutely everyone can easily understand.

A Closer Look At Ritalin™ / generic name = methylphenidate

Ritalin is a central nervous system <u>stimulant</u> *used to treat attention deficit disorder (ADD), attention deficit hyperactivity disorder (ADHD), and narcolepsy.*

- ***Nutrients known to be depleted: Vitamin B_{12}, vitamin C, and potassium.***

More common side effects may include:

Inability to fall or stay asleep, nervousness.

In children, loss of appetite, abdominal pain, weight loss during long-term therapy, and abnormally fast heartbeat are more common side effects.

Less common or rare side effects may include:

Abdominal pain, abnormal heartbeat, abnormal muscular movements, blood pressure changes, chest pain, dizziness, drowsiness, fever, hair loss, headache, hives, jerking, joint pain, loss of appetite, nausea, palpitations (fluttery or throbbing heartbeat), pulse changes, reddish or purplish skin spots, skin reddening, skin inflammation with peeling, skin rash, Tourette's syndrome (severe twitching).

This drug should not be prescribed for anyone experiencing anxiety, tension, or agitation, since the drug may aggravate these symptoms.

This medication should not be taken by anyone with the eye condition known as glaucoma, anyone who suffers from tics (repeated, involuntary twitches), or someone with a family history of Tourette's syndrome (severe and multiple tics).

This drug is not intended for use in children whose symptoms may be caused by stress or a psychiatric disorder.

<u>This drug should not be used in children under six years of age,</u> should not be used as treatment for severe depression of either external or internal origin and may exacerbate (worsen) symptoms of behavioral disturbance and thought disorder if given to psychotic children.

This medication should not be used for the prevention or treatment of normal fatigue, nor should it be used for the treatment of severe depression.

This drug should not be taken during treatment with drugs classified as monoamine oxidase (MAO) inhibitors, such as the antidepressants Nardil and Parnate, nor for the 2 weeks following discontinuation of these drugs.

<u>There is no information regarding the safety and effectiveness of long-term treatment in children</u>. However, suppression of growth has been seen with the long-term use of stimulants, so your doctor will watch your child carefully while he or she is taking this drug.

Blood pressure should be monitored in anyone taking this drug, especially those with high blood pressure.

Some people have had visual disturbances such as blurred vision while being treated with this drug.

Make sure you tell your doctor if you have any other medical problems, especially:

- *Alcohol abuse (or history of) or*
- ***Drug abuse or dependence (or history of)—<u>Dependence on methylphenidate may be more likely to develop</u>***
- *Epilepsy or other seizure disorders—The risk of having convulsions (seizures) may be increased*
- *Gilles de la Tourette's disorder (or family history of)*

- *Glaucoma or*
- *High blood pressure or*
- *Psychosis or*
- ***Severe anxiety, agitation, tension, or depression or***
- *Tics (other than Tourette's disorder)—Methylphenidate may make the condition worse*

The use of this drug by anyone with a seizure disorder is not recommended. Be sure your doctor is aware of any problem in this area. **Caution is also advisable for anyone with a history of emotional instability or substance abuse, due to the danger of addiction.**

Excessive doses of this drug over a long period of time can produce addiction. It is also possible to develop tolerance to the drug, so that larger doses are needed to produce the original effect.

Careful supervision is required during drug withdrawal, since depression as well as renewed overactivity can be unmasked. Long-term follow up may be needed for some patients. Reports of suicide after drug withdrawal have been reported.

Possible interactions:

- *Antiseizure drugs such as phenobarbital, Dilantin and Mysoline*
- **Antidepressant drugs** *such as Tofranil, Anafranil, Norpramin, and Effexor*
- *Blood thinners such as Coumadin*
- **Clonidine** *(Catapres-TTS)* [NOTE: Often prescribed with Ritalin™]
- *Drugs that restore blood pressure, such as EpiPen*
- *Guanethidine (Ismelin)*
- *Phenylbutazone*
- *Amantadine (e.g., Symmetrel)*
- *Amphetamines*
- *Appetite suppressants (diet pills)*
- *Bupropion (e.g.,* **Wellbutrin**, *Zyban)*
- **Caffeine** *(e.g., NoDoz)*
- *Chlophedianol (e.g., Ulone)*
- *Cocaine*
- **Medicine for asthma or other breathing problems**
- **Medicine for colds, sinus problems, hay fever or other allergies (including nose drops or sprays)**
- *Nabilone (e.g., Cesamet)*
- *Pemoline (e.g., Cylert)—Using these medicines with methylphenidate may cause severe nervousness, irritability, trouble in sleeping, or possibly irregular heartbeat or seizures*

- *Monoamine oxidase (MAO) inhibitor activity (isocarboxazid [e.g., Marplan], phenelzine [e.g., Nardil], procarbazine [e.g., Matulane], selegiline [e.g., Eldepryl], tranylcypromine [e.g., Parnate])—Taking methylphenidate while you are taking or less than 2 weeks after taking an MAO inhibitor may cause sudden extremely high blood pressure and severe convulsions; at least 14 days should be allowed between stopping treatment with an MAO inhibitor and starting treatment with methylphenidate*

- *Pimozide (e.g., Orap)—Pimozide is not used to treat tics that are caused by medicines. Before tics are treated with pimozide, the doctor should find out if the tics are caused by methylphenidate.*

The following additional information was obtained from literature review by Richard Scarnati, of an article titled ***"An Outline of Hazardous Side Effects of Ritalin™ (Methylphenidate)"*, published by *The International Journal of the Addictions*,** in which Scarnati listed a large number of adverse affects of Ritalin™ and provided published journal articles which reported each of these symptoms. **He claims that, for every one of the following Ritalin™ side effects, there is at least one confirming source in the medical literature:**

- *Paranoid delusions*
- *Paranoid psychosis*
- ***Hypomanic and manic symptoms, amphetamine-like psychosis***
- *Activation of psychotic symptoms*
- *Toxic psychosis*
- *Visual hallucinations*
- *Auditory hallucinations*
- ***Can surpass LSD in producing bizarre experiences***
- ***Effects pathological thought processes***
- ***Extreme withdrawal***
- *Terrified affect*
- *Started screaming*
- ***Aggressiveness***
- ***Insomnia***
- ***Since Ritalin is considered an amphetamine-type drug, expect amphetamine-like effects***
- ***Psychic dependence***
- ***High-abuse potential DEA Schedule II Drug***
- ***Decreased REM sleep***
- ***When used with antidepressants one may see dangerous reactions including hypertension, seizures and hypothermia***
- *Convulsions*
- ***Brain damage may be seen with amphetamine abuse***

As noted by retired medical director, Dr. Heinrich Kremer, of Barcelona Spain:

The effects of a long term Ritalin treatment are more harmful than the desired positive therapeutic effects. Long term Ritalin therapy proves to interfere enormously with personality development and physical maturity during childhood and teen years, with highly risky long-term consequences (http://www.shirleys-wellness-café.com/ritalin.htm).

And, at https://www.lawyersandsettlements.com/case//ritalin_heart_attack_stroke, it was reported that ***"Ritalin and other ADHD drugs have been linked, by FDA received reports, to heart attacks, strokes, hypertension, and some of these reported cases have led to death."*** According to this same website, *"If you or a loved one has suffered from a heart attack or stroke while taking Ritalin, you may qualify for damages or remedies that might be awarded in a possible class action lawsuit."* Call toll free (866) 866-5529 for a free Ritalin™ case evaluation. This might be at least one way to hold them accountable. Unfortunately, if you qualify, the damage has already been done. It's much easier to avoid the problem if it's not already too late.

Ritalin™ and Cancer

According to information compiled from http://www.cancer.gov, the website of the National Cancer Institute, and http://www.cancer.org, the website of the American Cancer Society, ***"Cancer is the leading cause of disease-related deaths in children under the age of 20. Every year, about 12,400 children and teens under the age of 20 are diagnosed with cancer, and approximately 2,300 die."***

With that in mind, we then need to consider the following study performed at the University of Texas Medical Branch at Galveston:

> *A new study found that* ***every one of a dozen children treated for attention deficit / hyperactivity disorder with methylphenidate*** [Ritalin™] ***experienced a threefold increase in levels of chromosome abnormalities – occurrences associated with increased risks of cancer and other adverse health effects.***
>
> *The researchers say that to their knowledge this is the first study addressing the potential chromosome-breaking effects associated with treatment of children with methylphenidate, the generic name for a group of drugs that includes Ritalin, Concerta, Metadate CD and others.*
>
> *The new Texas study involved researchers drawing blood from children diagnosed with ADHD before they began taking methylphenidate in order to get a baseline level of chromosomal abnormalities. Three months after the children had begun taking the drug, the researchers drew the children's blood and tested it a second time. Chromosomes are the bodies within cells that carry genes and genetic information. All 12 of the children whose before-and-after blood cells were studied, were treated with normal therapeutic doses of methylphenidate.*
>
> ***Most of the abnormalities found in the studied blood cells consisted of chromosome breaks "and a higher frequency of aberrations is reported to be associated with an increased risk of cancer down the line,"*** *said lead author Randa A. El-Zein, M.D., Ph.D., an assistant professor of epidemiology at M.D. Anderson who performed the blood studies using several techniques.*

> ***"It was pretty surprising that all of the children taking methylphenidate showed an increase in chromosome abnormalities in a relatively short period of time,"*** *El-Zein said* (http://www.newswise.com/p/articles/view/510069).

Dr. Samuel S. Epstein, M.D. feels that **the American Academy of Pediatrics' guidelines for treating behavioral disorders in children with Ritalin™, ignores evidence of cancer risks,** as follows:

Ritalin™ Prescribed For ADHD Increases Cancer Risk

> *Methylphenidate* [Ritalin™] *is the most widely prescribed of a class of amphetamine-like drugs used to treat ADHD.* ***Between 1991 and 1999, United States sales of methylphenidate increased more than 500 percent.***
>
> *Some 40 years after the drug was first marketed, carcinogenicity* ***tests were conducted at the taxpayers' expense by the National Toxicology Program, the results of which were published in 1995.*** *Adult mice were fed Ritalin over a two-year period at dosages close to those prescribed to children. The mice developed a statistically significant incidence of liver abnormalities and tumors, including highly aggressive rare cancers known as hepatoblastomas.*
>
> ***The American Academy of Pediatrics has endorsed the use of the drug*** **[Ritalin™].** *However,* ***the Academy ignores clear evidence of the drug's cancer risks of which parents, teachers and school nurses, besides most pediatricians and psychiatrists, still remain uninformed and unaware.***
>
> ***The National Toxicology Program concluded that Ritalin is a "possible human carcinogen,"*** *and recommended the need for further research.* ***While still insisting that the drug is safe,*** *the Food and Drug Administration admitted that these findings signal "carcinogenic potential," and required a statement to this effect in the drug's package insert. However,* ***these inserts are not seen by parents or nurses.***
>
> ***Apart from cancer risks, there is also suggestive evidence that Ritalin induces genetic damage in blood cells of Ritalin-treated children.***
>
> ***There is no justification for prescribing Ritalin, even by highly qualified pediatricians and psychiatrists, unless parents have been explicitly informed of the drug's cancer risks. Otherwise, prescribing Ritalin constitutes unarguable medical malpractice*** (http://www.ritalindeath.com/Ritalin-Cancer.htm).

Even though the results of the above study was published in 1995, (12 years ago, as of this publishing), the FDA still insists that "the drug is safe"! And although it seems as if a lot of tax payers' money and effort was invested to prove a drug such as Ritalin™ definitely poses a serious risk, their only response is to include a warning in the drug's package insert, which is normally discarded along with the fine print that few ever read. It is thus seldom considered, by those prescribing Ritalin™, but instead just provides a certain degree of protection to the drug manufacturer. You are then taking it at your own risk, as if you were forewarned, (even if your doctor didn't warn you)! It's a tactic the FDA can use to allow a dangerous drug to remain on the market, while protecting the manufacturer, by providing a disclosure that few ever see, or are aware of. It's basically a good way to discourage anyone from conducting studies to prove that drugs the FDA approved as safe, actually aren't, (something they would rather not admit to). As a result, many dangerous drugs remain on the market for years, exposing millions, while billions of dollars are being made by the developers, at the public's expense.

Ritalin's Cancer-Promoting "Inactive" Ingredients

Something few are actually aware of is, just a small amount of some substances, (added to medications, often just to provide a pleasing appearance), normally considered as "inactive", can easily prove to be anything but inactive.

The following information, obtained at http://www.rxlist.com/cgi/generic/methphen.htm, lists several **"inactive"** ingredients found in Ritalin™, (although they definitely are "active" - especially regarding promoting cancer). Following are **just three** of the "inactive" ingredients found in Ritalin™, and how they promote cancer:

- **F D & C Green No. 3 (10 mg tablets) - *"Possibly carcinogenic* [cancer causing]*."***
(http://www.purezing.com/living/living_toxins_commondyes.html)

- **Polyethylene glycol (PEG) - *"May contain ¼-dioxane which is a possible carcinogen, estrogen mimic and endocrine disruptor. Moderately toxic, and possible carcinogen.*** *Many glycols produce* ***severe acidosis,*** *central nervous system damage and congestion.* ***Can cause*** *convulsions,* ***mutations,*** *and surface EEG changes"* http://www.purezing.com/living/living_toxins_commondyes.html).

- **Mineral Oil** - ***"Causes testicular tumors in the fetus,*** *deposits accumulate in the lymph nodes and* ***prevents absorption of vitamin A from the intestines."***
(http://www.purezing.com/living/living_toxins_commondyes.html)

It is important to note that without the presence of vitamin A, protein cannot be utilized in the body. Vitamin A also enhances the immune system, and is a powerful antioxidant, (which prevents cancer), as well as being important for healthy skin, hair, bones, and teeth. And, insufficient vitamin A can cause a deterioration of the pituitary gland's basophil cells where the thyroid-stimulating hormone is formed, limiting the amount of iodine that the thyroid gland can absorb, and reducing the amount of thyroid hormone it produces. In the chapter on Hypothyroidism, you will learn the importance of adequate thyroid function, and the dozens of potential side effects associated with hypothyroidism, (many of them mimic "ADHD" symptoms).

Ritalin™ and Irreversible Brain Damage

According to an article published in the *International Journal of Risk & Safety in Medicine* (1999), as part of a study researched by Peter R Breggin, M.D., director at the International Center for the Study of Psychiatry and Psychology (ICSPP), titled ***"Psychostimulants in the Treatment of ADHD"***, a test performed in 1994 found that ***"MPH* [Methylphenidate or Ritalin™]** ***decreased the overall flow of blood by 23-30% into all areas of the brain."***

The article goes on to explain that Methamphetamine (M-AMPH) is FDA-approved for the treatment of behavioral disorders in children, although **it has long been demonstrated to cause neurotoxicity, including the destruction of brain cells**. The article states:

> ***Chronic exposure to M-AMPH can produce irreversible loss of receptors for dopamine and/or the death of dopaminergic and other neurons in the brain.*** **[Methamphetamine showed]** ***persistent neurotoxic changes in dopamine function (dopamine depletions of 55-85%), and also demonstrated dopaminergic cell loss of 40-50% in the substantia nigra*** (http://www.breggin.com/Newstimulants.pdf).

You can easily see why the dopamine depletion is a "major concern", as it could potentially contribute to the development of Parkinson's disease later in life. Parkinson's is a very degenerative disease that should be avoided at all costs. And the destruction of brain cells would likely result in a lower IQ in children, as well as a much greater risk for developing Alzheimer's disease later in life. So the question is, **why do we continue placing our children on such potentially dangerous stimulants?**

Ritalin™ and Cardiovascular Damage

According to statistics reported to the FDA MedWatch program between 1990 and 2000, (http://www.adhdfraud.org/commentary/1-6-02-2.htm), **there were 186 deaths from Ritalin™**! As noted by one mother: ***"One toy might be recalled if 1 or 2 children die from it. How many children have to die from these drugs before we realize and put an end to this horror?"*** The question remains, how many more children actually died from complications associated with Ritalin™, where the connection with Ritalin™ was not made?

Following is a true story, told by one mother (Monica), posted on her website (http://www.ritalindeath.com), regarding her son. It is an effort to expose the health risks, dangers, deaths, and suicides that are a direct result of the prescribing of Ritalin™ and other psychiatric drugs to children, as follows:

> *Our fourteen-year-old son Matthew suddenly died on March 21, 2000.* ***The cause of death was determined to be from the long-term (age 7-14) use of Methylphenidate, a drug commonly known as Ritalin.***
>
> *According to Dr. Ljuba Dragovic, the Chief Pathologist of Oakland County, Michigan,* ***upon autopsy, Matthew's heart showed clear signs of small vessel damage caused from the use of Methylphenidate (Ritalin).***

The certificate of death reads: "Death caused from Long Term Use of Methylphenidate, (Ritalin)."

I was told by one of the medical examiners that ***a full-grown man's heart weighs about 350 grams and that Matthew's heart's weight was about 402 grams.*** *Dr. Dragovic said* ***this type of heart damage is smoldering and not easily detected with the standard test done for prescription refills. The standard test usually consists of blood work, listening to the heart, and questions about school behaviors, sleeping and eating habits.***

What is important to note here is that Matthew did not have any pre-existing heart condition or defect.

We were not provided with information involving the dangers of using Methylphenidate (Ritalin) as "treatment" for Attention Deficit Hyperactivity Disorder. One of these dangers includes the fact that Methylphenidate, Ritalin causes constriction of veins and arteries, causing the heart to work overtime and inevitably leading to damage to the organ itself.

We were not made aware of the large number of children's deaths, that have been linked with these types of drugs used as "treatment."

While Matthew was taking Methylphenidate (Ritalin), at no time, were we informed of any test: echocardiogram, MRI. These types of tests could have detected the damage done to his heart. These tests are not considered "standard" in monitoring "treatment" of ADHD they are usually never administered to children. ***Sadly death is inevitable without the possibility of detection.***

According to an article by Gardiner Harris, printed in the *New York Times*, February 9, 2006, stimulants used to treat ADHD (such as Ritalin™ and Adderall™) must now carry a "black box" warning, regarding the dangerous effects these drugs have on the heart. A portion of the *New York Times* article states:

"I must say that I have grave concerns about the use of these drugs and grave concerns about the harm they may cause," said Dr. Steven Nissen, a cardiologist at the Cleveland Clinic and a panel member.

The votes* [to suggest that stimulants labels carry the "black box" warning – the most serious of the agency's drug-risk warnings] *came after the FDA medical officers described reports of 25 sudden deaths among people taking stimulants – the deaths were mostly children – and a preliminary analysis of millions of health records that suggested stimulants might increase the risks of strokes and serious arrhythmias in children and adults.

> ***The preliminary analysis suggested that the stimulants might increase heart risks more than twofold.*** *Such an increase may not be significant in children, whose heart risks are low, but could cause concern in adults, panel members said.*
>
> *The drugs' soaring popularity* [Ritalin™] *and increasing use in adults, panel members said, mean that the FDA should study them more closely and warn patients and doctors about the potential risks to the heart.*
>
> *Arthur A. Levin, director of the Center for Medical Consumers in New York City, and a member of the panel, said* ***"For us to sit around and talk about it, and for us to not make a very strong warning about the uncertainty of these drugs and their possible risks, would be unethical."***
> ***Dr. Thomas R. Fleming, a professor of biostatistics at the University of Washington and a panel member, said stimulants might be far more dangerous to the heart than Vioxx or Bextra, drugs that were withdrawn over the past two years because of their ill effects on the heart.***
>
> *Dr. Kate Gelperin, a medical officer in the Office of Drug Safety, noted that stimulants had long been known to increase blood pressure and heart rates. Other studies have shown conclusively that increased blood pressure leads directly to increased deaths from heart problems, she said.*
>
> ***"I want to cause people's hands to tremble a little bit before they write that prescription," Dr. Nissen said*** (http://amphetamines.com/methylphenidate/black-box.html).

Better yet would be, in my opinion, to assure that no doctor could legally ever write a prescription for Ritalin™. I concur with Dr. Fleming, as Ritalin™ is actually associated with "many more risk factors" than Vioxx™ and Bextra™. Why, then, is the FDA still allowing doctors to continue placing millions of children at risk, by prescribing Ritalin™?

Another horror story found on the Internet, tells of a 12-year-old boy who had been on Ritalin™ for only four years, as follows:

> *The child had from time to time been noted as having a rapid irregular heartbeat. This was considered not to be a problem at the time.* ***One day during the exertion of running the child fell to the ground with a very rapid and irregular heart beat, shortness of breath and chest pain.*** *He was rushed to a hospital where the Doctor who had put the child on Ritalin examined him.* ***The doctor assured the mother that there was no real problem with this incident and that it was caused by the Ritalin.*** *The mother was told to continue the Ritalin dose and that this type of incident* ***"will happen from time to time and you need not worry about it."***
>
> ***One week later, the child fell from his bicycle and died at the road side of a heart attack.*** *An autopsy performed on the child revealed the product of years of irregular and occasionally rapid irregular heart beat.* ***The child had a greatly***

enlarged heart due to the heart muscles working against each other during the phases of irregular beating of the organ.

(http://www.uhuh.com/education/ritpsych.htm#c.%20Hazardous%20Heart%20Attacks%20Caused%20by%20Ritalin)

Something else to consider, as mentioned previously, is that any manmade chemicals, including dyes added for aesthetics, can very well have a negative influence! According to information obtained at http://www.rxlist.com/cgi/generic/methphen.htm, Ritalin™ contains D & C Yellow No. 10 (in 5 mg and 20 mg tablets), which definitely produced cardiovascular effects in clinical trials, reported as follows: *"Oral administration to 122 patients with a variety of allergic disorders caused the following reactions:* ***general weakness****, heatwaves,* ***palpitations,*** *blurred vision, rhinorrhea* [persistent watery mucus discharge from the nose], ***feeling of suffocation,*** *pruritus* [an intense itching sensation] *and urticaria* [an itchy dry skin eruption]*"* (http://www.blackwell-synergy.com/doi/abs/10.1111/j.1365-2222.1978.tb00449.x).

So the question remains: Considering the many serious side effects associated with Ritalin™, would you possibly allow anyone to place your child on such a dangerous drug? Hopefully not! Not only that, but more adults have begun taking Ritalin™ as well. As a matter of fact, Americans use a full 90% of all Ritalin™ in the whole world! We are the largest consumers of "legal drugs" of any other nation, as well. Aren't we privileged to have access to so many different drugs? Not only that, but they're often even covered by our insurance. Such a blessing!

Natural Solutions For Treating "ADHD"

One Surprisingly Effective Approach – Behavior Modification

A possible "New Approach" for challenging children: ***"The Nurtured Heart Approach,"*** by Dr. Howard N. Glasser, Director of the *Children's Success Foundation*.

The following information can be obtained on the foundation's website at http://www.difficultchild.com/nharesearch.html:

It is a strategic family systems approach designed to turn the challenging child around to a new pattern of success. The approach is now used in hundreds of classrooms nationally, and its strategies have been adopted ```with substantial success as the school-wide discipline plan in several Tucson schools.

The Nurtured Heart Approach teaches significant adults how to strongly energize the child's experiences of success while not accidentally energizing his or her experiences of failure.

Traditional approaches for parenting and teaching can easily backfire with challenging children: they inadvertently reward children by providing more energy, involvement and animation when things are going wrong. Challenging children wind up being very confused because they perceive a high level of incentive for pushing the limits and for negative behaviors and little incentive to make successful choices. Often, the harder adults try applying these normal methods, the worse the situation becomes, despite the best of intentions.

The numbers speak for themselves:

Tolson Elementary School in Tucson Arizona, a Title 1 school of over 500 children (80% free or reduced lunch) has shown remarkable progress since beginning a school-wide Nurtured Heart Approach intervention in 1999. Prior to that many children were referred for ADHD assessments and were put on medicates. ***They had eight times the normal number of school suspensions per year as other schools in the district and teacher attrition was well over 50% per year.***

Since that time there has only been one child suspended, no children at all diagnosed as ADHD and no new children on medications. *Teacher attrition has dropped to less than 5% and special education utilization has dropped from 15% to 5%. Best of all, the school has gone from the worst in district as measured by standardized test scores to having dramatic and continuing positive progress. This data is in keeping with other informal observations noted when this approach has been applied in other school-wide applications.*

Dr. Shirli Ward researched *The Nurtured Heart Approach* for her doctoral dissertation in 1996, as reported on http://www.difficultchild.com/nharesearch.html, as follows:

Mothers reported significant improvements in their child's behavior related to the following: conduct, anxiety, communication, acute problems, and overall severity. In addition, in terms of their own well-being, mothers reported fewer depressive symptoms, decreased stress levels *and increased parenting effectiveness and satisfaction following treatment.*

These results were found to be consistent across the researched diagnostic categories of Attention Deficit Hyperactivity Disorder, Oppositional Defiant Disorder, Conduct Disorder and Depressive Disorder as well as for children for whom treatment was sought for general noncompliance and Adjustment Disorder.

Dr. Howard Glasser seems to be a talented doctor, who first introduced this approach in 1994, at his Center for the Difficult Child (CDC), located in Tucson, Arizona. He has experienced amazing success just by employing this one behavioral technique, which is apparently relatively easy to learn. For example, two masters degree students reached a high level of competency in only 2 months. The objective is for the therapist to work with parents of the problem child, (often just the mother). Due to the ease of training, and relatively short period of time required to learn the technique, in my opinion, this is training that all teachers could benefit from and should receive. They would then better understand how to deal with problem children when necessary, and how to advise the parents, rather than suggesting they be needlessly placed on dangerous medications, which is just a quick fix, and definitely not in the child's best interest.

A Recent Update On "The Nurtured Heart Approach"

The following update on this "highly effective" program, was obtained from an e-newsletter sent from "Parents Against TeenScreen" (this article is also available at http://www.tucsoncitizen.com/daily/frontpage/42934.php):

This Arizona article describes a public school that focuses on praising kids for their accomplishments and ***has very nearly done away with Ritalin****.*

[The proof is:] ***Only "Two of the 519 students are on medication for ADHD"!***

Students at Tolson Elementary School know how they should be treated. And they won't settle for less.

Things are peaceful now at the West Side school at 1000 S. Greasewood Road. But that wasn't always the case.

In 2000, when Maria Figueroa first came to the Tucson Unified School District school as principal, ***she spent most of her day on student discipline. Many pupils were medicated for attention disorders.***

Then she discovered Howard Glasser, a Tucson therapist who co-authored "Transforming the Difficult Child : The Nurtured Heart Approach."

The school dived head-first into the program, which teaches adults how to build up children using oral and written praises. Expectations are high, and children learn to interact with classmates and adults.

The program is strict, with immediate consequences for missteps, although little emphasis is placed on negative behavior. Instead, children get praise cards they may keep at school or take home for parents to see.

When Figueroa first came to Tolson, she writes, "once the lunch recesses began at 10:30 a.m., there was a constant line of at least 15 students waiting their turn to meet the principal to receive the sentences for hitting, cursing, racial slurring or other infractions."

Now the emphasis is on seeking out character to build an "inner wealth" of self-esteem.

At Tolson, praise notes are given daily. "We go through cases of them," Figueroa said. The result is happy students and teachers who don't want to leave the school.

"Teachers don't treat us bad," said fourth-grader Nick Gaitan, 10. "They don't yell at us and they give us lots of praise notes for things like perfect attendance, good citizenship, finishing our math or reading quietly. My mom likes it when I get them."

Glasser said when children receive positive attention, they don't seek the negative kind.

"I praise constantly and celebrate improvement," *said teacher Karen Pischansky, who now calls parents with positive news about their kids.* ***"I show the students I care about them and their education."***

And the students get it.

"When they see we pay more attention to their positive behavior, they respond," she said. ***"They feel successful."***

Fourth-grader Victoria Gavaldon, 10, pulls out 34 praise notes she has received this year. ***"It's really nice to know we've been doing a good job in class," she said. "It makes me feel like I want to do it more."***

That's what Glasser expects from his program. He created the approach to deal with children who had attention deficit hyperactivity and attention deficit disorders without using medication.

When kids are medicated, they are at the mercy of the drugs, *he said. "And the worst-case scenario is* ***the kid starts believing in the drug, not in himself."***

Educators discovered that ***the praising technique worked equally well with children who didn't have attention disorders.***

And it all but wiped out the use of medication *for the disorders in Tolson students.*

"Here, teachers are more likely to refer challenging students to GATE programs than to special education programs," Figueroa said referring to Gifted and Talented Education. "We have seven kids in special ed now and 59 in GATE. That's a complete reversal from a few years ago."

"They're finding that inner wealth. They're accruing a sense of greatness," *he said. "And this is not a static bank account of wealth.* ***In the best of worlds, it keeps growing and the child sees himself getting greater and greater."***

This is truly a success story, and a program that all schools could unquestionably benefit from. Would you rather your child was unnecessarily drugged with potentially dangerous drugs such as Ritalin™, or treated with the respect they deserve, and motivated to do better? The answer should be obvious.

Also noted, gifted children tend to misbehave when they are not adequately challenged, which is why the "Gifted and Talented Education" (GATE) program makes perfect sense, for gifted children. Although these children could easily have tremendous potential, that potential is all too often discouraged, and even suppressed with drugs, rather than developed. Who knows?

They could possibly become a great scientist, or even one of our future leaders! Could you imagine the influence that such drugs, (which many gifted and talented children diagnosed with ADHD are being place on), could possibly have had on the brilliant scientist Albert Einstein for instance? Both the SSRI antidepressants such as Prozac™, and stimulants such as Ritalin™, that many doctors are placing many children on, can contribute to brain damage!

All you have to do is watch the TV program *"The Nanny"* to get a feel for how some children quickly learn how to manipulate their parents, and basically gain control, which then becomes a problem for their teacher once they start school. Like "The Nanny," Dr. Glasser has developed a proven method to drastically change the behavior of "problem children." At times, the source of the problem is just the parents, who must be trained to tactfully and effectively maintain discipline. Unfortunately, parenting skills are not taught in school, although something parents should learn.

To locate a workshop being offered nearest you, either call 1-888-992-9399, or check their website at http://difficultchild.com/sp-bin/spirit?PAGE=26&CATALOG=5. There are also videos and audios available for anyone who would like to learn the procedure, called "Transforming the Difficult Child." The complete six-hour video is $99.95, and the two-and-a-half-hour audio is only $19.99. Dr. Glasser's book, *Transforming the Difficult Child*, can also be ordered directly from their fulfillment service by calling 1-800-311-3132.

Dr. Glasser's program, combined with identifying and resolving any allergies or nutritional deficiencies, should provide an effective plan for eliminating any "need" for resorting to medications. We would instead be producing healthy full-functioning children, free from depression, and behavioral problems. And, an improvement would soon be noticed in their grades as well.

A Possible Quick Fix For Food Allergies

As noted previously, if you suspect that you or your child is suffering from a food allergy, having your doctor order an ALCAT test, (which can identify many allergens), can be extremely beneficial. Once you have determined what food allergies you have, you may be able to turn off your chemical reactions by following the three-step procedure, as outlined by Dr. Joan Mathews Larson, Ph.D., (*Depression-Free, Naturally,* 2001), as follows:

> *First: A chemical ecologist can prepare a neutralizing dose containing minute amounts of the chemical to which you are sensitive. When this is placed under your tongue, the chemical sensitivity fades within minutes. At the same time, your immune system's ability to handle that chemical is strengthened.*
>
> *Second: Your doctor will recommend you take sodium and potassium bicarbonate in the form of Alka-Seltzer Gold or give you a prescription for alkali salts. These salts effectively* ***neutralize the excess acidity that develops in the body during allergic reactions.*** *Two tablets of Alka-Seltzer Gold help reduce the symptoms that occur from chemical exposure.*
>
> *Third: It is essential to avoid as much as possible the chemicals to which you are sensitive. Avoid chlorinated tap water* [and fluoridated water as well]. *Taking*

> *several capsules of antioxidants daily will help protect your brain from oxidation damage and heighten your immune system functioning* (pp. 244-245).

If you are unable to find a doctor to assist you with the above procedure, you might try the following. In his book *Nutrition and Mental Illness*, Dr. Carl C. Pfeiffer, Ph.D., M.D. suggests several vitamins that Dr. William Philpott found effective in reducing allergic symptoms, as follows:

> *Vitamins C and B_6 are probably the most effective. The patient on adequate vitamin C will have fewer allergic symptoms. B_6 should be given to the point of nightly dream recall, and the minerals calcium and potassium should be in plentiful supply in the diet. Zinc and manganese are also needed by the allergic patient. Elimination of the offending foods may be needed for several months* (p. 51).

You can try adding back foods you are allergic to after a few months, (especially if it's a food you really enjoy that would otherwise normally be healthy). Just re-introduce one allergic food at a time, and begin with small portions, and try not to eat it every day. Sometimes your body can gradually adjust to an offending food. Quite often, foods that people are allergic to are the foods they eat the most of, or most often.

Natural Supplements For Resolving "ADHD" Symptoms

1. **Essential Fatty Acids (EFAs).** As noted in the *Life Extension's Disease Prevention and Treatment, expanded fourth edition*, (1991/2004, pp. 143-147):

> ***Essential fatty acids (EFAs) are the most important nutrients to consider in the battle against ADHD.*** *One study found that* ***deficiencies in highly unsaturated fatty acids (HUFAs) cause the symptoms of ADHD. After 12 weeks of supplementation with HUFAs, researchers found major improvements in ADHD-related symptoms in children with specific learning difficulties.***

Additional evidence from volunteers, as reported in the German journal *Fortschritte der Neurologie-Psychiatrie*, suggests that ***"increased intake of these fats can reduce impulsive and aggressive behavior,"*** which are two commonly exhibited traits with ADHD (*Life Extension* magazine, July 2006, p. 48).

And further research, as announced in *The Australian* newspaper, reported on a double-blind study where 145 children, aged seven to 12, with ADHD, were given either *"a commercially available dietary supplement containing a combination of fish oil and evening primrose oil, in a ratio of four to one."* After fifteen weeks, when parents were questioned, children taking the active fish oil capsules, ***"showed improvements in attention, behavior and vocabulary"*** (http://www.theaustralian.news.com/au/common/story_page/0,5744,16279500%255E23289,00.html).

As mentioned, fish oil is one source of EFAs, (available in liquid or soft gels). Another source comes from flax, (either flax seeds or flax seed oil). In fact, Dr. Bruce West, D.C. feels that ***"Flax oil is the supreme source of essential fatty acids"*** (*A Special Report from Health*

Alert, 2001, p. 1). I would recommend either one-tablespoon each, or four large soft gels each, (both fish oil and flax oil).

2. **Valerian Root.** Although calming, this herb does not cause drowsiness, but instead relieves stress and anxiety, helps in staying focused, and is often beneficial for a child with ADHD. Valerian Root is fast acting, perfectly safe, and is also a very effective herb for relieving stress, (see Jeffrey's Story, in the chapter on "ADHD"). Valerian is inexpensive and should be available in your local health food store. Two capsules, twice daily, are normally adequate.

3. **Choline and Inositol (or DMAE).** According to Eva Edelman (*Natural Healing for Schizophrenia*, 1996/1998), *"Choline and inositol nourish and strengthen nerves and brain. They have been used to* ***help relieve anxiety and depression, and promote sleep."*** And, ***"DMAE, a potent form of choline, is reported to sometimes benefit behavior disorders, and frequently be effective in hyperactivity****"* (p. 31). DMAE is normally available at most health food stores. I would recommend one 150 mg capsule, twice daily. Incidentally, if cost is a concern, you might consider **lecithin granules**, (which are inexpensive), and the body can use to produce both choline and inositol. Lecithin also helps homogenize fats.

4. **Calcium and Magnesium.** Dr. Lendon Smith, M.D., pediatrician and director of the *Optimal Wellness Center*, was among the first to warn against sugar, white flour, and junk food known to contribute to sickness, hyperactivity, obesity, allergies, and many illnesses in children and adults. He also found that **all his ADD/ADHD patients were deficient in calcium and magnesium**, despite the fact that many were drinking a quart of milk a day. Dr. Smith then observed:

> *Apparently they could not absorb the calcium from the dairy products because of their sensitivity. The intestines were rejecting it.*
>
> ***About half of them had dark circles under their eyes (a give-away that they were eating something to which they were sensitive). In most cases, that sign indicated a dairy sensitivity.*** *If they had ear infections as infants, they were taken off milk.*
>
> *Apparently these people have some enzyme defect, genetic or nutritional, that prevented them from making norepinephrine, a stimulant, which we all now recognize is made to help the filtering device in the limbic system do its job* (http://www.mercola.com/2001/jan/7/lendon_smith.htm).

Dr. Smith treated his ADD/ADHD patients with **500 mg of magnesium and 1000 mg of calcium daily,** and observed:

> ***It took three weeks, but 80% of them were able to get off Ritalin or dextroamphetamine, or whatever stimulant they were on.*** *It did not work on all of them.* ***As time went by, I had them take vitamin B6 and essential fatty acids.*** *I found that if a stimulant drug had a calming effect, it meant that the child did not have enough norepinephrine (a stimulant) in his limbic system, and that* ***I***

> ***could help with a good diet and some supplements which should shore up the enzymes in his brain that make the neurotransmitters.*** (http://www.mercola.com/2001/jan/7/lendon_smith.htm)

If you stop to consider, **it's quite amazing that Dr. Smith was able to "get 80% of children off Ritalin" in only three weeks, just by something so simple as placing them on two inexpensive minerals, (calcium and magnesium)!**

5. **The B Vitamins (especially Vitamin B_6).** Not only is it Dr. Smith's opinion, but also according to Eva Edelman (*Natural Healing for Schizophrenia*), **vitamin B_6 has been long been used in the treatment of hyperactivity and learning disabilities.** I personally suggest taking a good vitamin B-100 complex daily, which should contain 100 mg of vitamin B_6. It's not advisable to take individual B vitamins, unless you are also taking the complete B-complex as well. Taking an additional 100 mg of vitamin B_6 daily should be OK if necessary.

6. **Zinc** is critical for the development of nerves and the production of neurotransmitters (i.e. serotonin, dopamine, etc.). The following information was obtained from Eva Edelman's *Natural Healing for Schizophrenia, second edition* (1996/1998, pp. 34, 56):

> ***Zinc is abundant in the brain hippocampus and may function as a neurotransmitter. It is needed in neuron development, neurotransmitter synthesis* [production]*, and copper chelation. It promotes resistance to stress, supports thyroid and insulin activity, as well as intellectual functioning,* [and] *helps moderate moods.***
>
> ***Zinc is used in treating histamine imbalances, and blood sugar disorders.***
>
> ***Deficiency can lead to headaches, lethargy, irritability, and behavior disorders.***

7. **PediActive™ - By *Nature's Plus.*** Available through *eVitamins* by calling (888) 222-6056 or by visiting http://www.evitamins.com/product.asp?pid=706.

> *Pedi-Active is a precisely calibrated formula designed for the active child. Each naturally sweetened, delicious chewable tablet supplies a complete profile of the most advanced neuronutrients available, including a diversified combination of phosphatidylserine, DMAE and activated soy phosphatides. Pedi-Active is a state-of-the-art nutritional supplement that naturally complements an active child's delicate system.*

In his article titled ***"Ritalin: Legally Sanctioned 'Speed',"*** Dr. Julian Whitaker, M.D. points out that ***"There are natural alternatives to both Ritalin and Concerta, but you're not likely to hear about them from most conventional doctors. And if the Federal Trade Commission (FTC) has its way, you won't be able to find these products in health food stores, either"*** (http://www.shirleys-wellness-café.com/ritalin.htm). Dr. Whitaker continues:

> *Late last year, the FTC charged Natural Organics, a company that markets* ***a natural alternative to Ritalin called Pedi-Active ADD,*** *with making unsubstantiated claims – despite the fact that Natural Organics has submitted some 200 studies, including 18 double-blind studies, in support of its claims. According to Natural Organics CEO Gerald Kessler, the FTC has failed to produce a single study supporting its allegations. Kessler questions the FTC's motives, and I agree –* ***it's not consumers the FTC is trying to protect, it's the profit-hungry pharmaceutical companies and their stockholders.***

8. **Goji juice – Also known as Chinese Wolfberry.** Studies have shown that **as a person's alkalinity changes, they also experience a reversal of their illness,** including cancer, high blood pressure, diabetes, chronic renal failure, obesity, high cholesterol, arthritis and other illnesses associated with physical or mental discomforts, **including attention deficit disorder, anxiety and depression.** The goji berry is sometimes referred to as the happy berry, as it's thought to elevate the mood. According to research by Dr. Victor Marcial-Vega, 90 percent of the patients he started on a goji juice regimen reversed their acid to alkalinity just by ingesting goji juice (*Breakthroughs In Health*, Vol. 1, Issue 1, p. 13).

If you recall, in her book *Depression-Free, Naturally,* (2001), Dr. Larson noted that excess acidity develops in the body during allergic reactions. Thus, goji juice should help reduce the allergic symptoms that result from eating foods you might be allergic to.

9. **BeCalm'd™ – by *NeuroGenesis, Inc.*** According to an undated *Bob Livingston Letter*, BeCalm'd™ is a clinically proven formula that has been used for years in clinics and hospitals. Taken on an empty stomach, **BeCalm'd™ enters the bloodstream in five minutes and crosses the blood-brain barrier in 30 minutes.** There are five primary fluids in the brain known as neurotransmitters. They are serotonin, dopamine, norepinephrine, opioid, and GABA (**G**amma **a**mino**b**utyric **a**cid). Acting together, the complex flow and exchange of these chemicals between brain cells controls how we feel about and view life at any given moment. BeCalm'd™ provides the brain with the nutrition it needs to reproduce its own supply of neurotransmitters naturally. According to their website:

> *BeCalm'd™ was developed through research at the University of Texas Health Science Center the work of several scientists at NeuroGenesis. Since 1984 Four Patents have been awarded. It is the ONLY product of its kind granted use of selected neurotransmitter enhancing ingredients providing nutritional support for:*
>
> *Increased Mental Focus* — *Limiting Anxiety*
> *Decreased Stress* — *Limiting Overeating*
> *Limiting Fatigue* — *Improved Sleep*
>
> ***BeCalm'd™ Raises the Serotonin Levels Naturally.***

[It might be worth noting here that Prozac™ does not produce or raise serotonin levels, but instead suppresses the reuptake of excess serotonin in the brain – an important issue.]

All the ingredients are natural and of the highest quality pharmaceutical grade and the amino acids are derived from plant sources. The capsules are NOT of a bovine extract.

Guaranteed: No filler, no sugar, no salt, no yeast, no preservatives or chemical additives, no artificial dyes or colors. Gluten free.

BeCalm'd™ consists of the following ingredients: Calcium, Magnesium, Vitamin B_6, Folic Acid, DL-Phenylalanine, L-Glutamine, and 5HTP (natural L-tryptophan). NOTE: The body uses 5HTP to produce serotonin. It's a precursor, one step closer to serotonin than L-tryptophan.

BeCalm'd™ is available through *Advanced Marketing* distributors at http://www.add-becalmd.com, or by calling 1-800-862-5033

10. Balance Formula One™. My friend, Dr. Sal Martingano, is a motivational speaker, who has been featured on Talk-Radio since 1988. He is also a healthcare researcher, and was mentored by Dr. James M. Allerton, the founder - formulator of Balance Formula One™. His relationship with Dr. Allerton spanned over a decade, and was ended only by Dr. Allerton's death in 1998. Under Dr. Allerton's mentoring, Dr. Martingano gained rare and privileged insights into the physiological rationale for the Balance Formula One™ product. Dr. Allerton's research demonstrated that **the hypothalamus was responsible for the hormones important for normal brain function.** And it was also Dr. Allerton's research that lead to the development of the unique formulation of specific nutrients found in Balance Formula One™. That formula fulfilled the nutritional requirements of the hypothalamus, and lead to the discovery that **psychotropic disorders can be effectively and safely corrected, without the use of potentially dangerous mind-altering drugs.**

Dr. Allerton's revolutionary concepts have stood the test of time, as Balance Formula One™ has helped countless numbers of both children and adults, eliminate any need for psychotropic drugs over the years, and has done so with an unparalleled level of success.

Dr. Allerton's research centered on the Hypothalamus because of its ability to produce the major neurotransmitters of the brain; Serotonin, Dopamine, Norepinephrine, GABA, acetylcholine, and others. Furthermore, the lateral portion of the hypothalamus instructs the body as to its needs, such as eating and drinking, and even how much of each substance is best. It basically helps control our eating habits, encouraging us to provide the food our body and brain need the most. **The hypothalamus also controls stress disorders, our level of anxiety or depression, as well as our behaviors.**

An important factor is: the neurotransmitters are not released from a "reservoir" of neurotransmitters within the hypothalamus, They are instead produced on an "as needed" basis. Lack of the appropriate nutritional requirements can result in **inappropriate hypothalamus function, often resulting in abnormal behaviors, such as lack of alertness, motivation, and mental focusing, as well as a host of behaviors, (such as ADHD),** that have been inappropriately classified by the profession of Psychiatry. Many typical hypothymaic disorders are included in the conveniently-created 374 "mental diseases", found in the *4th Edition of the Diagnostic and Statistical Manual* (*DSM*), also known as the Psychiatrist's Bible. I would suggest they go back to the original version of the Bible, which is based on fact, rather than fiction!

Dr. Allerton was fully aware of this movement, thus he dedicated his time, money and research into developing a formulation that would totally satisfy the nutritional requirements of the Hypothalamus.

Dr. Martingano claims:

> *My 18 years of work with Balance Formula One™ has proven that Dr. Allerton was correct in his assumption. With testimonials from* ***all aspects of correction of "mental disorders", from ADD to Post Partum Depression, the success rate of Balance Formula 1 exceeds 98%. We are losing our children to false diseases.*** *We are allowing the takeover of our medical system to drug therapy. It seems that* ***gone are the days of "common sense" given up to "dollars and cents". Much is at stake.*** *The mental sanity of the people of the world must be protected from pharmaceutical tyranny.*

Although everyone (child or adult) could benefit from the Balance Formula One™, it would be especially beneficial for anyone who had been taking Prozac™. Dr. Tracy, (one of the foremost authorities on Prozac™), has explained that just one 30 mg dose of Prozac™ causes a 200% increase in the level of the stress hormone cortisol. Thus, **anyone taking Prozac™ will have a highly elevated level of cortisol on a daily basis.**

Then according to the renowned neurologist and brain specialist, Dr. David Perlmutter, M.D., **elevated cortisol damages the HPA axis (hypothalamus, pituitary, and adrenal), where hormones are regulated, and long-term memories are stored.** All three organs in the HPA axis are responsible for hormone regulation. Dr. Perlmutter also noted that, those with Alzheimer's disease normally have elevated cortisol in their brain. **The hypothalamus is the master regulator, and thus one of the most critical organs for hormone regulation,** and thus the one that Dr. Allerton focused on with his Balance Formula One™.

The company claims the following:

Balance Formula One™ gives control over: Anxiety, Depression, Stress Related Disorders, PMS, ADD/ADHD, Hormone Regulation & more.

Benefits reported by users:

- *Makes my entire body feel calm and in control*
- *Normalizes pre-menstrual syndrome*
- *Can safely withdraw from drug abuse*
- *Stress related syndromes are gone forever*
- ***Depression no longer enters my mind***
- *No more sensations of Anxiety*
- ***Normalizes ADD/ADHD behavior***

Balance Formula One™ is quickly absorbed and clinical studies have demonstrated ***positive results often occur within as little as 15 minutes.***

> *Since Balance Formula One™ is a food concentrate, it can be used as part of the daily health regime of a child and requires no physician supervision.*
>
> *The ingredients in Balance Formula One™ are: Vitamin C, E, B1, B2, B6, B12, Niacinamide (Niacin), Pantothenic Acid, Choline, Zinc, Manganese, Calcium, Magnesium, Phenylalanine, Tyrosine, Valine, Leucine, Isoleucine, Thiamine, Folic Acid, PABA, Adrenal Tissue, Selenium, all produced under strict pharmaceutical guidelines.*

It was also noted that *"Evaluations of neurotransmitter levels has revealed that* ***approximately 84% of the population has some degree of neurotransmitter deficiency or imbalance."*** It's important to explain that, not only are the appropriate ingredients important, but the proper level and balance can be critical as well. That's especially true regarding supplements targeting the brain.

The typical dosage is two capsules, three times daily with meals, although for a child 70 pounds or under, it's usually one capsule, three times daily.

Based on many years of research, I might add that it's quite obvious that Dr. Allerton definitely put a great deal of extensive research, and dedication, into his formulation. It appears to be a very complex and broad-based formula that would reflect his obvious genius, and depth of nutritional knowledge. In such a formula, not just the proper ingredients are necessary, but also the optimum balance of ingredients is critical as well. This greatly increases its complexity.

In my opinion, Dr. Allerton's genius, combined with most pharmaceutical companies' outstanding marketing talent, would eliminate the justification for placing any child on unquestionably dangerous drugs. A symptom-free product with that kind of potential would obviously be a best seller. The only problem is, natural supplements (with that many ingredients) would not be nearly as profitable as a single chemical that was mass-produced, and marked up about 65,000% (average). And from my observation, marketing just didn't happen to be one of Dr. Allerton's talents, (and possibly not even one of his interests). Everyone doesn't aspire to become a billionaire. Unfortunately, it's those producing and aggressively marketing the toxic disease promoting, mind-altering drugs, that so many children are being exposed to, who have become billionaires. And worst of all, at our children's expense, (they have unfortunately become their innocent victims)! Never forget, that decision should be yours – "not your doctor's"! Once you complete this book, you will likely be far better informed than most doctors in the nation, regarding how to truly maintain both your mental health, and that of your child's, (and without resorting to dangerous drugs).

Balance Formula One™ can be purchased by calling (888) 762-8153, extension 434, or by visiting http://www.highway2health.net/store/balancef1_1.htm.

If some of the simpler inexpensive solutions, such as the B vitamins, calcium and magnesium, or EFAs such as flax and fish oil, prove ineffective, then Balance Formula One™ would be my choice. It targets the source of most mental and behavioral problems – the balance of hormones (calming and stimulating), controlled by the hypothalamus. The very same master hormone regulator that Prozac™ damages, due to the highly elevated cortisol it stimulates! Yet, Prozac™ is still many doctors' drug of choice for kids. They obviously need to be educated, because they are needlessly placing millions of kids at risk.

CHAPTER NINE

The Beginning Of The Inevitable "Domino Effect" – By Either Replacing, or Adding Additional Drugs To Ritalin™

According to research documented in 1997 by C. Whalen and B. Henker, (http://www.breggin.com/Newstimulants.pdf), **they were unable to find any *"long-term advantage"*** to taking Ritalin™, and they observed ***"It is often disheartening to observe how rapidly behavior deteriorates when medication is discontinued.*** *Apparently, whether a child is medicated for 5 days, 5 months, or 5 years,* ***many problems return the day after the last pill is taken."*** As drugs are only designed to treat symptoms, and do not address the underlying cause, or attempt to resolve it, that's what you should expect. Quite often, they actually worsen the underlying problem instead, (which was found to be true). This is obviously something we must stop doing, as there are many long-term risks, and absolutely no long-term benefits!

More Side Effects Result In More Prescriptions For More Medications

According to pediatric neurologist, Dr. Fred Baughman, what is happening is that ***"These children become for-profit receptacles for psychiatric drugs,"*** which has unfortunately become a reality (http://www.lawyersandsettlements.com/articles/pharma_lawsuits.html). And not only that, but **there is little proof (if any) that these "addictive, dangerous, and potentially deadly drugs" have any real benefit.** Unfortunately, there is plenty of proof (that keeps piling up) that the effects of these drugs leave devastating effects on our health, (and that of our children), sometimes lasting a lifetime.

For example, the following information, obtained on the Public Broadcasting website (http://www.pbs.org/wgbh/pages/frontline/shows/medicating/drugs/diller.html), explains:

> *"Rebound" is a term used to describe the worsening of symptomatic behavior after a drug has worn off.* ***Rebound from Ritalin is not uncommon; some parents feel that their child becomes even more "hyper" in the late afternoon or evening, as the drug wears off.*** *In studies of the phenomenon using Ritalin and Dexedrine, some but not all of the children showed some aspects of rebound, but none were so severely affected that stopping their medication was indicated. Dexedrine or longer-acting preparations of Ritalin are often recommended in situations where rebound persists.* ***Some physicians prescribe a second drug such as Clonidine*** **[in a class of drugs called Alpha$_2$ Agonists, used to treat hypertension]** ***to treat the rebound.***

As you are about to learn, Clonidine is one drug that can possibly interact with Ritalin™, although many doctors totally ignore that warning, and thus place their patients at unnecessary risk.

The following information, suggested by Drs. Carol E Watkins, M.D. and Glenn Brines, Ph.D., M.D., (both **definitely pro-drugs**), is available on their website (http://www.ncpamd.com/Stimulant_Side_Effects.htm). This is an excellent example of how **the**

majority of the "medical professionals" just prescribe more drugs to deal with the side effects of the very first drug (what I refer to as the typical domino effect):

> ***Stimulants are often used to treat AD/HD and other conditions.*** *The most common stimulants are methylphenidate (Ritalin, Concerta, Metadate-ER) and amphetamine (Dexedrine, Dexedrine Spansules, Adderall.)* ***We have been using these medications for years. Despite some dramatic media reports, the stimulants have a fairly good safety record.***

[MY NOTE: **I can't help but wonder where they acquired their information – likely the companies who produced the drugs. Although they are normally referred to as medical "professionals", you will soon discover that they are instead very unprofessional in the way the "practice" medicine!]**

> *Often we can treat annoying side effects so the individual can continue to take the stimulant. Too many people stop their medication instead of working with their physician to find a way to decrease side effects.*
>
> ***Often we can treat side effects so you can continue to take your medication.***
>
> ***Instead of stopping your medication, work with your physician to find a way to reduce side effects.***
>
> ***Reduced appetite:*** *Some people find that methylphenidate compounds have slightly less appetite suppression than amphetamine compounds.*
>
> ***Rebound:* *Some people who take short acting methylphenidate or amphetamine experience irritability or depression for an hour as the stimulant wears off. Sometimes this is worse than the individual's behavior before the medication was started.*** *Recently several new long-acting stimulant preparations have been released. Although the long-acting compounds often have less rebound, it may still occur in susceptible individuals.* ***Sometimes, we add a tiny dose of short-acting stimulant when the longer-acting stimulant wears off.***
>
> ***Jittery feeling:*** *Eliminate caffeine or other stimulant-type medications.* ***A small dose of a beta-blocker (a type of blood pressure medication) can block tremor or jitters.***

[MY NOTE: Beta Blockers lower the heart rate, which becomes a major concern during any physical activity. It will create an oxygen deficiency throughout the body, and especially the brain!]

> ***Sleep difficulty:*** *Sometimes the sleep problem is due to the AD/HD, not the medication. If the sleep problem is truly due to medication effect, we have several options.* ***Clonidine or guanfacine facilitate sleep.***

Irritability: ***Sometimes irritability may be due to the AD/HD or another psychiatric disorder. If the irritability is truly due to the stimulant, one might reduce the stimulant dose, switch to a different stimulant, add an SSRI, (Paroxetine, sertraline) an alpha agonist (Clonidine/guanfacine) or use another class of medications to treat the AD/HD.***

[MY NOTE: A lot of guessing seems to be going on in order to deal with a symptom that could very well be a side effect of the Ritalin™. The drugs recommend create a very dangerous combination of drugs that are contraindicated (not recommended) with Ritalin™.]

Depression: ***This may occasionally be a delayed effect of stimulant medication. It may be more common with the long-acting stimulants. If the depression truly is related to the medication, one may switch to another class of medications to treat AD/HD. These second-line medications would include the tricyclic antidepressants and bupropion (Wellbutrin.)***

Anxiety: *If an individual is anxious,* ***the stimulants can exacerbate the symptoms****. The treatment of this side effect is similar to that of depression.*

Blood glucose changes: ***Individuals with diabetes mellitus or borderline glucose tolerance may experience a rise in blood sugar. Such individuals can often take stimulants but may need closer monitoring of their diabetic control.***

[MY NOTE: If the patient is borderline diabetic, and remains on Ritalin™ or an SSRI antidepressant as recommended above, **they will soon become a full-blown diabetic.**]

Increased blood pressure: *Stimulants may cause increases in blood pressure or pulse. Some adults may opt to continue the stimulant and* ***add a blood pressure medication.***

[MY NOTE: There are serious complications associated with all blood pressure medications, especially a deficiency of oxygen to the brain. I cover this issue in considerable detail in my book *A Drug-Free Approach To Healthcare*, now available in a new *Revised Edition*.]

Psychosis or paranoia: *These are rare side effects. They may occur in an individual who is already* ***predisposed to a bipolar disorder*** *or another psychotic disorder. Psychosis may also occur when someone takes a stimulant overdose.*

[MY NOTE: Antidepressants such as the Prozac™ that many children are also placed on, are by far the greatest contributor to the bipolar disorder noted.]

Tics and stereotyped (repetitive) movements: *In the past we rarely gave stimulants to individuals with tics because we believed that the stimulant would make the tics worse. Recent data seems to indicate that low to moderate doses of amphetamine or methylphenidate do not exacerbate tics. If an individual has tics,* *or develops them while on a stimulant, it should be discussed with the prescribing physician. The patient and physician should then carefully weigh the risks and potential benefits or medication treatment.*

You can easily see, from the information found on this website, that some doctors insist on adding more dangerous drugs to deal with Ritalin's serious side effects, rather than just eliminating its use, and using a natural alternative, (something they never consider). This causes what I refer to as the typical domino effect, which often leads to even more serious drug complications. If you look earlier in the chapter on "ADHD", (when we first introduce Ritalin™), you will discover that some of the very drugs suggested on these M.D.s' website, **such as Clonidine and Wellbutrin™, are considered as risky for anyone taking Ritalin™!** Which, as noted, causes an increased risk for drug interactions. How can they possibly justify placing young children at that kind of risk?

Prescribing Additional Drugs To Deal With A Common Side Effect (Insomnia) (Just One Example)

A prime example of the "domino effect" becomes apparent when you look at a study reported by Medco Health Solutions, as follows:

> ***Among kids ages 10 to 19, use of sleeping pills jumped by 85 percent from 2000 to 2004, with spending on remedies by (or on behalf of) this group soaring 223 percent, Medco found*** (*The San Francisco Chronicle*, March 1, 2006).

and

> **[There was]** ***an 85% increase in the use of sleeping pills among children and young adults between 2002 and 2004*** **[only two years].** *According to the study, about 15% of the adolescents who took sleeping pills were also taking drugs to treat attention deficit (ADD) and hyperactivity disorder (ADHD).* ***Since those drugs*** **[stimulants, i.e. Ritalin™]** ***can cause insomnia, the sleeping pills may actually be little more than an attempt to counteract that side effect*** (http://www.yourlawyer.com/newsletter/read/61).

The October 1999 issue of *Archives of Pediatrics and Adolescent Medicine*, reported on a study from Michigan State University in Lansing, that reviewed the medical records on **223 Michigan children who had been diagnosed with ADHD at or before the age or 3,** and found that **Ritalin™ and Clonidine were the most frequently prescribed drugs** (http://www.sierratimes.com/06/03/13/70_224_245_243_78118.htm). Yet, the authors of the report point out that **most of the drugs used had never been tested for safety or efficacy on young children**. Not only that, but **giving Ritalin™ to children under six years is contraindicated (not recommended), although many doctors totally ignore warnings of drug interactions!**

And, **although studies dating as far back as 1995 found the combination of Ritalin™ and Clonidine to be lethal, and four sudden deaths were even reported due to cardiac complications in children taking Clonidine and Ritalin™ together, this combination continues to freely be prescribed** (http://www.scoop.co.nz/stories/HL0603/S00163.htm). In spite of the known risk, you likely noticed from the information you just read, that two "pro-drug" M.D.s actually **recommend adding Clonidine for insomnia or irritability, (two of Ritalin's side effects)**, and I am sure they are not the only doctors who are doing so.

What Else Do We Know About Clonidine (The Drug So Frequently Prescribed With Ritalin™)?

Actually plenty, as you will soon discover. First and foremost, as we just learned, studies have long confirmed that ***"The combination of Ritalin™ and Clonidine* [were found] *to be lethal."*** After checking out the side effects and warnings associated with Clonidine, one can't help but wonder why any doctor would possibly subject a child to such a serious risk; especially "at or before the age of 3" (as previously noted in the Michigan study). Clonidine alone can be risky, but as you will soon discover, when combined with Ritalin™, it can easily become a ticking time bomb, and sudden withdrawal especially could easily set it off.

From one source we find that:

> *Clonidine should not be stopped suddenly. Headache, nervousness, agitation, tremor, confusion, and* ***rapid rise in blood pressure can occur. Severe reactions such as disruption of brain functions, stroke, fluid in the lungs, and death have also been reported.***
> (http://www.pdrhealth.com/drug_info/rxdrugprofiles/drugs/cat1072.shtml)

Then from another source we learn that ***"Children may be more sensitive than adults to Clonidine. Clonidine overdose has been reported when children accidentally took this medication"*** (http://www.nlm.nih.gov/medlineplus/druginfo/uspdi/202152.html). The problem is, it's not just accidental, when their doctor prescribed Clonidine!

This is actually a prime example of what's often referred to as the "off-label prescribing" of a drug. Clonidine was only FDA-approved for treating hypertension (high blood pressure). It's obvious that young children would not be experiencing hypertension. Although there is absolutely no justification for allowing this very risky practice, **an M.D., (irrespective of his or her experience, or area of expertise), can prescribe a drug for pretty much anything that he or she might choose. There appears to be absolutely no accountability required,** and many drugs are all too often prescribed in "risky combinations", (such as Ritalin™ and Clonidine). So what's the excuse doctors use to justify prescribing it, (especially to young children)? As you will soon learn, (beyond question), **there are "absolutely no valid excuses", whatsoever!**

One excuse that our definitely **"pro-drug doctors"** thought they had found, was to deal with one common side effect associated with Ritalin™, **"sleep difficulty".** So let's see what Dr. Dale M. Edgar, Ph.D., with Stanford University, has to say in that regard. Dr. Edgar claims that Clonidine induces high-sustained levels of non-REM (N-REM) sleep for 2 – 4 hours, but **it then causes *"profound REM sleep inhibition"*!** They will basically be missing the most critical part of the sleep cycle, referred to as "REM sleep".

Then according to Dr. Ann Blake Tracy, we find that:

> ***REM [sleep] has proven to be specifically essential to good mental health. Full-blown psychosis can be produced by depriving a person of REM sleep over a period of time.***
>
> ***There is much evidence to indicate that suppression of REM [sleep] jeopardizes both the learning and memory functions of the brain.***
>
> ***The body and central nervous system rebuild structurally and functionally during REM sleep.*** *When REM is repressed protein synthesis in CNS* [Central Nervous System] *tissue is disrupted preventing this restorative process* (*Prozac: Panacea or Pandora?,* 1991/1994, pp. 186, 188).

We then learn that only two of the "**many undesirable side effects" associated with Clonidine just happen to be "insomnia" and "drowsiness"! And they prescribed the Clonidine for "sleep difficulty"**? Then, **the American Academy of Sleep Medicine reports**:

> ***"We know that depression is associated with sleep problems.*** *But what this study shows is that, in depressed youths, not all sleep problems are the same," said* [Xianchen] *Liu,* [M.D., Ph.D.]. ***"Insomnia and sleepiness is 'double trouble.' Youths having both of these had more severe depression than youths with just one sleep problem."***
> (http://www.sciencedaily.com/releases/2007/01/070101104155.htm)

As you likely noticed, Dr. Liu stressed that it was the combination of **insomnia and sleepiness, (or drowsiness), that is considered as "double trouble".** And now we now also know exactly why there was **an 85% increase in the use of sleeping pills among children in only two years.** Not only that, but as we discovered, **those same two side effects associated with Clonidine also lead to severe depression.** Incidentally, I forgot to mention that **"depression" is another side effect associated with Clonidine,** and we can now see why. Then, the severe depression would normally lead to a prescription for an antidepressant such as Prozac™. And not only does Prozac™ greatly increase the level of the stress hormone cortisol, but it also depletes 16 critical nutrients, and even appears to have more potential side effects than any other drug on the market, (575 listed with the FDA). And of course we can't forget that according to Dr. Tracy, every single molecule of Prozac™ actually contains three molecules of the environmental toxin fluoride. And then, **considering the fact that both Clonidine and Ritalin™ also inhibit the critical REM sleep, we do indeed have "double trouble".** What a terrible nightmare they are creating for our children, and just so some wealthy corporations can become even wealthier, and their CEOs can justify their multi-million dollar bonuses!

Combining Ritalin™ and Clonidine is one of the best possible ways I know of to effectively suppress the critical REM sleep, and increase the need for both sleep medication and antidepressants in the process. A brilliant marketing strategy that someone obviously deserves credit for, although I can't help but wonder if they're fully aware that they are basically playing Russian Roulette with our young children's lives! Actually it's even worse, as we're fully aware from research, that this dangerous combination greatly inhibits the critical physical and mental restorative process, which normally takes place during the REM sleep cycle! Thus, it's not actually Russian Roulette, but instead a sure thing. If our youth are our future, and we continue both destroying their health, and lowering their IQ at an early age, our future looks rather dismal. The sooner we intervene, and put a stop to the obvious corruption of our healthcare system, the more innocent children's lives (our nation's future) can be saved.

And of course we can't overlook the fact that **Clonidine is <u>also prescribed</u> by our "drug experts" for "irritability".** So let's see how Clonidine might possibly help in that regard. First, I might add that we don't all use the very same adjectives to describe certain behaviors. A typical example is the "374 different mental conditions" that psychiatrists have somehow identified, (quite a challenge for any group of "experts", I would say)! I can quite easily see that **some of the side effects associated with Clonidine could, to many observers, just be variations of irritability, such as: Agitation, nervousness, anxiety, and even restlessness.** Then we also have the **behavioral changes** noted, and I doubt very much that they are referring to any improvement in behavior. Then again, irritability could be just one of many possibilities regarding a change in behavior that they might experience. And keep in mind that we're talking about **giving a child a potentially dangerous drug, just to deal with the side effects of another dangerous drug, (which the child never really needed in the first place)!** Not only that, but **the "contrived condition" ADHD has absolutely no scientific basis whatsoever!**

Once again, we find that **Clonidine is actually adding to, rather than resolving, the irritability problem that it was prescribed for in this case.** Not only that, but there are some rather scary potential side effects we still haven't addressed. Some of Clonidine's potential side effects are especially risky for anyone taking Ritalin™! For example, **suddenly dying of a heart attack is a known risk that some children have experienced while taking Ritalin™.** Yet we find that ***"<u>a pounding heart beat</u>, <u>heart irregularities</u>, <u>and congestive heart failure</u>" <u>are three potential side effects associated with Clonidine</u>, which are of particular concern for anyone on Ritalin™.*** We can easily see why they would be considered as a risky combination!

Then we also have **"hepatitis", which is a serious liver condition** that would be an obvious concern, as a compromised liver could easily lead to an overdose of both Ritalin™ and Clonidine, (both considered as toxins by the liver). **The combining of drugs, (especially with liver damage), greatly increases the risk of drug overdose.** The liver recognizes both of them as the toxins they are, and thus attempts to metabolize and remove them.

And then we can't forget that **Clonidine was designed to lower the blood pressure,** which would be one more concern for a child who should obviously not have elevated blood pressure to begin with. So **we're basically <u>creating</u> "low blood pressure", yet we find that Ritalin™ causes constriction of veins and arteries, causing the heart to work overtime.**

And we find that **"irregular heart beat" is a side effect associated with both Ritalin™ and Clonidine!** Studies have found that when children die of a heart attack after several years on Ritalin™, they have a greatly enlarged heart. And **anyone with congestive heart failure, (one potential side effect associated with Clonidine), also has an enlarged heart, (an indication that the heart has been overworked, and is weakened).** Irregular heartbeat reduces the ability of the heart to efficiently circulate the blood, and deliver oxygen. Not only that, but it contributes to damage to the heart muscle, (leading to an enlarged heart). If you recall, **"fluid in the lungs" was one concern listed regarding Clonidine. That's normally the result of a weak heart, referred to as "Congestive Heart Failure". The condition reduces the efficiency of the lungs, and contributes to an oxygen deficiency.**

So we basically have two drugs, which many children are now commonly being placed on, contributing to both an irregular heartbeat, and an enlarged heart, (and thus a weak heart). That combination, added to constricted veins and arteries caused by Ritalin™, is a serious concern! Then if we're taking medication designed for lowering blood pressure (that wasn't really elevated to begin with), you are basically compounding an already bad condition, which would lead to **a major deficiency of oxygen, especially to the brain,** as it requires the most pressure to deliver blood (and thus oxygen) to the highest point – the brain.

You can now easily see why combining the two drugs, Ritalin™ and Clonidine, would be a "serious concern". Considering everything that we just discovered, the question is: **How could any doctor, in his or her right mind, possibly justify prescribing such a dangerous, (and basically useless), combination of drugs to "little kids"?** If there is any rational justification whatsoever, I would like to know what it is, and if not, **I see absolutely no reason why that highly questionable practice should not be discontinued immediately!**

The Next Step: Graduating From Ritalin™ To SSRI Antidepressants – How The Transition Gradually Takes Place

An article by Dr. Heinrich Kremer, titled *"Ritalin – Target Brain"*, further demonstrates how and why the "domino effect" takes place, as follows:

> *During the 60's, drug users in San Francisco discovered that* ***the euphoric effects of amphetamines could be greatly increased when intravenously injected, but were followed inevitably by sudden and deep depression phases.***
>
> *However,* ***the higher the overall feeling of pleasure attained, the deeper the depression was afterwards.*** *The fast developing amphetamine tolerance could, as with all narcotics, only be compensated with higher and higher doses and the habitual high doses actuated the compulsive longing for the stuff, the classic drug dependency scenario.*
>
> ***These circumstances finally resulted in making amphetamine and its derivatives, lawfully illegal narcotics.***
>
> ***From the extreme results of amphetamine use (deep depression, paranoia, hallucinatory psychosis, and excessive appetite suppression, with gross retardation),*** *one can induce which neurotransmitter function within the grain neurons are influenced by amphetamine and its derivations.*
>
> *The tolerance creation is explainable because of the decrease of sensitivity of the receptors.* ***These receptors become "immune", which explains the dramatic depressive collapse (crashing) following an amphetamine high.***
>
> ***The depressant effects of amphetamines are associated with the over activation of the serotonin receptors.***

> ***Depressive individuals with too little serotonin receptor activation often attempt serious, especially violent, suicide attempts or can be impulsively violent against others.* Long-term amphetamine use can therefore, lead to a tendency for violence against self or others because of the over activation of the serotonin receptors, thereby enhancing a desensitizing of the down regulating receptors.**
>
> ***The danger exists with higher Ritalin doses that the neurotransmitter reservoirs don't replenish fast enough because Ritalin forces a sudden drainage.*** *The result can be unexpected psycho-social and organic slips* (http://www.shirleys-wellness-café.com/ritalin.htm).

According to a study published January 18, 2005, research has proven that **children who take Ritalin™ may be at greater risk for depression when they become adults,** (resulting in a prescription of antidepressants), as stated in the following article:

Early Ritalin Use Could Lead To Depression In Adulthood

> ***Children who take the drug Ritalin may be at greater risk for depression when they become adults, according to work released at the annual American College of Neuropsychopharmacology (ACNP) conference in Puerto Rico. Misdiagnosis, combined with Ritalin use, can lead to clinical depression in adulthood,*** *according to a study conducted by the National Institutes of Health and McLean Hospital/Harvard Medical School.* ***Three to 12 percent of children suffer from hyperactivity, or attention deficit disorder.***
>
> ***Because most children show some of the behaviors of inattention and hyperactivity at times, the diagnosis of ADHD is a complex process that should involve specialists*** (http://www.newstarget.com/z003316.html).

Now you can see how Ritalin™ use can lead to a prescription for an SSRI antidepressant, such as Prozac™. Although SSRI antidepressants such as Prozac™ and Paxil™ attempt to elevate the level of serotonin in the brain, they do not actually produce serotonin. They just override the body's attempt to monitor and regulate the serotonin level in the brain. Incidentally, according to Dr. Glenmullen, **although the SSRI antidepressants are by definition "supposed to be" selective to serotonin only, that's not actually the case, as they also "suppress" another feel-good hormone (dopamine) by over 50%! That, in itself, is a major issue that he refers to as the "*Prozac backlash*".**

What Are The Many Benefits Associated With Dopamine (Which Prozac™ Is Known To Deplete)?

As dopamine plays such an important part in many different areas, any drug known to deplete dopamine "should be avoided" at all costs! First, it might be helpful to explain that dopamine is a neurohormone, (a hormone used in the brain). The release of dopamine is regulated by the hypothalamus, which is located in the brain. And as we have learned, just one

30 mg dosage of Prozac™ causes a 200% increase in the stress hormone cortisol. Then, according to the neurologist and brain specialist Dr. David Perlmutter, M.D., **elevated cortisol was found to damage the HPA (hypothalamus, pituitary, adrenal) axis in the brain, where hormones (including serotonin and dopamine) are regulated, and long-term memories are stored,** thus we can easily see a potential problem. Incidentally, the hypothalamus and pituitary, just mentioned, regulate the thyroid, and thus our metabolism as well.

And if someone just happens to be put on, and left on Prozac™ "for a lifetime", (which all too often happens), there is a serious concern. According to the late Dr. John Lee, M.D., ***"A lifetime of high cortisol levels may be a primary cause of Alzheimer's disease and senile dementia"*** (*What Your Doctor May Not Tell You About Premenopause*, 1999, p. 342).

So now let's take a look at some of the benefits of dopamine, (that Prozac™ so "generously depletes"), as follows:

> *In the frontal lobes,* ***dopamine controls the flow of information from other areas of the brain.***
>
> ***Dopamine disorders in this region of the brain can cause a decline in neurocognitive functions, especially memory, attention and problem solving.***
>
> *Reduced dopamine concentrations in the prefrontal cortex are thought to* ***contribute to attention deficit disorder*** *and* ***negative schizophrenia*** (http://en.wikipedia.org/wiki/Dopamine).

And while many children are being placed on Prozac™ or Paxil™, or some other SSRI antidepressant, due to some **"totally unscientific evaluation"**, we find that ***"Deficits in dopamine levels are implicated as one of several possible causes for attention-deficit disorder (ADD)"*** (http://en.wikipedia.org/wiki/Dopamine).

So Prozac™ not only dulls the emotions, (a common side effect), but it also reduces motivation, and the ability to experience pleasure, and as you just learned, **even contributes to attention deficit disorder (ADD), and possibly even schizophrenia in the process. Yet, more children are now being placed on SSRI antidepressants, (which just worsens the problem), than at any other time in history! If this is not a disaster about to happen, I don't know what is.**

How SSRI Antidepressants (And Their Depletion Of Dopamine) Can Actually Cause Depression

Another concern is the overstimulation of serotonin, along with the accompanying depletion of dopamine, (another serious concern). Especially if you consider that ***"drugs that reduce dopamine activity*** *(e.g., antipsychotics) have been shown to* ***reduce motivation*** *as well as cause anhedonia* ***(the inability to experience pleasure)"***, as stated in dictionary under the definition of dopamine (http://en.wikipedia.org/wiki/Dopamine).

The above symptoms help explain why "depression" is one potential side effect that some eventually experience, as Prozac™ gradually depletes their dopamine level, while also reducing serotonin receptors. Thus, we also find the following:

*Antidepressants appear to primarily enhance serotonergic neurotransmission during preliminary drug administration but **it takes several weeks for the antidepressant effect to be noticed.***

The late effect of antidepressants is thought to involve the indirect serotonergic modulation of dopaminergic neurotransmission.

Blocking the D_2 dopamine receptor is known to cause relapse in patients that have achieved remission from depression, and such blocking also counteracts the effectiveness of SSRI medication.

Interestingly, it's after being placed on antidepressants for a while, that people begin experiencing a relapse, and "depression soon returns". That's also about the time that some begin experiencing Parkinson's-like symptoms, as Parkinson's disease is also caused by a dopamine deficiency. One can't help but wonder if Prozac™ or Paxil™ could actually be at least one contributor to Parkinson's disease. It appears that Paxil™ is possibly even worse than Prozac™, in that regard, as it seems to contribute to uncontrollable movements even sooner than Prozac™.

The "newer legal" drugs such as Prozac™ and Paxil™ operate on the very same principle (overstimulation), and target the very same hormones that the "older drugs, now illegal" do. They all attempt to force us to feel better, although in an unnatural way. **There are always "serious consequences" associated with all "mind-altering drugs", be they legal, or illegal.** The bipolar disorder is a common side effect associated with SSRI antidepressants. The "high" caused by over-stimulation, is invariably followed by the typical "low", which is the time that most are more prone toward committing suicide. This is the very reason that antidepressants are known to increase the risk for suicide, (the higher the high – the lower the low will eventually be).

Prozac's Critical Nutrient Depletion Contributes To Depression

Just listing the following nutrients depleted by Prozac™ wouldn't begin to tell the whole story. Keep in mind that **for the sake of brevity, I'm only listing the benefits of the nutrients depleted that appear to be of greatest concern.** Only by understanding the many benefits that each nutrient provides, can you truly appreciate the importance of avoiding any drug, such as Prozac™, known to deplete them. Following are the **"16 nutrients"** depleted by Prozac™, along with their benefits:

1. **Vitamin B_1** – Reduces stress and anxiety; enhances energy and learning capacity. **Deficiencies can produce fatigue, poor coordination, forgetfulness, and irritability or nervousness.**

2. **Vitamin B_2** – Enhances vision, reduces eye fatigue, and strongly influences how well the thyroid gland synthesizes its hormones. **Deficiencies can produce dizziness, insomnia, slowed mental response, fatigue, and anxiety.**

3. **Vitamin B_3** – Enhances memory, prevents senility, and is helpful for schizophrenia and other mental diseases. Assists in normal functioning of the nervous system, and is essential to the good health of all glands, especially the thyroid. **Deficiencies can produce depression, dementia, dizziness, fatigue, insomnia, irritability, and low blood sugar.**

4. **Vitamin B_6** – Involved in more bodily functions than almost any other single nutrient. It affects both physical and mental health, and promotes red blood cell formation. It is required by the nervous system (stress resistance) and needed for normal brain function. **Deficiencies can produce anemia, headaches, depression, dizziness, fatigue, learning difficulties or memory loss. A thyroid gland deficient in vitamin B_6 has difficulty converting iodine into thyroid hormone.**

5. **Vitamin B_{12}** – Assists in cell formation, prevents nerve damage, and promotes normal cell growth. It assists in memory, concentration and learning, and maintains a healthy nervous system. It prevents insomnia by enhancing sleep patterns and REM sleep. **Deficiencies can produce anemia, chronic fatigue, weight gain, spinal cord degeneration, memory loss, depression, degeneration of nerves, moodiness or nervousness. Deficiency can also result in a significant reduction in the conversion of T_4 to T_3 thyroid hormones.**

6. **Folic Acid** – Assists in the formation of blood cells, prevents and treats folic acid anemia, regulates homocysteine levels and tissue functions, and maintains normal patterns of growth. It is considered a brain food, is needed for energy production, and is also a natural analgesic or painkiller. It assists in treating depression and anxiety, and maintains the nervous system. **Deficiencies can produce anemia, fatigue, insomnia, memory problems, paranoia, and weakness.**

7. **Vitamin C – Necessary for more than 300 metabolic functions in the body.** It is an antioxidant, and when combined with toxic substances (i.e. heavy metals, pollution), vitamin C can render them harmless, allowing them to be eliminated from the body. It enhances the immune system, thus promoting the healing of wounds and burns, preventing infection, and fighting bacterial infection. It assists the body with oxygen use, aids in the prevention and treatment of cancer, and assists in the production of anti-stress hormones. **Deficiencies can produce tooth loss, extreme weakness and fatigue, increases susceptibility to infection (especially colds and bronchial infections).**

8. **Vitamin D** – Prevents muscle weakness, enhances the immune system, prevents depression, and is necessary for healthy thyroid function. **Deficiencies can produce skeletal malformations, retarded growth in children, insomnia, visual problems, and insulin resistance.**

9. **Calcium** (an essential mineral) – Assists in neuromuscular activity and the entire nervous system. **Deficiencies can produce heart palpitations, muscle cramps, insomnia, nervousness, depression, or hyperactivity.**

10. **Magnesium** (an essential mineral) – **More than 300 enzymes are activated by magnesium, and low magnesium levels make nearly every disease worse.** It is responsible for the production and transfer of energy, thus reducing fatigue. It is necessary for healthy nerves and muscular tissues, as well as nerve transmissions and impulses. It is also a natural tranquilizer, known as the anti-stress mineral, and assists in the prevention and treatment of depression and PMS. **Deficiencies can produce weakness, fatigue, insomnia, nervousness, anxiety, confusion, irritability, depression, seizures, asthma, chronic fatigue, insulin resistance, type II diabetes, chronic stress, attention deficit hyperactivity disorder (ADHD), and poor memory.**

11. **Manganese** (a trace mineral) – Necessary in the syntheses of thyroxine, the principal hormone of the thyroid, relieves fatigue and nervous irritability, and improves memory. It promotes a healthy nervous system, a healthy immune system, assists with blood sugar regulation and energy production. **Deficiencies can produce confusion, convulsions, eye problems, hearing problems, heart disorders, irritability, memory loss, loss of muscle coordination, muscle contractions, sprains, strains, weak ligaments, tremors, abnormalities in insulin secretion, impaired glucose metabolism and pancreatic damage. Low levels of manganese are often found in people with epilepsy, hypoglycemia, and schizophrenia.**

12. **Selenium** (a trace mineral) – Protects the immune system, and is necessary for conversion of the T_4 thyroid hormone to the active form T_3 hormone. **Deficiencies have been linked to cancer, heart disease, exhaustion, infections, liver impairment, and pancreatic insufficiency.**

13. **Sodium** (a trace mineral) – Necessary for stomach, nerve, and muscle function, and assists in making the cell walls permeable. **Deficiencies can produce confusion, depression, dizziness, fatigue, headache, poor coordination, recurrent infections, muscle weakness, poor concentration, and memory loss.**

14. **Zinc** (a trace mineral) – Promotes mental awareness, and is a constituent of insulin. It is necessary for the conversion of the T_4 thyroid hormone to the active form T_3 hormone. **Deficiencies can produce delayed sexual maturation, fatigue, growth impairment, night blindness, decreased immune system (susceptibility to infection, recurrent colds and flu, slow wound healing), impaired memory, and propensity to diabetes.**

15. **Glutathione** (an amino acid compound) – Protects the liver from alcohol-induced damage. **Deficiencies can produce decreased immune system, lack of coordination, mental disorders, tremors, and contribute to oxidative stress, which plays a key role in the worsening of many diseases including Alzheimer's disease and Parkinson's disease.**

16. **Coenzyme Q_{10}** (CoQ_{10}) – Enhances the immune system, and is beneficial in treating obesity, diabetes, and anomalies of mental function (i.e. schizophrenia and

Alzheimer's disease). It boosts energy levels, and plays a critical role in energy production. It is also a natural antihistamine, thus it is beneficial for those who suffer from allergies, asthma, or respiratory disease. **Deficiencies can produce congestive heart failure, fatigue, and decreased immune system, and has been linked to diabetes, muscular dystrophy, and periodontal disease.**

As you can easily see, every single nutrient depleted by Prozac™ plays an important role in preventing the many undesirable physical, mental, and emotional conditions that often trigger a prescription for other nutrient-depleting medications, which basically compounds the problem.

What They Don't Tell You: Sarafem™ and Prozac™ Are Actually The Same Thing! (Generic Name = Fluoxetine)

It might be worth explaining that, Sarafem™ was created by Eli Lilly about the time the patent of Prozac™ was about to expire. Just before Sarafem™ was launched, a new disorder called Premenstrual Dysphoric Disorder (PMDD) was conveniently created, and entered in the *DSM* by the very creative psychiatrists.

You might say, it's exactly the same chemical as Prozac™, but in a pretty pink and lavender capsule with a feminine-sounding name. Eli Lilly could then begin charging more for Sarafem™ than Prozac™. And of course, far more women take antidepressants for various reasons, (the typical off-label prescribing). Thus, Sarafem™ will still be prescribed for the very same things that Prozac™ was, plus one new conveniently created condition, (or possibly the same condition, with a new name).

Although Sarafem™ contains the exact same chemicals as Prozac™, it also contains some inactive ingredients that are even more of a concern than the inactive ingredients in Prozac™. **While evaluating the "very active" inactive ingredients in Sarafem™, pay particular attention to the sodium lauryl sulphate (SLS), listed last, which is especially troubling.** So many women are being placed on, (and charged more for), Sarafem™ than they would be for Prozac™, although Sarafem™ is actually even worse.

Just be aware that all the potential side effects associated with Prozac™ also apply to Sarafem™, (and possibly even more, due to the additional "inactive ingredients" found in Sarafem™). As it's now considered an "entirely new drug" they can conveniently exclude some of the well-known side effects associated with Prozac™. And don't forget, Sarafem™ will also deplete the same 16 nutrients that Prozac™ does. So, let's see what they have to say about Sarafem™.

More common side effects may include:
Anxiety, diminished sex drive, inability to sit still, insomnia, nervousness, restlessness.

Less common side effects may include:
Agitation, confusion, emotional instability, loss of memory, sleep disorders, weight gain.

Rare side effects may include:
Symptoms of hypoglycemia (low blood sugar), including anxiety or nervousness, difficulty

in concentration, shakiness or unsteady walk, lack of energy; mood or behavior changes, overactive reflexes, racing heartbeat, restlessness, activity you cannot control.

In children and adolescents, less common side effects may also include: *Agitation, hyperactivity, mania or hypomania (inappropriate feelings of elation and/or rapid thoughts), personality changes (sometimes extreme), rage, suicidal thoughts.*

While you are taking fluoxetine you may need to be monitored for worsening symptoms of depression and/or suicidal thoughts especially at the start of therapy or when doses are changed. Your doctor may want you to monitor for the following symptoms: anxiety, panic attacks, difficulty sleeping, irritability, hostility, impulsivity, severe restlessness, and mania (mental and/or physical hyperactivity). These symptoms may be associated with development of worsening symptoms of depression and/or suicidal thoughts or actions.

Why is Sarafem Prescribed [as found at http://www.drugs.com/pdr/sarafem.html]:

Sarafem is prescribed for the treatment of depression*--that is, a continuing depression that interferes with daily functioning. The symptoms of major depression often include changes in appetite,* ***sleep habits, and mind/body coordination; decreased sex drive;*** *increased fatigue; feelings of guilt or worthlessness;* ***difficulty concentrating; slowed thinking; and suicidal thoughts.***

Sarafem is also prescribed to treat obsessive-compulsive disorder. *An obsession is a thought that won't go away;* ***a compulsion is an action done over and over to relieve anxiety. The drug is also used in the treatment of*** *bulimia (binge-eating followed by deliberate vomiting). It has also been used to treat other eating disorders and* ***obesity.***

In addition, Sarafem is used to treat panic disorder, *including panic associated with agoraphobia (a severe fear of being in crowds or public places). People with panic disorder usually suffer from panic attacks--feelings of intense fear that develop suddenly, often for no reason. Various symptoms occur during the attacks, including a rapid or pounding heartbeat, chest pain, sweating, trembling, and shortness of breath.*

In children and adolescents, Sarafem is used to treat major depression and obsessive-compulsive disorder.

Under the brand name Sarafem, the active ingredient in Sarafem is also prescribed for the treatment of premenstrual dysphoric disorder (PMDD), formerly known as premenstrual syndrome (PMS). *Symptoms of PMDD include mood problems such as* ***anxiety,*** *depression, irritability or persistent anger,* ***mood swings****, and tension. Physical problems that accompany PMDD include bloating, breast tenderness, headache, and joint and muscle pain. Symptoms typically begin 1 to 2 weeks before a woman's menstrual period and are severe enough to interfere with day-to-day activities and relationships.*

The "Inactive" Ingredients in Sarafem™ Are Actually "Very Active"!

According to the *Physician's Desk Reference, 55th Edition*, (2001), following are Sarafem's "inactive" ingredients, and their dangers:

- **F D & C Blue No. 1** - ***"A synthetic food dye, derived from petroleum distillates. Current studies suggest a small cancer risk"*** (*PDR, 55th edition*, 2001).

- **F D & C Yellow No. 6** - ***"Suspected of causing tumors in adrenal glands and kidneys. May cause allergies, hyperactivity, and chromosomal damage. Banned in Norway but not in the U.S."*** (http://www.purezing.com/living/living_toxins_commondyes.html).

  "Possible side effects are abdominal discomfort, allergies, hyperactivity, hives, kidney tumors, nausea and vomiting. This is derived from petroleum distillates" (http://www.purezing.com/living/food_articles/living_articles_fooddyes.htm).

  "Oral administration to 122 patients with a variety of allergic disorders caused the following reactions: ***general weakness, heatwaves, palpitations, blurred vision,*** **rhinorrhea [persistent watery mucus discharge from the nose],** ***feeling of suffocation, pruritus*** **[an intense itching sensation]** ***and urticaria*** **[an itchy dry skin eruption]***"*(http://www.blackwell-synergy.com/doi/abs/10.1111/j.1365-222.1978.tb00449.x).

- **F D & C Red No. 3** – ***"Linked to allergic reactions, skin rashes, hyperactivity and asthma so it may be a good idea to avoid them"*** (http://www.vegetarian-restaurants.net/Additivies/Artificial-Colors.htm).

  "History of causing thyroid tumors in animals." (http://www.purezing.com/living/living_toxins_commondyes.html)

  "Can cause sensitivity to light and thyroid hormone levels. May lead to hyperthyroidism. Consumption of Red No. 3, which has estrogen-like growth stimulatory properties and may be genotoxic, could be a significant risk factor in human breast carcinogenesis **[cancer causing]**.***"*** (http://www.purezing.com/living/food_articles/living_articles_fooddyes.htm)

- **Dimethicone** - ***"May promote tumors and accumulate in the liver and lymph nodes"*** (http://www.purezing.com/living/living_toxins_commondyes.html).

- **SLS (Sodium Lauryl Sulphate)** - ***"Builds up in heart, lungs, brain and liver and may cause damage to these organs. Damages immune system. Contains endocrine disruptors and estrogen mimics. Impairs proper structural formation of young eyes. May contain carcinogenic*** **[cancer causing]** ***nitrosamines.*** *This is a* ***detergent*** *derived from* ***coconut oil and may be labeled natural or even organic"*** (http://www.purezing.com/living/living_toxins_commondyes.html).

Another Antidepressant - Serzone™ Greatly Increasing The Potential For Liver Damage

We are all unique, (referred to as our bio-individuality). We all have genetic differences, and our diets normally vary considerably as well. Some of us take a lot of medications, while others take a lot of vitamins, (my preference). Our size, our age, the condition of our liver, and even our metabolism can all have an influence on our "effective dosage." The end result is: no two people will respond exactly the same to the very same dosage of a particular drug, (but especially drugs such as Prozac™).

Incidentally, we find the following regarding a close cousin to Prozac™, a newer drug called Serzone™, as announced on October 2, 2003:

> ***It has come to the attention of Health Canada that nefazodone (Serzone) has been associated with adverse hepatic events including liver failure requiring transplantation in Canada.*** *Following discussions with Health Canada, Bristol-Myers Squibb Canada has decided to* ***discontinue sales of nefazodone,*** *effective November 27, 2003* (http://www.mentalhealth.com/drug/p30-n05.html).

I would expect similar risks associated with Prozac™ or Paxil™, and especially for someone who also consumes alcohol, or possibly has the candida yeast infection. As we learned earlier, the candida turns your intestine into an internal brewery. And of course, Prozac's potentiation of alcohol by ten times, and Paxil™ by forty times, greatly increases the damage to the liver that alcohol is well known for. Then as we also learned, the potential for liver damage by the metabolite of alcohol (acetaldehyde) would be even greater. As Prozac™ and Paxil™ are so difficult to metabolize, the metabolism of both alcohol and acetaldehyde is considerably compromised. Thus a particular concern for both the liver and brain, as they will both be exposed to excessively elevated levels of both toxins, and for much longer as well.

Incidentally, Serzone™ just happens to be one of the sixteen drugs approved by the NFC for use with children under TeenScreen, which is inconceivable considering its potential for creating liver failure! And once again, it was approved with very little research or data to justify its use, considering its long-term dangers, as reported in the following article:

> *While the pre-marketing studies were restricted to patients with a DSM-III-R diagnosis of non-melancholic Major Depressive Disorder, it is expected that nefazodone* [Serzone™] *will be prescribed for patients with Dysthymia* [mild chronic depression]*, Major Depression, and Bipolar Disorder.*
>
> ***Although nefazodone*** **[Serzone™]** ***has mostly been studied for periods of administration of up to 8 weeks, it is expected that patients with long-standing depressions will take the drug for longer periods of time*** (http://www.dr-bob.org/tips/nefazodone.html).

If you noticed, they indicated that the studies were mostly **"up to 8 weeks"** long, which basically means 8 weeks **or less!** The problem is, most of the serious side effects begin showing up after long-term use, which is the very reason, in my opinion, that most drug companies conduct the shortest studies that the FDA will allow, and the FDA is "far too lenient" in that regard. Thus, the majority of testing is conducted on those who receive the drug after FDA approval. Unfortunately, those placed on drugs (such as Serzone™), which were approved on such short-term studies, are normally totally unaware of the fact. Once they experience liver failure (or some other major reaction), it could very well be too late. It's amazing just how little protection the FDA actually provides, allowing many to be placed on drugs "proven to be dangerous"! Unfortunately, few are aware of the facts, and our children will now be their guinea pigs!

The question is, does anyone truly care about what they are doing to our children? I certainly do, and I hope you do as well! I'm inclined to believe that, in the majority of cases anyway, it's likely the lack of knowledge, (the result of deliberate deception on the manufacturer's part), rather than a total lack of caring.

When One Drug Doesn't Work, "Why Not Try More"?

Following is an excerpt from *The Johns Hopkins Depression and Anxiety Bulletin* (Fall 2006 Issue) that verifies the very poor success rate patients have experienced with antidepressants, and the common "trial and error" approach of most doctors.

- *After failure on an antidepressant, the next step you and your doctor decide to take is **largely a matter of trial and <u>error</u>** based on your doctor's experience with other patients, your medical history, and your doctor's consultation with other mental health professionals.*

- ***One antidepressant treatment does not fit all. <u>You may need to try several antidepressants to find a drug regimen that works for you</u>.***

- ***At standard doses of the most commonly used class of antidepressants -- selective serotonin reuptake inhibitors (SSRIs) -- <u>30% of patients with severe depression achieve remission with the first antidepressant prescribed</u>.***

- ***It often takes 12 weeks to achieve an adequate response to an antidepressant,** not the standard four to eight weeks that most doctors and mental health specialists were previously using to guide decisions.*

- *If the first choice of an antidepressant does not provide adequate symptom relief, **switching to a new antidepressant is effective about 25% of the time.***

- *If the first choice of antidepressant does not provide adequate symptom relief, **adding a new antidepressant while continuing to take the first medication is effective in about one-third of people.***

- ***For people who don't respond to first-line therapy with an SSRI, adding a second drug to the SSRI drug regimen appears to be <u>slightly better</u> than completely switching medications.***

- ***For those who don't respond to switching to a new antidepressant or adding a second drug, trying a third medication can still help about one in five people.***

Although these potentially dangerous drugs are very slow to react, seldom effective, create many serious side effects, deplete some of the most critical nutrients, and are far less effective than natural solutions, they are most doctors' first (and only) choice. That shows the tremendous influence that the pharmaceutical industry has on how our healthcare is conducted, (and what is covered by your health insurance).

Unfortunately, this type of "remedy" continues to be routinely practiced, as confirmed in the following report from the combined annual meeting of the Pediatric Academic Societies and the American Academy of Pediatrics:

> ***Ritalin and Prozac, as well as various combinations of similar stimulants and antidepressants, are being prescribed together for an increasing number of children,*** *according to a new study presented here.*
>
> ***Among those children taking Prozac, Zoloft, Luvox or Paxil—collectively known as selective serotonin reuptake inhibitors (SSRIs)*** *and prescribed or depression, school phobias, bed wetting and eating disorders—in 1998,* ***30% were also taking Ritalin, Dexedrine or related drugs, presumably for attention-deficit disorder.***
>
> ***When the researchers considered those children on Ritalin or similar drugs, they found that 8% were also taking an SSRI.***
>
> *These findings are in addition to the overall trends showing* ***a steep increase in the number of children taking either drug type from 1990 through 1998.*** *By 1998, 10% of children aged 6 to 14 years were on Ritalin or stimulants, as were* ***1% of preschoolers had prescriptions for the drugs.***
>
> [According to Dr. Jerry Rushton of the University of Michigan in Ann Arbor, one hypothesis is that], "***The trends show over-diagnosis, the idea that 'if the child is not doing so well, then one drug didn't work, maybe we should try two or three' "*** (http://www.antidepressantsfacts.com/RitProChildren.htm).

This is an all too common, although dangerous, concept! And as you are about to learn, it is becoming even more and more common at an alarming rate!

Alarming Statistics – Covering Only Ten Months
The "Very Worst" Form Of Child Abuse, (And Worst Of All, It's Totally Legal)!

I'm just one of a fairly large group of mental health professionals, decision makers, and activists, that Vince Boehm communicates with, and keeps updated daily on the recent findings relating mostly to psychiatric drug abuse. Although our healthcare in general is far overdue for a major overhaul, by far the greatest abuse and most potentially dangerous is regarding all the mind-altering drugs being "aggressively promoted", especially as they are now targeting our innocent children. Children under the age of five have recently become their primary target. Young children are much more prone to experience an adverse drug reaction than an adult would, (at least 3 times as likely). That threat greatly increases when polypharmacy (prescribing multiple drugs) is the procedure. Polypharmacy is becoming more and more common, especially in recent years. The additional drugs are often prescribed just to treat the side effects of antidepressants such as Prozac™ and Paxil™ prescribed initially.

Ben Hansen is a psychiatric survivor and activist, that serves on the Michigan department of Community Health Recipient Rights Advisory Committee. Through the Freedom Of Information Act (FOIA), Ben was able to uncover condemning information that Eli Lilly has done its utmost to hide from the public. Following is an extract of an article written by Ben Hansen, originally intended for publication in *The International Center for the Study of Psychiatry & Psychology (ICSPP)* quarterly newsletter, forwarded to me by Vince Boehm:

> *The purpose of my FOIA lawsuit in Michigan is not simply to embarrass one pharmaceutical manufacturer –* ***my aim is to gain access to data that will blow the lid off the entire psychiatric drug industry****.* [MY NOTE: Something that in my opinion is far overdue!]
>
> *The lawsuit, "Ben Hansen vs. State of Michigan Department of Community Health," boils down to a fight over the release of records which show a list of each patient's psychotropic drugs by drug NAME, not just by drug CLASS. For example,* ***we know at least one Michigan Medicaid patient is currently on a total of 17 different psychiatric drugs, but the State of Michigan doesn't want us to know the names of the drugs in the 17-drug cocktail!***
>
> *For now I wish to share a sampling of the psychiatric prescribing data I've obtained so far. The numbers speak for themselves.*
>
> ***During a 10-month period from January 2006 to October 2006,*** *Michigan Medicaid statistics show:*
>
> - ***100% increase in children under age 18 on 3 or more mood stabilizers.***
> - ***100% increase in children age 6-17 on 4 or more psychiatric drugs.***
> - ***79% increase in adults on 5 or more psychiatric drugs.***
> - ***67% increase in adults on 3 or more psychiatric drugs.***
> - *49% increase in adults on 2 or more insomnia agents.*

- *45% increase in children under age 18 on a benzodiazepine for at least 60 days.*
- ***45% increase in children under age 18 on 2 or more antipsychotics.***

Keep in mind that **the above statistics reflect a period of "only 10 months"!** We could soon be in serious trouble if we allow the current trend to continue. Both the poor, and foster children, covered under Medicaid, experience the greatest abuse of all. Not only are more being needlessly placed on psychiatric drugs, but also multiple drugs, (greatly increasing the risk)! After all, they are totally free to the recipient, (a perfect selling point). **If their parents were fully aware of the "many dangers" they pose, you likely couldn't pay them enough to allow their children to be placed on such dangerous drugs,** especially if they were also aware that they are totally unnecessary, (something I can easily prove).

Drug companies such as Eli Lilly have been aggressively and very deliberately creating unbelievably scary statistics, (and they're not just numbers, but millions of innocent victims' lives at stake), and they have somehow been allowed to continue doing so for years! Isn't it about time we finally put a stop to such outright deception and corruption? **If the answer is yes, get involved, and be part of the solution!** You can bless many lives (including your own) by doing so, and although Eli Lilly, and PhRMA in general, have tremendous resources, collectively we do as well. If everyone in the nation were fully aware of the many facts that you are now learning, some of the companies producing these dangerous mind-altering drugs would soon be out of business! You can help make that become a reality.

As you are about to read, Mary Lou became part of the solution, when she took her health into her own hands. She eventually discovered that the majority of her uncomfortable symptoms, (including her asthma), were just side effects of her medications. And would you believe, it all started with Prozac™, one of the worst drugs on the market for depleting critical nutrients, and producing conditions such as diabetes and the bipolar disorder (which she developed). She eventually discovered what I already knew – absolutely none of her nine medications were appropriate, (not one)!

Mary Lou's experience is not just unique, but instead quite typical of what millions of adults in the nation today are also experiencing. I will be taking you through her medications and showing you what I refer to as the "typical domino effect" associated with all medications. Once a doctor convinces you that a drug such as Prozac™ is an appropriate solution, the process begins, and more drugs soon follow. Incidentally, it's very common for a doctor to prescribe a drug such as Prozac™ for anything that he or she might choose, (with absolutely no justification). It's something that drug companies encourage doctors to do. They don't even need to prove it works for the particular condition it is being prescribed for. So now I'll take you, drug by drug, side effect by side effect, from one medication to nine, and finally from nine to none!

CHAPTER TEN

Mary Lou's Story

Diagnosed With A Prozac™ Deficiency?
The Typical Domino Effect, Beginning With Prozac™
Sixteen Years and Nine Medications Later – Totally Drug-Free

By analyzing Mary Lou's story, step by step, we can better understand just how "**un**scientific" medicine has become. You will also be able to better appreciate why it's so critical that we not allow the same to happen to our children. As so many more children are now being placed on antidepressants at a much earlier age today, by the time they reach their mid 20s, they could very well be taking nine medications, as Mary Lou was, or possibly even more, depending on their doctor!

Following is an extract of Mary Lou's Story from my previous book, *A Drug-Free Approach To Healthcare, Disease Prevention – Not Symptom Suppression, Revised Edition* (2007). This portion of her true story documents the chronology of events that led to the prescribing of the nine medications she was taking. Incidentally, a common cause of depression, (especially with women), is a hypothyroid condition, which Mary Lou was actually experiencing prior to being placed on Prozac™. This condition was never diagnosed or resolved, but instead exacerbated by her two antidepressants, and lithium therapy. She was eventually prescribed the wrong form of thyroid medication (Synthroid™), which seldom resolves the condition, although the form that is normally prescribed most by traditional doctors. So, now we'll determine exactly what led to all those medications.

Why Was Mary Lou Placed On All Those Medications?

We will begin with the very first drug (Prozac™), which not only contributed to her addiction for alcohol, but also kept it going. Then, Prozac™ also initiated its award-winning performance of nutrient-depletion! With a total of **"sixteen nutrients depleted,"** it should definitely be at the top of the class. If you then consider that the list of nutrients depleted includes mostly the very important ones, it would likely be a candidate for first prize! Mary Lou eventually developed the bipolar disorder, as well as diabetes, (both common side effects of Prozac™). For the bipolar condition, she was placed on a potentially dangerous form of lithium (lithium carbonate). If you want to see just how dangerous, be sure to read the chapter on Bipolar Disorder, later in this book.

Two primary issues of concern are: (1) both lithium and Prozac™ are known to suppress the thyroid, and (2) both contribute to diabetes (basically double jeopardy). You will also discover that there are some even worse potential side effects associated with lithium carbonate than with Prozac™, (and that's saying something!). Just a few are: **permanent kidney scarring, other kidney damage, liver disorders, coma, blindness, and even death**. There are many others, but these are just some of the more serious ones. A rather scary drug I would say, and just to deal with one of the side effects associated with Prozac™. Paradoxically, Prozac™ and lithium actually have opposing actions in the brain, as Prozac™ is actually a stimulant, while lithium is a well-known suppressant. That being true, they would basically tend to "cancel each other out", as well as suppressing the thyroid, while contributing to diabetes in the process! Why not just stop taking both, (something Mary Lou eventually did)? It would certainly make more sense, and eliminate the potential of a great deal of unnecessary side effects, as well as the depletion of sixteen important nutrients just from Prozac™ alone.

Incidentally, that is not the end of the antidepressant story. Not only the bipolar disorder, but even **"depression" is a potential side effect associated with Prozac™.** Apparently that was also true in Mary Lou's case, as her doctor somehow deemed it necessary to **place her on another antidepressant called Desyrel™!** You will also find a warning of potential interactions when combining either lithium carbonate or Desyrel™ with Prozac™, which her doctor apparently overlooked, as he combined both with Prozac™. That could easily pose a major threat for a serious drug interaction, especially if alcohol was also consumed (one more contraindication). Although Prozac™ is well known for producing cravings for alcohol, doctors all too often ignore that concern, in spite of the warning against drinking alcohol while on Prozac™! And as we have learned from Dr. Tracy, Prozac™ potentiates alcohol ten times, thus one drink basically equates to drinking ten, which greatly increases the potential risk from drinking alcohol. One can't help but wonder just how much time was invested in evaluation before such a potentially dangerous combination of medications was prescribed, and especially for anyone known to have an alcohol addiction, (which Mary Lou at one time had, and Prozac is well-known for keeping the addiction going).

Now that we've covered the drugs Mary Lou had been placed on for depression, we will look at those prescribed for cardiovascular concerns. We will begin by evaluating the cholesterol-lowering drug Zocor™. There are many excuses used to justify prescribing this class of drugs. One such excuse is high blood pressure, which just happens to be one potential side effect associated with both of the antidepressants she was taking. Another is diabetes, which both Prozac™ and lithium carbonate are known to contribute to, (and something Mary Lou developed). I might add that during this time, Mary Lou was still dealing with an unresolved hypothyroid condition. Two common conditions associated with low thyroid function are depression (thus the Prozac™ solution), and elevated cholesterol (and thus Zocor™).

So, Mary Lou definitely qualified for, and was prescribed Zocor™, which would then lead to a whole series of cardiovascular problems. The first normally experienced is elevated blood pressure. So then, blood pressure medication was in order. Actually, not one but two medications were prescribed to deal with the problem. One was the ACE inhibitor Lisinopril, and the other was the diuretic (water pill) hydrochlorothiazide. We now have another serious concern regarding possible interactions when combining the ACE inhibitor (blood pressure medication) and the diuretic hydrochlorothiazide, (especially when combined with lithium). Mary Lou was unfortunately prescribed all three. Lithium is well known for the excessive excretion of both water and sodium through the kidneys, thus greatly increasing the risk of dehydration. Then, not only does the diuretic she was placed on contribute to dehydration, but one potential side effect of the ACE inhibitor is also dehydration! Under the circumstances, why in the world would any doctor in his or her right mind, possibly prescribe a diuretic that not only removes water (increasing the risk for dehydration), but also wastes many important vitamins and minerals in the process?

I asked Mary Lou if she knew why her doctor chose to include the diuretic with her ACE inhibitor. She said her doctor indicated it was common practice to do so, although most people are not also taking lithium. I can't help but wonder how many doctors actually take the time to evaluate the potential for drug interaction when new medications are added. In Mary Lou's case, that consideration was apparently just an oversight, although this appears to be a common problem in medicine today, rather than just the exception. (How about your doctor?)

This finally brings us to one more class of drugs: those prescribed to treat asthma. Not just one, but actually three of them were prescribed for Mary Lou! My first thought was: What in the world could possibly create such a serious case of asthma that would require the use of three different medications to control? As we are now fully aware, no drug created could possibly resolve any condition (that's not what drugs do), so a lifetime of controlling the symptoms is the only option.

From past experience, I suspected that her other medications might possibly be contributing to the problem, and was I right! It appeared that every single one of her other medications in it's own way, could very well to be contributing to the problem.

Following are the six culprits (her other medications) and the potential side effects associated with each that would lead to breathing difficulties:

1. Prozac™ - Trouble in breathing.
2. Lithium - Tightness in chest.
3. Desyrel™ - Chest pain and shortness of breath.
4. Zocor™ - Upper respiratory infection
5. Lisinopril™ - **Asthma,** bronchitis, and painful breathing.
6. Hydrochlorothiazide - Difficulty breathing, inflammation and fluid in the lung.

We also find some additional concerns regarding all three asthma medications:

- First, **two of three list high blood pressure as possible side effects.**
- Then, **the drug Alupent™ lists worsening or aggravation of asthma as one possibility.**
- Then, both Albuterol and Intal™ list allergic reaction as a potential side effect. The problem is, allergic reactions are known to stimulate the production of histamine.
- Elevated histamine in turn, results in a constriction of the bronchial tubes in the lungs, and can thus contribute to asthma.
- Then, according to the Prozac™ authority Dr. Ann Blake Tracy, Prozac™ causes constriction of the bronchial tubes and arteries, (aren't drugs fascinating?).

Albuterol appears to be the worst of all. It is **not only one of the two that can contribute to <u>hypertension</u>**, but also twenty other **major concerns** as follows:

* **Depression**
* **Aggression**
* Agitation
* Allergic reaction
* Anxiety
* Coordination problems
* **Diabetes**
* Drowsiness
* Excitement
* Fluid retention and swelling
* Heart palpitations
* **Increased blood pressure**
* **Increased difficulty breathing**
* **Irritability**
* Nervousness
* Overactivity
* Rapid heartbeat
* Respiratory infection or disorder
* Restlessness
* Sleeplessness

Not only that, but **the above are only "20 of the 67" potential side effects associated with Albuterol use**, (just one of three medications Mary Lou was taking for asthma). Those in bold print are those that appear to be the most serious, although they are all an obvious concern.

Mary Lou was basically in disbelief as she reviewed the potential side effects associated with each drug she had been taking. As she began identifying each one that she had been experiencing, it was such a relief to her to learn that it was actually the side effects from her medications that were responsible for the many symptoms she had been suffering from for so many years. Once the problem had been identified, the solution was quite obvious. When she discovered that Zocor™ was totally unnecessary, and the basic contributor to the elevated blood pressure she was taking medications for, and many other problems such as muscle pain and fatigue, it was the very first to go. Her next focus was the Prozac™ that had caused the bipolar disorder she was also given lithium for. Then there was the diabetes that normally results from the long-term use of Prozac™. Also, the issue that Prozac™, along with lithium, actually contributed to a worsening of her original low thyroid condition.

And finally, because the fluoride in Prozac™ not only suppresses the thyroid function but is also an enzyme inhibitor, her liver would be less efficient in detoxifying all her medications (basically toxins), causing her to experience more side effects from all her medications (which she did). Prozac™ is well known for increasing the side effects of all other medications. Then, we can't overlook the issue of the continual cravings for all addictive substances, but especially alcohol, which was being stimulated by Prozac™.

It soon became apparent that the underlying cause of her alcohol addiction, and the many symptoms she had experienced for years, were mainly caused by her medications (and the depletion of nutrients they created). Needless to say, armed with that knowledge, she was super-motivated to get off her medications, and as soon as possible. And in only two months, Mary Lou was totally drug-free!

Due to her sixteen years of Prozac™ use, I recommended she follow a more conservative withdrawal program. I suggested she immediately stop her cholesterol medication (which absolutely no one needs). This immediately brought her blood pressure into the normal range again. I then suggested that she stop drinking fruit juices and reduce her intake of sugar and starches, to maintain normal blood sugar, and then begin taking the following:

1. Drink two ounces of mangosteen juice, three times daily.
2. Drink ten 8-ounce glasses of water daily.
3. Take one teaspoon of Celtic sea salt (course crystals) daily.
4. Take two high potency coenzyme vitamin B-complex capsules daily.
5. Take two 200-mcg capsules of chromium picolinate, twice daily.
6. Take four 1,000 IU soft gel flax seed oil daily.
7. Take a multi-mineral, containing calcium, magnesium, and zinc.

Although I gave Mary Lou the nutritional guidelines to follow, she took the initiative to eliminate her medications on her own, once she learned the facts. Incidentally, she also attributed part of her success to prayer; a resource we all have available, and obviously one that we can all afford. God doesn't charge for His services, although they have tremendous potential.

An Explanation of Recommended Supplements

✓ The mangosteen is a broad-spectrum adaptogen with a wide range of benefits, such as reducing sugar cravings, stabilizing the blood sugar, and mood elevation. Dr. Templeman discovered that in his practice, he was able to replace twenty-two medications with the mangosteen juice. I might add that at the time of Mary Lou's withdraw, I had not yet learned about the amazing benefits of goji juice or noni, also broad-spectrum adaptogens. The goji berry is sometimes referred to as the happy berry, as it seems to elevate the mood. It also helps stabilize both the blood pressure and blood sugar.

✓ The water and Celtic sea salt combined provide an alternate source of energy for the brain, reducing the need for carbohydrates. Celtic sea salt also contains the natural form of the trace mineral lithium (helpful for the bipolar disorder), and iodine (crucial for normal thyroid function).

✓ A vitamin or mineral deficiency (caused by Mary Lou's NINE prescription medications) can lead to many disorders, including both mental and behavioral. The coenzyme form of B-complex vitamins should be the most effective, as the conversion in the liver is bypassed. The combination of antidepressants and alcohol would tend to reduce the efficiency of anyone's liver. Then if you were taking nine medications, as Mary Lou was, the liver's efficiency would be compromised even further.

✓ The chromium picolinate reduces the insulin resistance. The flax seed oil helps restore the insulin and serotonin receptors. It is also excellent for the bipolar disorder as well.

✓ I also recommended she request that her doctor replace her thyroid hormone Synthroid™, (which seldom works), with the natural Armour™ thyroid, (which seldom fails).

In 60 days, all nine of her medications had been successfully eliminated, and she indicated that she hadn't felt so good in years. It's quite obvious that Mary Lou (like so many others) definitely didn't need any of the medications she had been taking for so many years (sixteen years on Prozac™!). We can also see that the majority of her medications were to treat side effects associated with the drugs she was already taking. Drugs basically create the need for more drugs, (the typical domino effect).

Nutrient Depletion Contributes to the Domino Effect

Following are the nutrients being depleted by the nine medications Mary Lou had been taking, followed by the number of drugs responsible for depleting each. **Those in bold are considered some of the most important and widely used. The nutrients that can contribute to depression when deficient are identified with an asterisk.**

Once you understand the tremendous benefit of each nutrient depleted, you can better appreciate the important part each plays in your overall health, and why it should be an absolute top priority to begin eliminating your dependence on the medications responsible for creating this unnecessary depletion. The potential for a serious deficiency basically increases with each drug's contribution to the problem, as well as the many unpleasant side effects associated with each.

Vitamins Depleted:	Minerals Depleted:	Other Depletions:
Vitamin A – 1	* Calcium – 3	**Coenzyme Q_{10} – 5**
Vitamin B_1 – 1	* Iron – 1	* Essential Fatty Acids – 2
Vitamin B_2 – 1	* **Magnesium – 4**	Glutathione – 1
* Vitamin B_3 – 1	Manganese – 2	
* **Vitamin B_6 – 4**	Phosphorus – 3	
* **Vitamin B_{12} – 3**	* Potassium – 3	
Vitamin C – 5	Selenium – 1	
Vitamin D – 6	* Sodium - 4	
Vitamin E – 1	**Zinc – 4**	
Vitamin K – 1		
Choline – 1		
* **Folic Acid – 3**		
* Inositol – 1		

Although Mary Lou is just one example, many others are taking even more medications. So, what is your story? And most importantly, will it have a happy ending? Just remember, you (not your doctor) are in charge of, and responsible for your health! Your health is not only your responsibility, but also your right, and something you must never forget.

Incidentally, Mary Lou is just one example. I have helped many others eliminate their dependence on medications over the years, (often medications they would likely have been left on for the remainder of their lives). Those who took the initiative, and made the decision to end their lifetime dependency on medications, were amazed to discover it was not only possible, but also surprisingly easy. For Mary Lou, it was a pleasant experience to finally be free from the many side effects associated with the medications she had unnecessarily been taking. I say unnecessarily, as she felt so much better than she had in all those years while on her medications. It was a real eye-opener to Mary Lou, when she discovered that following her doctor's advice for so long was the basic underlying cause of the many unexplained conditions and symptoms she had been experiencing all those years.

Remember, just because your doctor places you on a medication, doesn't necessarily mean it's appropriate. In my opinion, medications are seldom, if ever necessary. Medications are the greatest contributor to poor health, (often even worse than a poor diet). Our body recognizes medications as the toxins they truly are. Why not just eliminate them to begin with, and save your liver the trouble? At least to me, (and your body), it certainly makes much more sense.

CHAPTER ELEVEN

What's Prozac™ Doing To Our Kids?

How Young Is Too Young?

According to the Alliance for Human Research Protection (AHRP), there are currently at least seven different programs that fund and promote mental health screening, and at least two of these are specifically involved with infant mental health screening. And just **how do they determine if a "preschool age" child is depressed?** As pointed out by AHRP:

> *If psychiatric experts and groups like the US Surgeon General and the authors of the Diagnostic and Statistical Manual admit, respectively, that the diagnostic criteria for adult mental illness are "value judgments based on culture" and "subjective,"* ***how can one accurately identify problems in non-verbal infants?*** (http://www.ahrp.org/cms/content/view/404/31/)

Information published by the Mayo clinic, report that **the three signs of depression** to watch for are: ***"listlessness, decreased interest in playing, and cries easily and more often than usual"*** (http://mayoclinic.com/health/antidepressants/DN00007). Sounds a lot like constipation or colic to me, (possibly a change in diet is in order). Or another possibility is the mother's mood, which seems to have an influence on the infant, long before it learns to express its feelings. Young children are very sensitive to their mothers' emotions, (something she should be aware of).

Child psychiatrist Dr. Joan Luby, and colleagues at Washington University in St. Louis, published research in the *American Academy of Child and Adolescent Psychiatry*, (http://www.msnbc.msn.com/id/12037118/page/2/), which *"has* ***helped to scientifically validate that children as young as preschool age can suffer from depression, anxiety and other mood disorders."*** Also, the following was reported in the *Wall Street Journal* (October, 24, 2006, p. D1), as follows:

> ***A widely used mental health and development diagnostic manual for infants was revised last year*** *for the first time since 1994* ***to include two new subsets of depression, five new subsets of anxiety disorders (including separation anxiety and social anxiety disorders) and six new subsets of feeding behavior disorders (including sensory food aversion and infantile anorexia).***

And thanks to such "research", a study preformed by Zito and colleagues, and reported in the February 23, 2000 issue of the *Journal of the American Medical Association* (*JAMA*) ***"that found a 300% increase in the rates of psychotropic drug use of two to four year old children between 1991 and 1995, also showed three thousand prescriptions for the antidepressant Prozac in infants less than one year old"*** [That's totally inexcusable!] (http://www.ahrp.org/cms/content/view/404/31/).

Prozac™ - A Primary Contributor To Diabetes In Children!

From extensive research on SSRI antidepressants, I'm convinced that the medications children are being placed on are beyond a doubt contributing to their diabetes. You will learn, not only exactly how they contribute to diabetes, but also cancer. The proof I was looking for is: What percentage of the children being placed on diabetes medications, had been taking an antidepressant first, or possibly had their mother been on an antidepressant before they were born, (or both). My guess is, this would include by far the majority of the children. These statistics, along with my findings, could prove to be very valuable in putting a stop to the very aggressive promotional campaign by the drug companies, who are currently targeting our children and their mothers. Unfortunately, to date I have not been successful in obtaining those statistics. However, the following was reported in the *San Diego Union-Tribune*, April 4, 2006 (http://www.signonsandiego.com/news/health/20060404-1407-kids-diabetesdrugs.html):

> ***The number of prescriptions for the treatment or prevention of Type 2 diabetes in children doubled in the four years ended in 2005, according to a new study released by Express Scripts Inc., a pharmacy benefit manager.***
>
> *The rapid rise in prescriptions for the Type 2 diabetes has significance for the U.S. health system, experts said, because* ***diabetics often suffer serious and expensive medical complications such as blindness, limb amputations and kidney failure.***
>
> ***If patients develop diabetes earlier, their complications may also begin earlier.***
>
> ***Type 2 diabetes has been known as "adult-onset diabetes" because it is typically found in middle-aged or older adults, but the survey suggests that children with or at risk of the disease is becoming more common,*** *said Dr. Ed Weisbart, chief medical officer of Express Scripts Inc., which conducted the study.*
>
> ***Pharmacy benefit manager Express Scripts studied prescription claims for at least 3.7 million children aged 5 to 19 in its membership over four years.*** *Use of such treatments was most prevalent in teenagers from 15 to 19 years old.*
>
> ***Emily Cox, Express Scripts' senior director of research,*** *said she was expecting the study to show an increase in prescriptions because of all the publicity surrounding the obesity epidemic in the United States. Still, Cox was surprised by the intensity of the rise.*
>
> ***"You don't usually see a doubling of use in prescriptions in this short of a time," Cox said.***

This report immediately caught my attention, because it actually proved exactly what I had expected. As the rate of mothers placed on, and often left on, antidepressants throughout their pregnancy had dramatically increased, many children are being born hypoglycemic, and already predisposed to develop type II diabetes. Then as more children (at a much younger age) have been placed on the antidepressants as well, we should expect to experience a rapid escalation of children with diabetes, which was reflected in the statistical results of this huge 3.7 million study conducted by Express Scripts, Inc. It appears the attempt was to correlate the increase in the rate of diabetes in children, to childhood obesity, which antidepressants just happen to contribute to as well. The elevated blood sugar caused by antidepressants contributes to both diabetes and obesity, (and by far the majority of diabetics are overweight).

Not only are the known serious medical complications associated with diabetes such as blindness, limb amputations, and kidney failure, a major concern, (as mentioned in the *San Diego Union-Tribune* article, but scientists recently uncovered yet another.

They discovered *"that sperm from diabetic men have greater levels of DNA damage than sperm from men who do not have the disease. They warn that such DNA damage might affect a man's fertility"* (http://www.sciencedaily.com/releases/2007/05/070503075304.htm). Professor Sheena Lewis, scientific director of the Reproductive Medicine Research Group states ***"Our study shows increased levels of sperm DNA damage in diabetic men.*** *In the context of spontaneous conception,* ***sperm DNA quality has been found to be poorer in couples with a history of miscarriages."*** They warn that ***"The incidence of type 1 and type 2 diabetes is increasing rapidly worldwide,"*** and it's easy to see why. The dramatic increase in the prescribing of drugs such as Prozac™ and Zyprexa™, known to contribute to diabetes, (to even young children), is unquestionably a major contributor to the problem.

The obvious question is, what influence might drugs such as Prozac™ or Zyprexa™ (that the mother might be taking) have regarding her son acquiring diabetes at an early age? Often when a mother is taking a drug such as Prozac™ for example, the infant is born with low blood sugar, which eventually develops into diabetes. As an adult, he might find it difficult to get his wife pregnant, (due to damaged DNA), and if the pregnancy was successful, the chance for a miscarriage would still be greater. That might help explain why fertility clinics are becoming so popular the last few years. There has been a dramatic increase in the prescribing of antidepressants and antipsychotics that contribute to diabetes. And worst of all, they are now starting way earlier, by targeting pregnant mothers and "very young" children.

The Dilemma – An Obvious Conflict Of Interest About Express Scripts, Inc.

> *Express Scripts is a company dedicated to making the use of prescription drugs safer and more affordable for plan sponsors* ***and over 50 million members and their families.***
>
> ***We're one of America's largest pharmacy benefit managers,*** *providing the pharmacy benefit for millions of people nationwide through employers, managed-care plans, unions and governmental entities.*
>
> *Our headquarters is in St. Louis Missouri.*

We have major administrative offices in multiple states, including Minnesota, Pennsylvania, Arizona, New Jersey and Florida.
We have pharmacy and customer service operations in 10 states.
We have Canadian operations in Quebec and Ontario.
We employ a work force of more than 13,000 people.
(http://www.express-scripts.com)

The primary problem is, **Express Scripts Inc. sells drugs, (lots of drugs), and the missing statistics I was looking for is the medications these children were taking before they acquired diabetes.** I was already convinced that I knew the answer; I just need the statistics to prove that it was the antidepressants that so many children are needlessly being placed on, and at a very young age I might add. **Another telling statistic was the age group where the greatest increase was recognized (15 to 19 year olds). It makes perfect sense, as it normally takes a few years for these drugs to cause diabetes, but you can rest assured it will happen, especially after a few years of continuous use.** Another concern is, scientists have just recently discovered that **acquiring diabetes by the age of 17 will considerably shorten your life span, (actually from 17 to 20 years shorter)!** That's not just an issue for our children, but a concern for adults as well. So now we are not only needlessly putting our children on unnecessary and dangerous antidepressants, which often leads to the very debilitating diabetes, but their life span will be "considerably shorter" as well. Not only that, but their quality of life would be "greatly reduced" by their diabetes, which could lead to loss of eyesight, kidney failure, and possibly even amputation.

I have attempted to contact Emily Cox, but found it was impossible to contact her directly by phone or email. The only person I was ever able to talk to was the senior manager of public affairs, and she would only forward my phone number and email address to Emily, and first wanted to know why I wanted to talk to her. I explained that I was a doctor, and from years of research, was aware of the underlying problem behind the rapid increase in childhood diabetes. She then wanted to know what I thought the problem was. It appeared as though she might not have Emily contact me if I didn't divulge that information, so I reluctantly did. You can easily see the potential problem of a definite conflict of interest. It's quite obvious that my discovery could eventually result in a drastic reduction in the sales of two classes of medications they had been selling, (antidepressants and diabetes medications), and would likely prefer to continue selling. As of this printing, I have yet to hear from Emily Cox, the researcher with Express Scripts, Inc., and don't really expect to.

Another Study Conducted By Scripts, Inc. – The Other Statistic – "Twice As Many Children On Antidepressants"

Then to my amazement, I came across the statistics that would basically validate my suspicions. And interestingly, they actually came from the very same source: Express Scripts, Inc. Just a study conducted three years earlier, (although also covering the same time frame of four years). Most importantly, it was conducted by the same company, using the very same database, which means they should have been comparing the same basic group of children.

April 2, 2004—
Antidepressant drug use is up, especially among kids age 5 and younger.

The new numbers come from the databases of Express Scripts inc., the third largest U.S. pharmacy benefit manage. The sample includes nearly 2 million kids aged 18 and younger covered by medical insurance from 1998 to 2002.

For these children antidepressant use is up 100%.

"In teenagers, antidepressant use is really exploding," [Tom] *Delate* [Express Scripts' director of research] *tells WebMD:* ***"Antidepressant use among the very young is increasing even more rapidly.*** *Their rate of use is much lower than among older children – but* ***we're seeing a doubling of population using it."***

Serotonin-specific reuptake inhibitors – SSRIs such as Celexa, Luvox, Paxil, Prozac, and Zoloft – are more commonly prescribed for child patients than other antidepressants.

Paxil use increased 113% in girls and 91% in boys from 1998 to 2002.

So ***is it good, or bad that more kids are being treated with antidepressants? The scariest thing is that nobody knows,*** *says Robert Findling, MD, director of child and adolescent psychiatry at University Hospital, in Cleveland and chair of the American Academy of Child & Adolescent Psychiatry's research committee* (http://www.webmd.com/content/article/85/98399.htm).

It would definitely be scary if no one really knew whether placing more kids on antidepressants was good or bad, as Dr. Findling indicated. Fortunately, I know beyond a doubt, it's a "very bad" idea, and hopefully you soon will as well.

It's quite amazing that the exact same statistics applied, and in the same time frame as well, (only four years' time)! **Twice as many children were taking antidepressants, and twice as many were also placed on diabetes medications. There is unquestionably a direct relationship: The prescribing of antidepressants, followed in a few years by diabetes medication.**

Ideally, would be acquiring the complete statistics showing not only what antidepressants the children were taking, but also at what dosage, as well as how long. That could help prove the connection, and show which drugs actually pose the greatest risk. Some children are eventually placed on antipsychotics for the bipolar disorder (caused by drugs such as Prozac™) as well. The antipsychotic drug Zyprexa™, also produced by Eli Lilly, is quite often prescribed now for the bipolar disorder, and in most cases, children remain on Prozac™ as well. Zyprexa™ appears to be one of the worst drugs on the market for creating both diabetes and obesity, and often does so in a relatively short period of time. The question remains, how long can we allow them to knowingly continue giving drugs to our children, proven to contribute to diabetes, and do absolutely nothing about it?

Dr. Findling is at least "partially correct", as many in the nation have been deceived beyond a doubt, and thus either they or their children (or sometimes both) have been placed on antidepressants by their doctor. Even many doctors are under the false impression that their patients could somehow benefit from them. The most difficult task of all is finding a way to alert all those at risk, regarding the many dangers associated with their antidepressants. My book is an attempt to do just that. By far, the greatest challenge is getting my book, and thus the valuable information, to all those at risk. It's rather scary when you consider just how extensive the problems associated with these drugs can be, and how many young children are being placed on them in increasing numbers, (twice as many in only four years)! That shows just how effective the current very aggressive drug promotion campaign, targeting our kids, has unquestionably been.

Statistics From Another Source That Help Validate My Theory

Medco Health Solutions, Inc., one of the nation's leading pharmacy benefit managers, in partnership with the School of Public Health at The University of Medicine and Dentistry of New Jersey, recently proposed an area of research regarding ***"the potential link between the use of certain medications for severe behavioral disorders and the onset of diabetes."*** (http://www.medco.com/medco/corporate/home.jsp?ltSes=y&articleID=CorpAlertUMDNJ). This was brought about by national studies indicating that **the prevalence of diabetes increased 63 percent in the United States between 1999 and 2003 (only four years), while the number of people taking medications to treat severe behavioral disorders has increased by 34 percent over the past three years.** According to Dr. Roger Anderson, Ph.H., senior vice president and chief pharmacist for Medco of New Jersey, "***Recent studies suggest anti-psychotic medications may increase the risk of diabetes."*** Dr. Anderson then goes on to note that: ***"Considering the growing use of behavioral medications and the increasing rates of diabetes, a detailed investigation of the potential association between the two would be invaluable in shaping public policy and quality of care.***"

Another Medco study was recently published, (and posted on the *Forbes* website) with even newer statistics, as follows:

> ***Huge Increase in Diabetes Drug Use Among U.S. Adolescent Girls***
>
> ***From 2001 to 2006, the number of girls ages 10 to 19 in the United States taking drugs for type 2 diabetes increased by 167 percent, while use of chronic medicines for psychotic behavior and insomnia roughly doubled among girls and boys in the same age group,*** *according to a study by prescription benefit manager Medco Health Inc. of New Jersey.*
>
> *Experts said the study findings raise questions about mental and physical health problems in American youth and whether it's appropriate to give children drugs meant for adults, the AP reported.*
> (http://www.forbes.com/forbeslife/health/feeds/hscout/2007/05/16/hscout604669.html)

I totally agree with Dr. Anderson, and I believe he will find that is exactly what I have concluded, and am attempting to prove in this text. I have just broadened my scope to prove they also contribute to cancer, and brain damage as well. And interestingly, one class of antidepressants in particular (the SSRIs such as Prozac™, Paxil™, Zoloft™, and Celexa™), is a major contributor to all three. Just think, **by eliminating these antidepressants, (that are not any more effective than a placebo), we could greatly reduce the rate of birth defects,**

diabetes, cancer, lower IQs in children, and even earlier Alzheimer's disease in adults! And most importantly, it "should be so easy to accomplish"! Unfortunately, by far the greatest deterrent of all, is the tremendous influence of the huge pharmaceutical industry, with their extensive financial resources. Yet, if there's a will, (which I have), there is always a way, (which I "will" find).

The American Diabetes Association did report one study in their journal *Diabetes Care* (2005, issue 28, pp. 1063-1067), which found that between the ages of 20 and 50, *"people with newly diagnosed diabetes were 30% more likely to have had a history of depression than people without diabetes,"* and then went on to say that there was no way to account for these people with a history of depression, unless they sought treatment for their depression. And if someone were being "treated" for depression, wouldn't this mean they were likely "treated" with antidepressants?

So, from this information we can likely conclude that people with newly diagnosed diabetes were 30% more likely to have first been depressed, (and probably "treated" with antidepressants), than people without diabetes. The question posed in the article is: ***"What are the implications of the study? Young adults who have a history of depression*** **[and get treated for depression]** ***are more likely to get type 2 diabetes than people who don't have a history of depression*** **[and don't get treated for depression].** *More studies are needed to see how depression and type 2 diabetes are related."* I believe we already have ample proof that there is a definite connection between SSRI antidepressants and some atypical antipsychotic medications, and diabetes. My question is: What are we going to do with that knowledge? It's often stated that "knowledge is power", (when applied), and that becomes our responsibility, now that we know.

Antidepressants, Antipsychotics, and Stimulants - Major Underlying Contributors To "Childhood Obesity"

I'm glad this issue is finally being brought to the public's attention, as it obviously must be addressed before this serious trend continues to worsen. The fact that these drugs are also a contributing factor to childhood obesity, is something that very few are actually aware of. As you may have noticed, the study reported by Scripts, Inc. was attributing children acquiring diabetes, to their being overweight. We must ask ourselves the obvious question: What in the world could possibly cause children to begin acquiring diabetes, (at double the rate), and do so in only four years' time? And, do you really believe that our children's dietary and exercise habits would have somehow changed that drastically over the past four years? I believe not. At least, according to the news media, they have been improving the menus in some school cafeterias, as well as increasing the exercise programs in the schools. They have also been giving parents suggestions regarding things they can do to encourage their children to eat healthier, and exercise more. Yet, no consideration is ever given to one of the greatest contributors to obesity, (the drugs they are unnecessarily being placed on).

As mentioned at the beginning of this book, the Bush-appointed New Freedom Commission on Mental Health (NFC) has a preferred drug program in place that lists what drugs are to be used on children found to be "mentally ill." The approved list includes the following 16 drugs: *"Paxil, Zoloft, Celexa, Wellbutrin, Zyban, Remeron, Serzone, Effexor, Buspar, Risperdal, Zyprexa, Seroquel, Geodon, Depakote, Adderall, and Prozac."* Incidentally, I wonder if "sixteen" is somehow be a magical number, as that just happens to be how many nutrients that Prozac™ depletes as well!

Although these drugs, approved for use with children by the NFC, (although somehow without FDA approval for children), have numerous potentially dangerous, and possibly even deadly side effects, few are aware that "weight gain" is also a potential side effect associated with most of the drugs on that list. In fact, on a list of the 200 most prescribed drugs, 160 of them (81%!) actually listed "weight gain" as a potential side effect. It is no wonder that *"American children are increasingly becoming overweight,"* (which not only contributes to diabetes, but other concerns as well).

Following are some prime examples of the weight gain caused by some of the medications that many children (and adults) are being placed on:

✓ **The atypical antipsychotics such as Seroquel™, Risperdal™, Geodon™, and Zyprexa™, (all on the NFC-approved list),** actually cause weight gain. In fact, an article written for *USA Today* (May 2, 2006) by Marilyn Elias, reported about a Russellville Missouri teen that ***"gained about 100 pounds in a year"*** while taking one of these atypical antipsychotics (http://usatoday.com/news/health/2006-05-01-atypical-drugs_x.htm).

It is important to note that **although Seroquel™ and Zyprexa™ have the greatest potential for contributing to rapid weight gain, all antipsychotic medications have been shown to produce weight gain**. As noted by Marilyn Elias in her *USA Today* article, according to Benedetto Vitiello, chief of child and adolescent psychiatry at the National Mental Health Institute, the most serious problem of all caused by these medications is weight gain, and Vitiello notes that ***"The effect varies by drug, but kids typically put on twice the pounds they should in their first six months on atypicals."***

The article goes on to quote research psychiatrist Christoph Correll, of Hillside Hospital in Glen Oaks, New York, who states that ***"In the first three months on the drugs, children add about 2 to 3 inches to their waistlines."*** The article also points out that ***"A lot of this is abdominal fat, which increases the risk of diabetes and heart disease. Obese children are twice as likely as normal-weight children to have diabetes, according to a new University of Michigan study."***

✓ **The antianxiety medication Buspar™,** although not a member of the benzodiazepines family, **lists weight gain and alcohol abuse as potential side effects** (http://www.dr-bob.org/tips/nefazodone.html).

✓ **With the SSRI antidepressants (Paxil™, Zoloft™, Celexa™, Effexor™, and Prozac™), unexplained weight gain is listed among the leading side effects. Paxil™ is linked to some of the biggest weight gains,** with one in four patients adding at least 7 percent to their body weight, and some even report weight gain in the double digits (http://www.postgazette.com/pg/04137/316522.stm). According to Dr. Ann Blake Tracy, **they all create cravings for both sugar and alcohol.**

✓ **The following comments were posted by users of the antidepressant Remeron™**, at http://www.crazymeds.org/remeron.html:

- ***"You get intense hunger for the wrong foods, and with that comes weight gain,*** *dry mouth and constipation.* ***Then you want to sleep a lot.*** *It's like you may as well be smoking pot when you take Remeron."*

- ***"You will literally eat sugar straight out of the bag to satisfy your cravings for sweets and carbohydrates."***

- *"Remeron is not for mild to moderate depression, it's for people who are seriously depressed, who are willing to put up with the weight gain and the sleeping because those side effects suck much less than the dark pit of depressive despair one finds oneself in."*

- *"Just don't mix Remeron with Zyprexa as your choice of antipsychotic and antidepressant. One woman was recently prescribed that combination as an inpatient in a Canadian hospital. She reported on the bipolar support forum on about.com* ***how she ballooned up in weight, from 103 pounds to 162 pounds, in about six weeks, and carrying that on a 5' 1" frame. She gained a pound and a half a day, eating hospital food!"***

✓ **All anticonvulsants, including Depakote™, promote weight gain, increase appetite, and elevate insulin. Any drug that elevates insulin will promote type II diabetes.**

✓ **Adderall™** is just one stimulant used to treat ADHD, and as noted by Dr. Diana Schwarzbein:

> ***Stimulants cause insulin levels to rise too high****, which stimulates an excessive rush of stored serotonin – a temporary rush – which is quickly used up. Then, because serotonin levels drop rapidly, you begin to feel down again.* ***This depletion sets up a vicious cycle:*** *You experience the symptoms of low serotonin, and* ***in response you eat an excess of carbohydrates or use stimulants to obtain the rush or serotonin again*** (*The Schwarzbein Principle*, 1999, p. 42).

Using Fluoride For Behavioral Modification In Prisoners (and our children) – The Secret Ingredient In Prozac™ Has Actually Been Around For Years!

As stated by the UK National Pure Water Association:

> ***Fluorides have been used to modify behaviour and mood of human beings. It is a little known fact that fluoride compounds were added to the drinking water of prisoners to keep them docile and inhibit questioning of authority, both in Nazi prison camps in World War II and in the soviet gulags in Siberia*** (http://www.johnsonton-independent.com/).

Is this possibly the primary objective of placing so many children on Prozac™, which contains fluoride, or exposing millions to fluoride, by placing it in their drinking water? If so, are we basically drugging them into submission, and just for the sake of convenience?

According to a report by the Florida Statewide Advocacy Council, ***"an investigation in Florida found that*** **[of]** ***1,180 kids in foster care, 652 were on one or more psychotropic***

drugs" (http://www.records@psychsearch.net). There is something drastically wrong when **"over half the children" in foster care were placed on psychotropic drugs!**

And as if that's not enough, it appears as though the drugging of children in foster care is everywhere, as reported in an on-line article by Evelyn Pringle titled ***"TeenScreen – Another Gross Distortion,"*** as follows:

> *In October, 2004, the Texas inspector general for the Health and Human Services Commission said his office* ***interviewed staff at three state licensed wilderness camps, which provide care for foster children, and found that the average child arrives on four or five psychotropic drugs.***
>
> *After investigating the issue of drug use with foster kids, in an April 2004 report, Texas Comptroller, Carole Keeton Strayhorn, blasted the agency for* ***giving children drugs so "doctors and drug companies can make a buck"*** (http://www.sierratimes.com/05/07/30/pringle.htm).

The question is: Who is looking out for their best interest? Obviously – no one! They deserve the very same quality of care and concern as other children do, yet they're obviously not getting it! Although one drug can be dangerous enough, "four or five" can be outright scary!

Even worse, Dr. John Breeding, an Austin psychologist, claims he has seen cases in Texas where **some foster children were placed on as many as 17 drugs and says drugs are being used as chemical restraints. He wants all SSRIs and neuroleptic drugs banned from use on children,** warning that *"The SSRIs are extremely harmful and addictive; and can cause or exacerbate suicidal or homicidal tendencies; withdrawal is painful and dangerous"* (http://www.sierratimes.com/05/04/26/pringle.htm). **Placing children on that many drugs is, in my opinion, by far the very worst form of child abuse!**

I totally agree with Dr. Breeding, although I would tend to go a step further, and suggest that **"they be totally banned for all human use", (as cocaine, LSD, and heroin were).** They are all dangerous stimulants, operating on the same basic principle, (as the drugs that are now classified as illegal once were), and capable of contributing to the very same diseases and conditions in adults that they can in children.

In the April 1997 issue of *Life Extension* magazine, the editor, Saul Kent, wrote an editorial titled ***"What's Wrong with Prozac?"*** regarding the book titled *Talking Back to Prozac* by Peter R. Breggin and Ginger Ross Breggin. In that editorial, Kent noted that: *"Peter R. Breggin is a psychiatrist – formerly a consultant with the National Institute of Mental Health – who is a long-time critic of drug-based psychiatry. Ginger Ross Breggin is a writer and Director of Research and Education at the Center for the Study of Psychiatry."* According to Kent:

> *One of the most startling accusations the Breggins level is that* ***Prozac is a chemical cousin of amphetamine and cocaine-drugs which also inhibit serotonin reuptake.*** *It is those properties, the Breggins believe,* ***that make Prozac dangerous. And dangerous it is. Ordinary people have done things such as getting out of bed in the middle of the night and hanging themselves after taking it. There are numerous reports of 'speed'-like behavior and***

> ***aggression.*** *People have reported having nightmares where people are coming at them with knives, or they are going to kill others or themselves.* ***One woman, put on the drug for weight loss, ended up trying to shoot herself in front of her children.*** *(Her husband got the gun away from her). According to the Breggins,* ***this type of behavior is consistent with what people sometimes do on cocaine or "speed." Is Prozac legalized "speed"?***

If you just stop to think about it, these dangerous drugs are being forced on our children, (especially foster children). It's not the children who decide they need the drugs, and often it's not even the parents, who can even get in trouble for attempting to get their children off them due to their reactions, (which should be a warning sign). All too often, their doctor increases the dosage, changes medications, or even worse, adds another, just compounding the problem.

Prozac's Dangerous Dark Side – When Your Mind Is No Longer Your Own

Although the many potential side effects associated with SSRI antidepressants such as Prozac™ are a real concern, they actually pale in comparison to some of the true-to-life experiences Dr. Tracy discovered during her research. The best way to describe them is: Out right scary, and **"definitely not worth taking the risk!"** In her book *Prozac: Panacea or Pandora?* (1991/1994, pp. 157 – 270), Dr. Tracy shares just a few of the hundreds of experiences her patients encountered while they were on Prozac™, as follows:

> ***"My wife told me that while she was on Prozac she could have killed me once or twice. Yet she is the most gentle, kind and sympathetic person I've ever known in my life!*** *Contrary to what Lilly would have to say about it, it was not a pre-existing condition. Everybody has ups and downs and depression and so forth, but this is different.* ***This is a thousand times worse than the original problem they took the Prozac for to begin with."***

> *"I would wake up each morning thinking,* ***'Oh God, I'm still alive! I have to live another day of this hell of wanting to die!'*** *I thought of running into trees at a high rate of speed."*

> ***"During the month I spent on Prozac I could think of nothing but various ways of killing those closest to me*** *– my family, my mom, my dad and my brothers and sisters." (****A very sweet and sensitive 14-year-old girl*** *who took herself off Prozac because of these thoughts it was causing her).*

> ***"I felt I had to kill myself but I could not leave my family alone. I planned how I would accomplish the deaths of my husband and children in detail. How could I ever have had such thoughts?!"***

> ***"Throughout my life I have always been known as 'Mr. Mellow,' but the rage I felt on Prozac helped me to understand how someone could murder another."***

"I became obsessed with dying. I thought dying was the only way out, and I never contemplated suicide before that time."

"Nothing mattered to me, especially my life or anyone else's. I didn't care about anyone or anything!"

"I've been a reformed alcoholic for twelve years, but while on Prozac I started craving alcohol again!"

"I thought I had someone else's brain in my body!"

"After using LSD in my past, I can tell you that taking Prozac is like taking half a hit of LSD, except that it also made me angry and aggressive."

"Although it was completely out of character for me, the compulsion to drink was so strong after starting on Prozac that it became impossible for me to drive past a bar."

"I wanted to stop using Prozac, but I was addicted. How could I be addicted to a drug that my family practitioner gave me?"

"I felt as though I was on a combination of speed and cocaine."

"Wicked! That's exactly how you feel on Prozac, wicked, just plain wicked!"

As my father often said: *"If something seems too good to be true, it probably is!"* That certainly applies to Prozac™, which is obviously not a panacea as advertised, but instead, a Pandora, as Dr. Tracy discovered, and something that unfortunately far too many have learned the hard way, from their own personal experience. I would hope that you might learn from their experiences, and assure that our children will never be subjected to such dangerous drugs, although as we can see from the above, they pose a serious threat to adults as well.

School Shootings – The Antidepressant Connection
Replacing Your Brain With That Of A Monster
The Question Is – Who Is Truly To Blame?

Is it just accidental that the majority of children involved in school shootings were on antidepressants?

In the following accounts of school shootings, you will discover that sometimes the particular antidepressant was labeled as "unknown". In those cases, someone obviously knew, although the company producing the drug suppresses that information if at all possible. The following information was obtained at http://www.ssristories.com/index.php.

SSRI Stories

This website is a collection of 1500+ news stories with the full media article available, *mainly criminal in nature, that have appeared in the media or that were part of FDA testimony in either 1991, 2004 or 2006, in which antidepressants are mentioned. These stories have been collected over a period of years by two directors of the International Coalition for Drug Awareness (ICFDA). They experienced firsthand the drugs' power to harm and want to save others from the fate that befell them. Their focus has been on Selective Serotonin Reuptake Inhibitors (SSRIs), of which Prozac was the first, launched in December 1987. Other SSRIs are Zoloft, Paxil (Seroxat), Celexa, Sarafem (Prozac in a pink pill), Lexapro, and Luvox. These drugs are widely employed as first line treatment for depression. Other antidepressants included in this list are Remeron, Anafranil and the SNRIs Effexor, Serzone and Cymbalta as well as the dopamine reuptake inhibitor antidepressant Wellbutrin (also marketed as Zyban).*

Following are 24 school shootings, or attempts, influenced by antidepressants, as listed on the website:

What & Where	Drug	Date Reported
1. School Knife Attack in Indiana **Teen Knife Attacks Fellow Student	**"Meds for Depression"**	**12-06-2006**
2. School Hostage Situation in North Carolina **Teen Holds Teacher & Student Hostage with Gun	**"Antidepressant Withdrawal"**	**11-28-2006**
3. School Shooting in Colorado **Man Assaults Girl: Kills One & Self	**"Antidepressant"**	**09-30-2006**
4. School Shooting in Canada **Young Man Kills 1 & Self, Injures 19: Being Treated For Depression	**"Med for Depression"**	**09-19-2006**
5. School Shooting in North Carolina **Teen Shoots at Two Students: Kills his Father	**Celexa Antidepressant**	**08-30-2006**
6. School / Assault in Tennessee **Teen Attacks Teacher at School	**Zoloft Antidepressant**	**02-15-2006**
7. School Shooting in Minnesota **10 Dead, 7 Wounded: Dosage Increased One Week before Rampage	**Prozac – Antidepressant**	**03-24-2005**
8. School Violence in Pennsylvania **Teen Uses Knife to Attack Fellow Classmate	**"Antidepressants"**	**02-09-2005**
9. School Shooting Threat in New Jersey **Over-Medicated Teen Brings Loaded Handguns to School	**"Meds for Depression"**	**10-19-2004**
10. School Shooting in New York **Student Shoots Teacher in Leg at School	**"Meds for Depression"**	**02-18-2004**

What & Where (continued)	Drug	Date Reported
11.School Shooting Threat in Michigan **Teen Threatens School Shooting: Charge is Terrorism	**"Antidepressant"**	**05-31-2003**
12.School Machete Attack in Pennsylvania **Man Attacks 11 Children & 3 Teachers at Elementary School	**"Meds for Depression"**	**09-26-2001**
13.School Hooting in California **Teen Shoots at Classmates in School	**Celexa/Effexor Antidepressants**	**04-19-2001**
14.School Hostage Situation in Washington **Teen Holds Classmates Hostage with Gun	**Paxil/Effexor Antidepressants**	**04-15-2001**
15.School Shooting in Pennsylvania **14 Year Old Girl Shoots & Wounds Classmate at Catholic School	**Paxil – Antidepressant**	**03-10-2001**
16.School Hostage Situation in California **17 Year Old Takes Girl Hostage at School: He is Killed by Police	**Prozac/Paxil Antidepressants**	**01-18-2001**
17.School Shooting in Colorado **COLUMBINE: 15 Dead, 24 Wounded	**Luvox/Zoloft Antidepressants**	**04-20-1999**
18.School Shooting Treat in Idaho **Teen Fires Gun in School	**"Antidepressant"**	**04-16-1999**
19.School Shooting in Oregon **Four Dead, Twenty-Five Wounded	**Prozac Antidepressant Withdrawal**	**05-21-1998**
20.School Stand-Off in Idaho **14 Year Old in School Holds Police At Pay: Fires Shots	**Zoloft – Antidepressant**	**04-13-1998**
21.School Shooting in South Carolina **15 Year Old Shoots Two Teachers, Killing One: Then Kills Himself	**Zoloft – Antidepressant**	**10-12-1995**
22.School Shooting in Texas **Man, Angry Over Daughter's Report Card: Shoots 14 Rounds Inside Elementary School	**"Antidepressants"**	**09-20-1992**
23.School Shooting in Michigan **School Teacher Shots & Kills His Superintendent at School	**Prozac Antidepressant**	**01-30-1992**
24.School Shooting in Illinois **29 Year Old Woman Kills One Child, Wounds Five: Kills Self	**Anafranil Antidepressant**	**05-20-1988**

Number Twenty-Five?

Although not mentioned on this particular website's list, the most recent shooting (as of publication of this book anyway) was the horrible massacre at Virginia Tech College, which took place April 16, 2007. According to reports published by the *Chicago Tribune "Investigators believe Cho* [the shooter] *at some point had been taking medication for depression"* (http://www.cbsnews.com/stories/2007/04/18/earlyshow/main2698195.shtml).

Retired psychiatrist Nat Lehrman is the former Clinical Director of Kingsboro Psychiatric Center, a large psychiatric hospital in Brooklyn, New York. He is also a former assistant Clinical Professor of Psychiatry at Albert Einstein and SUNY Downstate Colleges of Medicine. Following is Dr. Lehrman's opinion, regarding "Mental health services and the Virginia Tech massacre", as printed in the April 25, 2007 edition of *Newsday*:

> *More mental health services, and even involuntary mental health screenings, have been proposed to prevent repletion of the Virginia Tech massacre. But mass murderer Cho Seung Hui did get mental health care in a hospital. He then rejected further treatment.* ***The drug-only treatment he got may well have aggravated his disturbance.***
>
> *Medication, often with little or no meaningful human contact, has now almost entirely replaced that older care pattern. And that's what Cho got.* ***And anti-depressant drugs, like those he was given, can themselves intensify suicidal and homicidal thoughts and behavior.***
> *When considering the effectiveness of mental health services, we should recognize that* ***in the fifty years since drugs began to be psychiatry's main treatment modality, there has been a five-fold increase in the fraction of mentally disabled in the population.*** *Before hurrying to expand mental health services, we should examine more critically the results of current treatment methods.*

To date, I have yet to learn what drugs Cho had been placed on. It appears that information has been deliberately withheld. I'm sure the companies producing the drugs are fully aware, but they would rather you weren't. They are deliberately ignoring the obvious, that the majority of those involved in school shootings were on one or more mind-altering drugs, (as you have just learned). They are instead attempting to use it as an excuse to expand the current mental health screening program to include college students!

Dr. Ann Blake Tracy has served as a consultant on high-profile cases of antidepressant-induced shootings, including Columbine and Andrea Yates, as well as appearing on programs including *20/20*, *Dateline*, and *60 Minutes*. Her feelings regarding the shooting at Virginia Tech were published in the *Modesto Bee* (April 29, 2007), as follows:

> *The murderous rampage that left 33 people dead at Virginia Tech has stirred countless emotions: sadness and anger, fear and hatred, grief and disgust.*
>
> *When Dr. Ann Blake Tracy heard the details, she felt many of those same emotions.* ***As terrible as it sounds, after nearly 20 years researching links between violent crime, suicide and antidepressants, Tracy is surprised only that it doesn't happen more often.***
>
> *In her experience, when it comes to investigating high-profile shootings, antidepressants are as common as the presence of loneliness, despondence and rage.*

> ***"I'm just so tired of seeing people die, I could scream,"*** *Tracy said during a phone interview.* ***"It's happening daily in this country. It's so massive, it's just unreal.*** *We've got so many school shootings now, I can't even begin to keep up with them all. And the reason is so incredibly obvious. You don't have to look at much to figure it out."*

I can't help but wonder what choice many patients might make if their doctor first provided them with alternative options, rather than just Prozac™ alone, "especially if the facts about each was also divulged", as you have just learned.

Should Prozac™ Maintain Its Legal Status and Continue Being Promoted For Children's Use?

I'll Provide You With The Facts and Let You Decide!

✓ We should first point out the very extensive list of potential side effects (575 listed with the FDA), the 16 nutrients Prozac™ depletes, and the many important benefits of each nutrient depleted, as well as the above-average potential for producing drug interactions with other medications a person might also be taking.

✓ The fact that all drugs are basically designed to suppress a particular symptom such as depression, and normally create other symptoms in the process, is an important issue that should be stressed. Then, as the underlying condition is not actually being addressed or truly resolved, it will likely continue to worsen. Also, when symptoms are suppressed, how could you possibly know if the condition was ever resolved?

✓ A very important issue is that Prozac™ disrupts the enzyme action in the body, the brain, and the liver, and it does so in more than one way:

1. First, thyroid suppression, caused by the elevated stress hormone cortisol, reduces the metabolism (and thus the body temperature). The lower the body temperature, the less efficient the action of all 3,000 of the body's enzymes will be. Dr. E. Denis Wilson, M.D. was able to prove that was true in lab tests, (just one degree makes a big difference).
2. Second, the overstimulation of the adrenals, caused by the elevated stress hormone cortisol, caused by Prozac™, for an extended period of time, causes the adrenals to become enlarged, resulting in a hair-rigger response (often an over-reaction to any stimulus). And, according to Dr. James F. Balch, M.D., it has been proven that those with enlarged adrenals are more inclined to be depressed.
3. Third, the fluoride in Prozac™ is an environmental toxin, classified as a halogen, similar in structure to iodine. It can thus fit into iodine receptors, blocking iodine in the thyroid, further reducing the thyroid's efficiency, as well as providing the same results that having a deficiency of iodine would exhibit. In his book *Iodine – Why You Need It – Why You Can't Live Without It* (2004, p. 22), Dr. David Brownstein, M.D. explains why iodine is so important:

> ***Every cell in the body contains and utilizes iodine.*** *The thyroid gland contains a higher concentration of iodine than any other organ of the body.* ***Large amounts of iodine are also stored in many other areas of the body including the cerebrospinal fluid <u>and the brain</u>*** *(Adrasi, E. Iodine concentration in different brain parts. Analytical and Bioanalytical chemistry. November 13, 2003).*
>
> ***<u>In the brain, iodine concentrates in the substantia nigra, an area of the brain that has been associated with Parkinson's disease.</u>***
>
> ***<u>Iodine is essential for the normal growth and development of children. Severe iodine deficiency can result in severe mental deficiency and deafness, as well as delayed physical and intellectual development.</u>***

4. Fourth, the fluoride in Prozac™ is known to directly inhibit enzyme action in both the liver and brain. It has actually been proven, in many different studies over the years, that children, who live in areas where iodine is deficient in the soil, were found to have lower IQs than those in areas with sufficient iodine. This proves that adequate iodine is critical for healthy brain function. When an extreme iodine deficiency exists, the children often experienced mental retardation.

✓ And then we can't forget that according to Dr. Glenmullen, **Prozac™ also suppresses the very critical hormone dopamine by over 50%,** which basically compounds the problem even further. **You can't over-stimulate one hormone, such as serotonin, without influencing another, such as dopamine**, (what Dr. Glenmullen refers to as the "Prozac backlash"). What a nightmare for someone, from the long-term use of a drug that absolutely no one really needs!

✓ Then if you recall, Dr. Sherry Rogers, M.D., in her book *Detoxify or Die* (2002), states that **every molecule of Prozac™ (fluoxetine) actually contains** ***"three molecules of toxin fluoride"!*** And that: ***"Fluoride is a potent enzyme inhibitor,"*** **and is** ***"<u>Known to cause excessive calcification, not only in arteries but joints and ligaments, and contributes to many forms of cancer</u> and osteoporosis."***

✓ Also take into consideration the fact that the **elevated serotonin reduces the sensitivity of its receptors,** just as **the fluoride in Prozac™ also damages the receptors for "all neurotransmitters"**.

✓ And the fact that, **according to the *Physicians Desk Reference, 55th edition*** (2001, p. 1127), **Prozac™ contains the following dangerous and "very active" inactive ingredients:**

- **F D & C Blue No. 1** – *"A synthetic food dye,* ***derived from petroleum*** *distillates. Current studies suggest* ***a small cancer risk****"* (*Physicians Desk Reference, 55th edition,* 2001, p. 1127.)

- **F D & C Yellow No. 6 – *"Suspected of causing tumors in adrenal glands and kidneys. May cause allergies, hyperactivity, and chromosomal damage. Banned in Norway*** *but not in the U.S."* (http://www.purezing.com/living/living_toxins_commondyes.html). As well as *"Possible side effects are abdominal discomfort, hives,* ***kidney tumors,*** *nausea and vomiting"* (http://www.purezing.com/living/food_articles/living_articles_fooddyes.thm). And, in other studies Prozac™ was found to cause the following reactions: *"general weakness, heatwaves, palpitations, blurred vision, rhinorrhea* [persistent watery mucus discharge from the nose], *feeling of suffocation, pruritus* [an intense itching sensation] *and urticaria* [an itchy dry skin eruption]*."* (http://www.blackwell-synergy.com/doi/abs/10.1111/j.1365-2222.1978.tb00449.x)

- **Polyethylene glycol (PEG)** - *"May contain ¼-dioxane* ***which is a possible carcinogen, estrogen mimic and endocrine disruptor.*** *Moderately toxic, and possible carcinogen* [cancer causing]. *Many glycols produce* ***severe acidosis, central nervous system damage*** *and congestion.* ***Can cause convulsions, mutations, and surface EEG changes"*** (http://www.purezing.com/living/living_toxins_commondyes.html).

- Also, the oral solution of Prozac™ contains Alcohol 0.23%.

✓ Another very telling statistic that shows just how potentially dangerous these mind-altering drugs can really be involves the increased incidence of school shootings, which parallels the dramatic increase in children being placed on these dangerous drugs, **(a 500% increase in 6 years)!**

✓ **Not only that, but** in more than one double-blind study, **placebos were found to be more effective than Prozac™ in resolving depression.**

✓ And according to an article titled *"Kids on Drugs,"* by Dr. Lawrence H. Diller, M.D. (author of *Running on Ritalin,* 2006), ***"In the only study demonstrating the effectiveness of Prozac in children when the patients and doctors didn't know which pill was taken, 60 percent of the improvement in depressive symptoms was attributed to the placebo effect!"*** (http://archive.salon.com/health/feature/2000/03/09/kid_drugs/)

The good news is, (as we will soon discover), we have many natural ways for resolving depression, which also provide additional health benefits in the process, and are far more effective than the placebo, which is something you can't say for Prozac!

But first, we'll take a look at just how corrupt, and totally unscientific, our drug approval process has become. You will learn how the approval of Prozac™ was fast-tracked by incorporating a small group of participants, for an unbelievably short period of time. Not only that, but the doctor who conducted one of the main studies the FDA used for Prozac's approval had been accused of fraud in other trials!

You will learn how Eli Lilly used the national media to promote Prozac™ as a perfectly safe "wonder drug" that nearly everyone could benefit from. Sounds a lot like their promotional campaign for LSD over 30 years ago. Their tactics haven't changed much, nor have their drugs!

I guess I'm getting ahead of myself, and possibly giving away the plot of a very troubling, although true story. So turn the page and we'll examine the politics of Prozac™.

CHAPTER TWELVE

The Politics of Prozac™

A Major Promotional Campaign By Eli Lilly:
Prozac™ - The New Wonder Drug!
(Very Similar To The Claims They Also Once Made For LSD)

In March 1990, Prozac™ was on the cover of *Newsweek*, boasting that the *"medical breakthrough"* had already been prescribed for so many conditions in addition to depression that *"even healthy people have started asking for it."* And, *New York magazine* called Prozac™ a ***"wonder drug,"*** while the *National Enquirer* described it as a ***"miracle diet pill".*** On yet another cover of *Newsweek*, it was announced, ***"Beyond Prozac: How Science Will Let You Change Your Personality with a Pill."*** It does sound a lot like another "wonder drug" - LSD, which Eli Lilly also blessed us with, and aggressively promoted back in 1956! They only pull these dangerous drugs when they are forced to, regardless of their dangers.

SSRI antidepressants are now prescribed for many conditions other than the original FDA-approved diagnosis of depression. An M.D. can, (entirely at his or her own discretion), prescribe pretty much any drug, for just about anything he or she might choose, and without any FDA approval for the specific condition it was prescribed for.

Dr. Jay Cohen, author of *Over Dose: The Case Against The Drug Companies*, tells us that the *"drug companies have marketed SSRI antidepressants vigorously not only to psychiatrists, who are supposed to have some expertise with these drugs, but also to family practitioners, pediatricians, gynecologists, internal medicine specialists, and anyone else who can pen a prescription"* (http://www.sierratimes.com/06/11/25/75_7_242_70_12181.htm). Dr. Cohen goes on to point out that *"this doesn't mean that they possess in-depth knowledge of SSRIs or their actions and toxicities."*

In fact, a study reported in the June 2006 issue of the *Journal of Clinical Psychiatry*, performed at the University of Georgia, found that ***"75% of the people prescribed antidepressants received them for a reason not approved by the FDA"*** (http://www.sieratimes.com/pf.php).

And from his experience, Dr. Joseph Glenmullen, M.D., in his book *Prozac Backlash* (2000), agrees that ***"as many as 75% of patients are needlessly on these drugs for mild, even trivial, conditions"*** (p. 11). To the already long list of conditions treated with drugs, Dr. Glenmullen says doctors prescribe these SSRIs for such complaints as: ***"anxiety, obsessions, compulsions, eating disorders, headaches, back pain, impulsivity, drug and alcohol abuse, hair pulling, nail biting, upset stomach, irritability, sexual addictions, attention deficit disorder, and premenstrual syndrome"*** (p. 14).

Yet, according to Dr. Tracy, **anxiety, obsessions, compulsions, impulsiveness, irritability, (and especially drug and alcohol abuse), are the exact same side effects associated with the SSRI antidepressants that these patients had been placed on by their doctors in the first place!** In essence, **antidepressants actually contribute to some of the very conditions they are often prescribed for** (quite amazing, I would say).

So, why do so many doctors continue ignoring the evidence? By the time you complete this book, you will begin to realize what a serious threat that can be for those who had been needlessly placed on these "very serious" medications. Dr. Tracy brings up an interesting point, when she asks the question:

> ***Why Do Doctors Seem To Have Such A Need To Defend Drugs?***
>
> ***Does it somehow validate the worth of their profession because if we didn't need drugs, perhaps we would no longer need them to supply those drugs?*** *Many doctors are telling their patients, who have developed complaints such as* ***seizures, hypoglycemia, diabetes, cancer, pancreatitis, rashes, bronchitis, kidney problems, blood platelet disorders, liver abnormalities,*** *etc.,* ***that their use of Prozac had no connection – even though there are medical evidences linking all these as possible side-effects of the drug****. [Warnings about these possible adverse reactions are listed in the* ***Prozac package insert and multitudes of adverse reaction reports made to the FDA.]*** (*Prozac: Panacea or Pandora?*, 1991/1994, p. 98).

How Prozac™ Got Past The FDA, and The Totally Corrupt Drug Approval Process

Consumer Reports, January 1993, published **an in-depth research report on Prozac™, Xanax™ and Halcion™. The conclusion: <u>These do not work!</u>** *Consumer Reports* stated **Prozac™, Xanax™ and Halcion™** **<u>all have histories of extensive potential for hazardous side effects, including death</u>** (*Breaking Your Prescribed Addiction*, Sahley & Birkner, 1998, p. 19).

In order to better understand the rationale behind this situation, it might be beneficial to evaluate the politics of Prozac™. Why these dangerous drugs are still legal obviously doesn't seem logical, especially in spite of the proven potential for serious physical and mental damage associated with their use, and no proven benefit over a placebo!

One problem stems from the drug approval process, which is the result of the budget priorities established by the FDA (where most of the funding is allocated). As most studies regarding the safety of a particular drug are actually conducted by the company that created the drug, the results of the study would thus be expectedly biased in favor of the drug's approval. This was recently confirmed in an *ABC News* report, as follows:

> ***A survey of clinical trials revealed that when a drug company funds a study, there is a 90% chance that the drug will be perceived as effective, whereas a non-drug-company-funded study will show favorable results only 50% of the time.*** *It appears that money can't buy you love, but it can buy any "scientific" result desired* (*Life Extension* magazine, August 2006, p. 70).

When allowed to conduct their own clinical trials, (as they are now doing), the companies employ every trick in the book to assure they will receive the drug approval they are looking for, which was reflected in the above report. The studies are seldom of sufficient duration necessary to identify any long-term risks. If they so choose, they could easily recruit younger people for the clinical trial, (those who are healthier, and not taking any other medications), although by far, the greatest risk would involve the seniors, who are already on several other medications, or very young children, (basically those that the majority of the prescriptions for most drugs will be written for.

Another problem is, according to Dr. Glenmullen, although the FDA only reviews about 25 new drugs a year, a professional staff of 1,500 doctors, scientists, toxicologists, and statisticians are assigned to review the results of studies already conducted by the companies themselves, on these 25 new drugs. Yet **they allot a staff of only five doctors and one epidemiologist to monitor the safety of more than 3,000 drugs already approved, and being prescribed for millions of patients!** The commonly held belief is that the drug approval studies are far from adequate to effectively determine their safety, suggesting that the FDA would rather not know about the results of a flaw in the approval process. As Dr. Glenmullen suggests, it would make more sense to assign a larger portion of the staff to evaluating the complaints filed, and long-term side effects from the 3,000 drugs being prescribed daily to millions, which should be obvious to anyone.

According to the United States Census Bureau, statistics indicate that there were 288,368,698 people in the United States as of July 2002. Then according to Dr. Ann Blake Tracy, during a lecture in Anaheim, California, on November 16, 2002, one in every 3½ people in the nation were currently on antidepressants. If Dr. Tracy were correct, that would translate to **more than 84 million people! And that was over four years ago!** That just shows the tremendous income potential for the pharmaceutical industry, and helps explain the motivation behind their aggressive marketing tactics. Unfortunately, that includes the continuous effort to suppress the many dangers associated with these very risky drugs that they are so aggressively promoting.

Come to find out, this is not just a "nationwide" issue, but is instead worldwide! Robert Verkaik, a Legal Affairs Correspondent for *The Independent News* in the United Kingdom, in an article dated December 4, 2000, talks about a retired teacher, Reginald Payne, in Cornwall in the United Kingdom, who **within 11 days of being on Prozac™, suffocated his wife and threw himself off a cliff near their home.** The family claims that **the pharmaceutical giant Eli Lilly, which manufactures the drug, was negligent in failing to warn Payne of the risk of side effects, which are said to include suicide, violent behavior, violent and aggressive thoughts, and homicidal tendencies.** Lawyers for the Payne sons were expected to go to the High Court in Britain sometime in 2001, to try to prove that the drug is to blame for the deaths of their parents. At the time, Verkaik wrote *"If successful, it could open the floodgates for hundreds of other families who believe Prozac played a role in the deaths of loved ones."* This article also brings to light that, as of December of 2000, Prozac™ was being taken by 500,000 people in Britain, (and Americans were taking far more medications than the British).

Leah Garnett of the *Boston Globe*, in an article dated May 7, 2000, wrote that evidence had come to light revealing Eli Lilly's internal documents, some dating to the mid-1980s, indicating that the pharmaceutical giant had known for years that its best-selling drug could cause suicidal reactions in a small but significant number of patients. Among the findings, Garnett wrote:

> ***Three years before Prozac received approval by the US Food and Drug Administration*** *in late 1987, the German BGA, that country's FDA equivalent, had such serious reservations about Prozac's safety that it refused to approve the*

antidepressant based on ***Lilly's studies showing that previously non-suicidal patients who took the drug had a five-fold higher rate of suicides and suicide attempts than those on older antidepressants, and a three-fold higher rate than those taking placebos.***
Another expert opinion is by:

Dr. David Healy, an expert on the brain's serotonin system and director of the North Wales Department of Psychological Medicine at the University of Wales, estimated that ***"probably 50,000 people have committed suicide on Prozac since its launch, over and above the number who would have done so if left untreated."***

And the reality is, as stated by Saul Kent, *Life Extension* magazine editor, *"A meticulous dissection of FDA documents reveals that* ***there is no proof that Prozac works better than tricyclic antidepressants – or that it works at all"*** (*Life Extension* magazine, April 1997).

This was re-confirmed when researchers at Northwest Clinical Research Center in Bellevue Washington compared the superiority of drugs prescribed for both depression and anxiety, over a placebo, with several studies conducted on each class of medication. Clinical trial data from the nine antidepressants approved by the FDA between 1985 and 2000 was evaluated. These trials comprised of 100,030 depressed patients. Similarly, the clinical trials data from the 13 anxiolytics (drugs to treat anxiety) approved by the FDA between 1985 and 2000 were examined. These trials consisted of 8,340 anxious patients. **Less than half (48%) of the patients who received antidepressants showed any superiority over those receiving a placebo. And, among the patients treated with drugs for anxiety, again only 48% showed superiority over the placebo** (*International Journal of Neuropsychopharmacology*, September 2002, pp. 193-197).

A more recent study was conducted at the Ottawa Health Research Institute in Canada, published in the February 2005 issue of the *British Medical Journal*, which reviewed **more than 700 clinical trials involving 87,650 patients**. The results *"determined that* ***even patients who were not depressed to begin with, and were taking SSRIs for other reasons, were more than twice as likely to attempt suicide as patients given placebos."***
(http://www.sierratimes.com/06/07/22/71_158_154_172_87990.htm)

All these studies strongly suggest that **conventional medications for treating depression and anxiety are actually less effective than a placebo.** My conclusion is, all patients should actually benefit more from a placebo, than they would from expensive potentially dangerous medications, (based on the study results). The placebo effect has long been recognized in medicine, and often the more confidence a patient has in their doctor, the greater the placebo effect would likely be. How many more studies must be done, and how many more times must we waste money (and lives) proving this? Drug companies often get drug approval for medications that are no more effective than a placebo would be. Unfortunately, although placebos are perfectly safe, and don't create side effects or deplete nutrients, that obviously doesn't apply to the medications they are managing to somehow receive FDA approval for.

How Did Prozac™ Possibly Get FDA Approval?

According to the previously mentioned editorial by *Life Extension* magazine's editor, Saul Kent, apparently, the Breggins discovered that ***"One of the main studies the FDA used in approving Prozac is based on data from only 11 patients! And it was conducted by a doctor who has been accused of fraud in other trials"*** (April 1997).

In addition, ***"None of the studies lasted for more than 6 weeks, and patients frequently rated Prozac as no better than placebo.*** *There are millions of people taking this drug, trusting that clinical trials proved its safety, its efficacy, and long-term benefit, yet there is apparently no such data."* Another important issue pointed out in the *Life Extension* article is:

> ***None of the patients who participated in the Prozac studies were suffering from severe depression.*** *While some of this type of thing might occur in a large study, what the Breggins show is that* ***juggling the data, and "cookin' the books" was the norm for the Prozac studies. One can only conclude that the real clinical trials for Prozac are being done on the American public – without its knowledge.***

Then in his book *Prozac Backlash*, Dr. Glenmullen poses the question: **In light of such serious reported side effects: *"One might ask why the public has not been made more aware"*?** He goes on to state that *"The answer lies in the lack of adequate public health policy for monitoring long-term side effects of prescription drugs"* (p. 20). Dr. Glenmullen claims that the FDA does have an approval process for new drugs coming to market, but only assurance of short-term safety:

> ***The tests typically last for only six to eight weeks, whereas the most serious, long-term side effects of drugs take years, sometimes decades, to emerge.*** *Under these circumstances, prescribing an entirely new class of agents to millions of people is* ***nothing short of an ongoing human experiment.***

Since the FDA doesn't seem to have the resources for a systematic program for monitoring late-appearing drug reactions, the agency is forced to rely on random, spontaneous reports from individual doctors. As a result, there is no tracking of thorough information on long-term side effects available, even to doctors. Instead, someone would need to sift through hundreds of medical journals to track down spontaneous case reports. Dr. Glenmullen quotes the 1998 book *Prescription for Disaster*, by Thomas Moore. The book details **the intense pressure Congress is under from lobbyists for the pharmaceutical industry to weaken rather than strengthen drug testing and monitoring.** In his book, Thomas Moore goes on to say **the nation's *"flawed monitoring system"* gives people an *"illusion of safety"* when, in fact, serious drug problems *"tend to be slow, insidious, and difficult to see."***

Dr. Candice Pert recognized the monsters she created, (and monsters they are!), and it's these monsters that Dr. Pert referred to that we are addressing. Just the fact that, according to Dr. Tracy, there are 575 potential side effects listed with the FDA, should be a clue as to the inherent potential dangers associated with Prozac™. The obvious question is: why in the world are these "mind-altering stimulants" (similar in action to cocaine), still on the market today and considered legal? And why are so many well-meaning doctors and psychiatrists still misinformed regarding how dangerous these drugs can potentially be? Most difficult of all to comprehend, is how the companies who produce these drugs, knowing how dangerous they can be, continue suppressing the fact, while aggressively promoting them (even to pregnant women and our children). They have to be totally void of any conscience!

And somehow, Eli Lilly officials continue to defend Prozac's effectiveness, saying its track record is backed by the fact that *"it is still the most widely prescribed drug of its kind."* In a statement given by Jeff Newton, an Eli Lilly spokesman, he actually wrote: *"There is no credible evidence that establishes a casual link between Prozac and violent or suicidal behavior. There is, to the contrary, scientific evidence showing that Prozac and medicines like it actually protect against such behavior"* (http://www.Pssg.org).

However, according to the *Boston Globe*, (May 7, 2000), internal documents showed that **in 1990, Eli Lilly scientists were pressured by corporate executives to alter records on physician experiences with Prozac™, changing mentions of suicide attempt to *"overdose,"* and suicidal thoughts to *"depression".*** As a result, researchers say that most U.S. doctors do not know to warn patients of the potentially dangerous side effects which, according to published literature on the topic, can be alleviated with sedatives or by going off the drug (http://www.pssg.org). German regulators, who eventually approved Prozac™ for use in that country, require a warning label about the risk of suicide and suggest the concurrent use of sedatives when necessary.

Eli Lilly has aggressively sought to discredit researchers who have published data linking its product to suicide. One such example is Dr. Glenmullen, author of the book *Prozac Backlash*. According to the *Boston Globe*, Dr. Glenmullen, a clinical instructor in psychiatry at Harvard Medical School and a clinician at the Harvard University Health Services, wrote the book because he was alarmed by the number of patients who were reporting severe side effects from the serotonin-boosting antidepressants including Prozac™, Paxil™, Zoloft™, and Luvox™. ***"The two most upsetting side effects were patients becoming suicidal on the drugs, and the development of disfiguring facial tics,"*** he said in an interview.

After obtaining hundreds of pages of FDA documents through the Freedom of Information Act, as well as internal Eli Lilly memos that are part of the public record in lawsuits filed against the drug company, Dr. Glenmullen wrote that **Eli Lilly had tried to downplay side effects of Prozac™ for years. Eli Lilly began a campaign to discredit the author,** and alerted newspapers and TV stations about the book, **saying that Harvard Medical School professors were unfamiliar with his work and didn't recognize his name, although Dr. Glenmullen is a graduate of Harvard Medical School, and was a clinical instructor in medicine at Harvard at the time!**

Chief among Dr. Glenmullen's critics is Massachusetts General Hospital's Rosenbaum, a professor of psychiatry at Harvard Medical School, who, in a written statement sent to the *Globe* (Garnet, 2000), **calls *Prozac Backlash* a *"dishonest book"* that is *"manipulative"* and *"mischievous."*** But Rosenbaum's objectivity has also been questioned. Not only was his 1991 study on Prozac™ and suicide criticized by at least two sets of researchers as well as the FDA; documents obtained by the *Globe* show that **Rosenbaum's relationship to Eli Lilly is a cozy one: he has served as a Prozac™ researcher and sat on a marketing advisory panel for Eli Lilly before Prozac™ was launched.**

Now let's look at some very important issues we have learned so far:

1. According to Dr. Ann Blake Tracy, *"As of October, 1993, 28,623 complaints of adverse side effects had been filed with the FDA, including 1,885 suicide attempts and 1,349 deaths"* (*Prozac: Panacea or Pandora?*, 1991/1994, p. 55).

2. In the *Journal of the American Medical Association*, the FDA commissioner, David Kessler indicated that ***"only about 1 percent of serious events are reported to the FDA"*** (*Prozac: Panacea or Pandora?*, Tracy, 1991/1994, p. 55). Notice he said **"serious events"**. If we then consider that the statement was made by the FDA commissioner himself, **that would translate to 2,862,300 adverse reactions, and 188,500 actual suicide attempts, and 134,900 actual deaths associated with Prozac™! These figures are unheard of in the history of the FDA – never have they seen anything that compares.**

3. We need to keep in mind that although these figures are unbelievably serious, **they were actually taken from statistics that, as of this writing, are more than 13 years old,** and as the prescribing of Prozac™ by doctors is continuing to escalate at a rapid pace, they could easily have doubled, or even tripled since then.

4. In an audiotape produced in 1999, titled *Help! I Can't Get Off My Antidepressants!,* Dr. Tracy states that one person in seven in our nation was currently on antidepressants. Although she didn't state how many were on antidepressants six years prior, when the statistics she quoted in her book *Prozac: Panacea or Pandora*? (1991/1994) were current, I am sure the percentage she quoted would reflect a much larger percentage of the population.

5. Then on November 16, 2002 in a lecture by Dr. Tracy at the *Symposium for Health Freedom* in Anaheim, California which I attended, she stated that since the 9/11 incident, the figure had actually doubled from "one in seven" to "one in 3½", and this shows the potential rate of acceleration when we consider that the rate of prescriptions actually doubled in approximately 3 years, and apparently precipitated by just one incident.

6. Another concern Dr. Tracy pointed out in her Anaheim lecture, was that in the four years from 1995 to 1999, in regards to **children under 6 years of age, Prozac™ use increased by an astounding 580%! And this was before Prozac™ had been approved by the FDA for use by children.**

7. And finally, the decision by the FDA in February 2003 to approve Prozac™ for use by children. That would certainly indicate an obviously disproportionate appropriation of staff by the FDA to evaluate the 3,000 drugs they approved, or a just overt corruption in a regulatory organization established to protect the public from dangerous drugs. Although both appear to apply, I personally feel that corruption is the true source of the problem.

And Now They've Approved One More Reason To Prescribe Prozac™ - "Intermittent Explosive Disorder" (IED)

As discussed in the first chapter of this book, one of the newest "mental disorders" to be announced is Intermittent Explosive Disorder (IED), which is defined as involving *"multiple outbursts that are way out of proportion to the situation,"* which can include road rage, temper outbursts that involve throwing or breaking objects, threats, aggressive actions and property damage, and even spousal abuse. These findings were released in the June 2006 issue of the *Archives of General Psychiatry.*

According to Dr. Emil Coccaro, chairman of psychiatry at the University of Chicago's medical school, *"there's a biology and cognitive science to this,"* and he goes on to claim that "*the disorder involves inadequate production or functioning of serotonin, a mood-regulating and behavior-inhibiting brain chemical.* ***Treatment with antidepressants, including those that target serotonin receptors*** **[referring to SSRI antidepressants such as Prozac™]*, is often helpful"*** (*The Washington Post,* June 6, 2006). You will now learn why following Dr. Coccaro's recommendations not only doesn't make a bit of sense, but could also be outright dangerous!

One unacceptable behavior identified that would qualify a person for being diagnosed with IED would be "road rage". And another is "aggressive actions", for which Dr. Coccaro recommends treating with antidepressants that target serotonin receptors, (translated, that means drugs such as Prozac™ and Paxil™). Yet, in her book *Prozac: Panacea or Pandora?* (1991/1994), Dr. Ann Blake Tracy claims that "*The rage and violent feelings are often referred to by the patients as:* ***'indescribable', 'an anger unlike I have ever felt before', 'only two weeks on Paxil I cannot believe I did not kill myself or someone else'."*** Then one of Dr. Tracy's patients shares the following experience: ***"After being on Prozac for one week I had an argument with another motorist and attempted to run over him with my car!"*** Additionally, one study reported in the *Journal of Clinical Psychiatry* (September 1989), revealed that ***"Prozac caused akathisia, or drug-induced insanity in 10 to 25% of patients. Symptoms of akathisia include hallucinations, aggression, self-destructive outbursts, terror, anger, hostility, hatred, and rage"*** (*Breaking Your Prescribed Addiction*, Sahley & Birkner, 1998, p. 86).

As you can easily see, we have sufficient proof that **the very drugs that Dr. Coccaro recommends for treating IED, actually "cause IED"!** According to Dr. Tracy, uncontrollable rage, which is totally out of character, is surprisingly common with people on these SSRI antidepressants. We know that the majority of the children involved in the school shootings, (an obvious sign of rage), were actually taking the very same serotonergic antidepressants that Dr. Coccaro recommended for those with IED. **Dr. Coccaro's observation is actually typical of far too many psychiatrists' "totally unscientific" conclusions, such as the 374 mental conditions they somehow managed to conveniently "create"!** As a result, psychiatrists can now quite easily identify some "abnormal condition" in nearly everyone, which of course would require prescribing some mind-altering drug in order to treat. **Talk about "drug pushers", (and worst of all, it's entirely legal)!**

Incidentally, Dr. Tracy actually attributes the increased rate of road rage to the ever-increasing number of people being placed on very same antidepressants that Dr. Coccaro recommends for those with an uncontrollable temper, (quite a contradiction, I would say). Dr. Tracy claims that due to the over-stimulation of stress hormones that the SSRI antidepressants produce on a daily basis, they tend to create an inappropriate response (over-reaction) to even minor stresses.

I couldn't help but wonder what prompted Dr. Coccaro to conclude that the serotonergic antidepressants would be an appropriate solution, and whose payroll he might possibly be on, so we did a little detective work, and guess what we discovered? You likely guessed it: ***"Dr. Coccaro reports that he receives research grants and serves on the speaker's bureau or as a consultant to Eli Lilly and Co., Abbott Laboratories, GlaxoSmithKline, and Forrest Laboratories"*** (http://www.infoshop.org/pipermail/infoshop-news/2006-June/005654.html). **The very same companies who are responsible for producing the drugs he is promoting!** Could it possibly be just a coincidence? I would guess not. It appears that he is just one of may doctors willing to come to some pre-determined conclusion for a price, and I'm sure it's not just a nominal fee. I have met Dr. Tracy and am familiar with her work, and I can assure you that she is definitely not on any pharmaceutical's payroll. If she were, she would likely be promoting them as Dr. Coccaro does, rather than warning you of their "many dangers", as I am also doing.

It's quite obvious that Dr. Coccaro could not have fully researched the facts before arriving at his proposed solution, if he truly believed what he said. If you noticed, he never provided any real science to back up his conclusion. Unfortunately, one announcement is often all it takes to promote another inappropriate use for a dangerous class of drugs, and it's a perfect marketing strategy. Then, as ridiculous as it might seem, "it actually works!" It then gets written up in major news publications, including medical journals, and often the news media picks up on it, and then it's announced to the whole world via the national news, often followed by a commercial for the drug. Unfortunately, few are aware that the "scientific study" is actually funded, and well controlled, by the very same companies that just happen to be producing the drugs that are being recommended for some new mental condition that doctors, such as Dr. Coccaro, conveniently helped them create.

CHAPTER THIRTEEN

Understanding Hypothyroidism – A Major Underlying Cause of Depression

Many of the symptoms associated with hypothyroidism (a suppressed thyroid condition) are very similar to those that the dangerous drugs such as Ritalin™ or Prozac™ are often prescribed for, with depression, behavioral disorders, and mood swings, being the most common. Cold hands, cold feet, and fatigue are also common hypothyroid symptoms, with more than forty other conditions or symptoms also identified, that are often associated with hypothyroidism.

The basic problem is: A low thyroid condition results in the reduced action of all 3,000 enzymes in the body. This then opens the door for several different prescriptions to deal with each of the potential symptoms that often result, from a low thyroid condition. Depression is one of the most common symptoms, which all too often results in a prescription for an antidepressant. Unfortunately, most medical doctors fail to take the time necessary to properly diagnose the underlying problem, resulting in some symptom-suppressing drug instead.

In my opinion, it's not just accidental that the established protocol that doctors were trained to follow, will not properly identify, (or treat), the very common hypothyroid condition. That basically results in the potential for many different thyroid-related symptoms that thus go unresolved. And of course, symptom-suppressing drugs, (with their own side effects), are the typical solution, which makes a perfect marketing tool for promoting a lot of "unnecessary medications".

As women are ten times as likely as men to experience the hypothyroid (low thyroid) condition, they normally experience by far the greatest potential for unnecessary "drug abuse". And as depression is a common side effect, that would explain why far more women are placed on antidepressants. The greatest concern is, millions of women are placed on, (and often remain on), antidepressants throughout their pregnancies, which as we learned, greatly compromises the development of the fetus, and contributes to many serious birth defects.

If I'm aware of this serious problem, then you can rest assured that the pharmaceutical companies are fully aware as well. Could you imagine the millions of women, and children especially, that are suffering needlessly, (often for a lifetime), just because of their doctor's training? These doctors are unknowingly being trained as "drug pushers" for the pharmaceutical giants. As Dr. Bruce West so aptly states: ***"Drugs for everything, and nothing but drugs for anything!"***

Your Medications Could Very Well Be Suppressing Your Thyroid

On our list of the 200 most commonly prescribed medications, of the 180 medications that were evaluated to determine nutrient depletion, **all but four (nearly 98%) were found to deplete nutrients necessary for healthy thyroid function. Those nutrients are listed below, along with the drugs or conditions known to deplete them.**

1. **Vitamin A** – depleted by steroids and corticosteroids, NSAIDs (i.e. ibuprofen), laxatives (mineral oil), estrogen and oral contraceptives, caffeine, aspirin, all cholesterol-lowering drugs, including statins and bile acid sequestrants (i.e. Questran™, Colestid™), antiseizure medication (i.e. barbiturates, phenytoin), antibiotics, antacids, and alcohol.

2. **Vitamin B_1 (thiamine)** – depleted by alcohol, antacids, antibiotics, antiarrhythmic agents (i.e. digoxin), antiseizure medication (i.e. barbiturates, phenytoin), caffeine, diuretics, estrogen and oral contraceptives, smoking, SSRI antidepressants, sulfa drugs, sugar, cooking (heat), food processing methods, and physical and mental stress.

3. **Vitamin B_2 (riboflavin)** – depleted by sulfa drugs, steroids and corticosteroids, muscle relaxants, mineral oil and laxatives, estrogen and oral contraceptives, diuretics, diabetes medication, antidepressants (SSRI and tricyclics), antiseizure medication (i.e. barbiturates, phenytoin), antibiotics, alcohol, antacids, sugar, ultraviolet light, physical and mental stress.

4. **Vitamin B_3 (Niacin)** – depleted by sulfa drugs, SSRI antidepressants, steroids and corticosteroids, sleeping pills, estrogen (and oral contraceptives), caffeine, antibiotics, alcohol, sugar, and physical and mental stress.

5. **Vitamin B_6 (pyridoxine)** – depleted by vasodilators (i.e. nitroglycerin), sulfa drugs, steroids and corticosteroids, smoking, sleeping pills, estrogen (and oral contraceptives), diuretics, diabetic medication, caffeine, asthma medications, antidepressants and MAO inhibitors, antibiotics, alcohol, sugar, heat (canning & roasting), and physical and mental stress.

6. **Vitamin B_{12}** – depleted by sulfa drugs, SSRI antidepressants, smoking, sleeping pills, proton pump inhibitors (i.e. Nexium™), muscle relaxants, mineral oil and laxatives, Histamine H_2 blockers (i.e. Tagamet™, Pepcid™, Zantac™), estrogen (and oral contraceptives), diuretics, diabetic medications, all cholesterol-lowering drugs, including statins and bile acid sequestrants (i.e. Questran™, Colestid™), calcium deficiency, caffeine, antiseizure medication (i.e. barbiturates), amphetamines and diet pills, antibiotics, and alcohol.

7. **Vitamin C** – depleted by steroids and corticosteroids, NSAIDs (i.e. ibuprofen), muscle relaxants, estrogen and oral contraceptives, diuretics, diabetic medication, antihistamines, asthma medications, aspirin, anticoagulants, antidepressants (most), antiseizure medication (i.e. barbiturates, phenytoin), antibiotics, analgesics, amphetamines and diet pills, alcohol, caffeine, cooking (heat), high fever, smoking, physical and mental stress.

8. **Vitamin D (Calciferol)** – depleted by steroids and corticosteroids, smoking, muscle relaxants, mineral oil (laxatives), Histamine H_2 blockers (i.e. Tagamet™, Pepcid™, Zantac™), estrogen (and oral contraceptives), diuretics, diabetic medication, all cholesterol-lowering drugs, including statins and bile acid sequestrants (i.e. Questran™, Colestid™), asthma medications, aspirin, antiseizure medication (i.e. barbiturates,

phenytoin), antibiotics, antidepressants, antiarrhythmics (i.e. digoxin), antacids, analgesics, alcohol, cooking (heat), light, high fever, physical and mental stress.

9. **Vitamin E (tocopherol)** – depleted by NSAIDs (i.e. ibuprofen), all cholesterol-lowering drugs, including statins and bile acid sequestrants (i.e. Questran™, Colestid™), Orlistat™ (fat-blocking weight loss agent), mineral oil (laxatives), estrogen and oral contraceptives, aspirin, antibiotics, alcohol, heat, frying, oxygen, freezing temperatures, air pollution, inorganic iron, and chlorine.

10. **Iron** - a trace mineral, depleted by NSAIDs (i.e. ibuprofen), mineral oil and laxatives, narcotics, histamine H_2 blockers (i.e. Tagamet™, Pepcid™, Zantac™), choline magnesium trisalicylate (an anti-inflammatory), all cholesterol-lowering drugs, including statins and bile acid sequestrants (i.e. Questran™, Colestid™), Carisoprodol™ (pain reliever), **thyroid medication,** caffeine (especially the tannic acid in coffee and tea), aspirin, antibiotics, antacids, high phosphorus diet (bran), excess sweating, heavy bleeding (i.e. menstruating women, bleeding ulcers), candida yeast infection, phosphate food additives and EDTA (**e**thylene**d**iamine **t**etraacetic **a**cid – a food preservative).

11. **Magnesium** – an essential mineral, depleted by steroids and corticosteroids, SSRI antidepressants, NSAIDs (i.e. ibuprofen), Immunosuppressants, high levels of zinc, estrogen and oral contraceptives, diuretics, diabetic medication, all cholesterol-lowering drugs, including statins and bile acid sequestrants (i.e. Questran™, Colestid™), antiseizure medication (i.e. barbiturates, phenytoin), antifungal medication, antibiotics, antiarrhythmic agents (i.e. digoxin), antacids, alcohol, Albuterol and other bronchodilators, antihypertensive (blood pressure lowering) drugs (including ACE inhibitors, beta blockers and calcium channel blockers), large amounts of fats, sugar, refined flour, fluoride, soft water consumption, and physical and emotional stress.

12. **Manganese** – a trace mineral, depleted by steroids and corticosteroids, SSRI antidepressants, diuretics, caffeine, alcohol, excess sugar, and heavy consumption of meat or dairy products.

13. **Potassium** – an essential mineral, depleted by steroids and corticosteroids, sodium bicarbonate (Alka Seltzer™), smoking, Parkinson's disease medication, NSAIDs (i.e. ibuprofen), muscle relaxants, laxatives, immunosuppressants, diuretics, caffeine, antiarrhythmic agents (i.e. digoxin), anti-anginal drugs used for heart disease (i.e. Norvasc™, Procardia™), asthma medication, aspirin, anti-inflammatories, antifungal medication, antibiotics, amphetamines and diet pills, alcohol, Acetazolamide™ (a carbonic anhydrase inhibitor), ACE inhibitors and other blood pressure lowering drugs (including beta blockers), excess sugar and refined foods, large amounts of licorice, and physical and mental stress.

14. **Selenium** – a trace mineral depleted by steroids and corticosteroids, SSRI antidepressants, excess zinc or copper, caffeine, alcohol, food processing, high fat foods, infection, injury, blood loss, aging, and physical and mental stress.

15. **Zinc** – a trace mineral depleted by steroids and corticosteroids, SSRI antidepressants, NSAIDs (i.e. ibuprofen), HIV medication, Histamine H_2 blockers (i.e. Tagamet™, Pepcid™, Zantac™), estrogen (and oral contraceptives), diuretics, caffeine, all cholesterol-lowering drugs, including statins and bile acid sequestrants (i.e. Questran™, Colestid™), antibiotics, antiseizure medication (i.e. barbiturates, phenytoin), antacids and ulcer medication, aspirin, alcohol, ACE inhibitors and other blood pressure lowering drugs (including beta blockers), diarrhea, perspiration, kidney disease, cirrhosis of the liver, food processing, physical and mental stress, a diet high in fiber, and the consumption of hard water. Zinc levels are also lowered by diabetes.

16. **Tyrosine** – a non-essential amino acid depleted by estrogen and oral contraceptives.

How SSRI Antidepressants Contribute To Thyroid Suppression

SSRI Antidepressants, such as Prozac™, Paxil™, Zoloft™, Celexa™, etc., are in my opinion, some of the greatest contributors to thyroid suppression. Although a low thyroid often contributes to depression, and one reason that many are inappropriately place on antidepressants, the SSRI antidepressants themselves just worsen the condition. Following are a few potential ways that SSRI antidepressants can contribute to hypothyroidism.

✓ **Nutrient Depletion!** Prozac™ and other SSRI antidepressants deplete ELEVEN of the 16 nutrients listed as being necessary for proper thyroid function!

✓ **Fluoride.** According to Dr. Sherry Rogers, M.D., every single molecule of Prozac™ just happens to contain three molecules of fluoride! The problem is, among other things, fluoride is a known thyroid suppressant, by disrupting iodine necessary for thyroid function.

✓ **Stress Hormones.** The stress hormone cortisol is another thyroid suppressant associated with Prozac™. As just one 30 mg dose of Prozac™ increases cortisol by 200%, it thus causes your body to respond as though you are stressed every single day! This elevated stress hormone not only suppresses the thyroid, but also contributes to elevated blood sugar leading to diabetes (a major cardiovascular risk factor).

✓ **Insulin resistance / Diabetes.** The increased level of blood sugar, stimulated by the elevated cortisol, not only **contributes to hypoglycemia, insulin resistance and thus type II diabetes**, but it also contributes to damage to the arteries in the process. And of course, once the insulin resistance in general is well established, we have another problem: **Insulin resistance in the liver.** Then the enzyme in the liver that is necessary for efficient thyroid hormone conversion becomes less efficient due to the insulin resistance, as it is dependent upon an adequate level of glucose for that process.

✓ **Bipolar Disorder and Lithium.** As Dr. Tracy noted, an antidepressant is basically a stimulant, such as cocaine, which also raises the level of serotonin in the neurons. Any unnatural stimulation of any hormone results in a rebound effect. In the case of Prozac™, it causes a shutting down of some serotonin receptors, or resistance to serotonin from the continual overstimulation caused by Prozac™. It in turn suppresses dopamine, which then often results in an imbalance of neurotransmitters, known as the bipolar disorder. This then leads to the prescribing of lithium carbonate.

✓ **Lithium carbonate.** Just two of the many potentially serious side effects associated with the drug lithium carbonate, normally prescribed for the bipolar disorder, (a side effect often caused by drugs such as Prozac™), are **permanent kidney scarring,** and **goiter (an enlarged thyroid gland).** As we know, that is caused by a deficiency of iodine, necessary for producing the thyroid hormone. **One thing lithium is well known for is its ability to bond to and remove iodine from the thyroid, (actually similar to fluoride in that regard).** For that very reason, high doses of lithium are often prescribed in order to treat hyp**er**thyroidism (above-normal thyroid), in order to **"reduce the thyroid function".** The problem is, by far the majority of people are actually suffering with hyp**o**thyroidism (low thyroid), rather than elevated thyroid.

So, not only does Prozac™ suppress the thyroid, but the lithium carbonate prescribed for the bipolar disorder (caused by the Prozac™), suppresses the thyroid as well, basically compounding the problem. As you can see, Prozac's influence is actually wide spread.

✓ **Protein-binding / Detoxification.** SSRI antidepressants are highly protein-binding, and thus very difficult for the liver to metabolize. This problem is basically self-perpetuating. The more the thyroid function is suppressed, the lower the metabolism will be, and thus the less efficient the detoxification of all drugs in the liver will be as well. First, keep in mind that the liver considers drugs such as Prozac™ as a toxin. Then second, due to the reduced metabolism, and the reduced enzyme action associated with the reduced body temperature, as well as fluoride's enzyme suppressing action, you should likely begin getting a considerably higher dosage of your antidepressant, as well any other medications you may be taking. Thus, you would be **greatly increasing the risk of a possible drug overdose!** Then an overdose of an SSRI antidepressant such as Prozac™ or Paxil™ can at times be life threatening, as they are inherently dangerous drugs.

For those who might also have trouble metabolizing proteins, this could be an extremely dangerous combination, with the potential for a deadly build up of drugs and toxins in the system. The only real solution is to get off the SSRI antidepressant! This becomes evident when you consider the autopsy report of a young woman, who stabbed herself to death after being on the SSRI antidepressant Paxil™ for just **two weeks**: ***"Her autopsy revealed a high blood level of Paxil, which reflects poor metabolization, a feature common in many SSRI suicide cases"*** (http://www.sierratimes.com/05/08/13/24_164_252_187_48525.htm). With these drugs, you are basically playing Russian Roulette, (you never really know what to expect).

There are so many variables that can come into play, that no one really knows for sure exactly how he or she might respond to such potentially dangerous drugs. It's bad enough to take your own life, as some have done on these drugs, but could you imagine taking the life of an innocent loved one, as many have also done? It would be horrifying, once you realized what you had done! Although Andrea Yates, a caring mother who drowned her 5 children, is a prime example, there are many others. Actually, far too many to allow the aggressive promoting of them for our young innocent children, (who trust in our judgment). Not only that, but they seldom have a choice in the matter. Our choice in their behalf is extremely critical, and must be based on the unbiased facts, which hopefully you now have. Although I plan to write many more books in the future, I believe the information in this book could be the most critical, as well as timely. As a result, completing it has become my top priority, and it has thus become a day and night project, as many innocent lives are at stake!

Other Potential Causes of Hypothyroidism (Low Thyroid)

1. **Iodine deficiency.** Maintaining sufficient iodine levels is essential for an adequately functioning thyroid. Unfortunately, an iodine deficiency is apparently all too common, and as stated by Dr. David Brownstein, M.D., in his book ***Iodine! Why You Need – Why You Can't Live Without It*** (2004), after testing hundreds of patients, he discovered that **more than 90% exhibited laboratory signs of an iodine deficiency.** Incidentally, fluoride (Prozac™) will cause an iodine deficiency. **(NOTE: For more detailed information regarding the thyroid, please see the last chapter of this book, under Additional Technical Information.)**

Dr. David G. Williams suggests a simple self-test to determine if you are iodine-deficient, as outlined in the June 2004 issue of his *Alternatives* newsletter. He admits that it's not 100% accurate, although it is easy to do, inexpensive, and works very well as a simple screening tool.

Just dip a cotton swab or ball into USP tincture of iodine (available at most any drugstore), and paint a 2-inch circle of iodine on a soft area of skin such as your stomach or the inner part of your thigh or arm. If the yellowish stain disappears in less than one hour, your body is lacking in iodine. If the stain remains for more than four hours, it is an indication your iodine levels may be adequate.

2. **Bromine** is a member of the halogen group, (a heavy metal), and contributes to an iodine deficiency as well. It has been proven that **bromine *"Will replace chloride and accumulate, will also be taken up by* [the] *thyroid gland instead of iodine,* [causing] *adverse effects on* [the] *brain and thyroid function"*** (http://www.hypoglycemia.asn.au/articles/rich_sources_nutrients.html).

And Dr. Brownstein notes the following:

> *When bromide* [the reduced form of bromine] *binds to the thyroid gland, it is not only a toxic element,* ***it worsens an iodine deficient problem.***
>
> *Bromine intoxication (i.e. bromism) has been shown to cause delirium, psychomotor retardation,* ***schizophrenia****, and hallucination. Subjects who ingest enough bromide feel dull and apathetic and have* ***difficulty concentrating****.* ***Bromide can also cause severe depression, headache, and irritability.***
>
> ***Recent research has demonstrated that some symptoms of bromide toxicity can be present with low levels of bromide in the diet*** (*Iodine: Why You Need – Why You Can't Live Without It,* 2004, p. 78).

Bromine is often used as a dough conditioner in baked goods, as well as a clouding agent in many popular drinks. Toxicity of bromine has been reported from ingestion of some carbonated drinks (i.e. Mountain Dew™, AMP™ Energy Drink, some Gatorade™ products), which contain brominated vegetable oils (*Clinical Toxicology*, 1997, pp. 315-320). Bromine is **still used today in many prescription medications** (i.e. those that treat asthma, and bowel and bladder dysfunction).

3. **Dehydration.** According to Dr. F. Batmanghelidj, M.D., author of *Your Body's Many Cries For Water*, dehydration reduces thyroid function. The body actually recognizes dehydration as stress, which is a known thyroid suppressant.

4. **Stress.** Stress hormones not only suppress the thyroid, but will also contribute to elevated blood sugar leading to diabetes. Stress (both physical and mental) also depletes the important mineral selenium, which is necessary for healthy thyroid function. This becomes obvious if you consider that **TEN (over half!) of the 16 nutrients necessary for healthy thyroid function are depleted by stress!**

5. **Bad Fats (Trans-fatty acids)** are found mostly in hydrogenated or partially hydrogenated oils. In his book *Overcoming Thyroid Disorders* (2002), David Brownstein, M.D. tells us that:

> *These foreign substances (trans-fatty acids) are actually incorporated into the cell membranes. This will* ***disrupt the normal functioning of the cells of the body, blocking the utilization of essential fatty acids. This can lead to the development of many chronic illnesses, including immune system dysfunction and hormonal imbalances, particularly thyroid imbalances*** (p. 181).

The nutrient depletion caused by bad fats, most importantly produces deficiencies of the fat-soluble vitamins A, D, E, and K, (all important, but especially for anyone with a low thyroid). Insufficient vitamin A can cause a deterioration of the pituitary gland's basophil cells where the thyroid-stimulating hormone is synthesized, limiting the amount of iodine that the thyroid gland can absorb, and reducing the amount of thyroid hormone it produces. Vitamin D is required for healthy thyroid function, and vitamin E has been shown to protect against at least 80 diseases, including the ability to prevent heart attacks. And as we learned earlier, vitamin K also serves many important functions, especially escorting calcium to the bones, rather than the arteries.

6. **High Protein Diet**. This concern is explained best by Broda Barnes, M.D., taken from his book *Hypothyroidism: The Unsuspected Illness* (1976), as follows:

> ***A diet high in protein requires additional thyroid for its metabolism.*** *There were no symptoms of hyperthyroidism in spite of the extra thyroid until the diet was cut back to a normal amount of protein. Then typical hyperthyroidism* [elevated thyroid] *appeared and the extra thyroid had to be discontinued.*
>
> ***It seems clear that a diet quite high in protein utilizes available thyroid hormone. Two studies in the medical literature indicate that excess protein lowers the basal metabolism*** **[thyroid function]** (pp. 273-274).

7. **Iron deficiency.** An iron deficiency can impair the body's ability to manufacture the thyroid hormone. Antibiotics, antacids, aspirin, all cholesterol-lowering drugs, and caffeine, as well as strenuous exercise, heavy perspiration, or heavy bleeding, often deplete iron.

8. **Selenium deficiency.** It has been found that **selenium-deficient individuals are almost always hypothyroid**. In fact, David Brownstein, M.D. states that ***"I have found significant numbers of patients in my practice who have selenium deficiencies, with resultant hypothyroid symptoms. When these deficiencies are improved, their hypothyroid symptoms often improve"*** (*Overcoming Thyroid Disorders*, 2002, pp. 65-66). **Selenium is a trace mineral that can easily be depleted by SSRI antidepressants,** caffeine, infection, and stress, or even a high fat diet.

9. **The Female Gender.** Approximately 90% of those who are hypothyroid are women. One reason is that the female liver is less efficient in producing the most active form thyroid (T_3 thyroid) than the male liver. Also, women have considerably more estrogen than men, and estrogen is a known thyroid suppressant.

10. **Elevated estrogen.** David Brownstein, M.D. (*Overcoming Thyroid Disorders*, 2002) explains that ***"Any orally prescribed estrogen will result in an increase in thyroxine binding globulin (TBG) which will decrease the amount of thyroid hormone that is available for the body to use."*** And he goes on to note that ***"I have seen many women with hypothyroid symptoms improve their condition when they stop taking their oral synthetic hormone replacement therapy"*** (p. 60).

Birth control pills also contain estrogens, and will thus substantially decrease the amount of thyroid hormone available to the body, just as estrogen replacement therapy (ERT) does, often leading to a hypothyroid condition. Dr. Brownstein comments regarding birth control pills, as follows: ***"I have successfully treated numerous women who have many of the signs of hypothyroidism by simply having them eliminate their use of birth control pills"*** (p. 60).

Although estrogen performs an important function during the childbearing years, its level should reduce following menopause. Even if a woman has had a total hysterectomy, and no longer has ovaries, her fat tissue, and even her adrenals are still capable of producing estrogen.

Estrogen and oral contraceptives also deplete **TWELVE of the 16 nutrients previously listed as necessary for healthy thyroid function!**

11. **Soy.** Unfermented soy products can mimic the effects of the female hormone, producing elevated estrogen levels, and resulting in thyroid suppression. In fact, one study found that ***"daily soy consumption resulted in symptoms of hypothyroidism*** *(i.e., malaise, constipation, sleepiness) and goiters* ***in 50% of the subjects,"*** and yet ***"These hypothyroid symptoms resolved one month after stopping the soy ingestion"*** (*Overcoming Thyroid Disorders*, David Brownstein, M.D., 2002, p. 63).

12. **Simple sugars.** A diet consisting of too many simple sugars initiates a downhill spiral, beginning with insulin resistance, and eventually resulting in Type II diabetes and hypothyroidism. **Sugar also suppresses the immune system, and contributes to the depletion of SEVEN of 16 nutrients previously listed as necessary for healthy thyroid function!** Sugar has absolutely no nutritional value – just empty calories. Incidentally, sugar just happens to be candida's favorite food, as well as cancer's.

13. **Overstimulation.** Adrenal exhaustion can result from overstimulation with substances such as caffeine, sugar, or aspartame (NutraSweet™). The elevated stress hormone cortisol,

(also caused by SSRI antidepressants such as Prozac™), suppresses the thyroid as well. Both stress and stimulants, over a long term, can result in adrenal fatigue, which can be very debilitating.

14. **Beta-Blockers,** such as Atenolol, Carvedilol, Propranolol, Metoprolol, commonly prescribed to treat hypertension (high blood pressure), suppress thyroid function. In a lecture given at a bariatric [obesity] conference in Los Vegas, Nevada, on the care and testing of the thyroid, Dr. Neal Rouzier, M.D., author of *Natural Hormone Replacement* (2001), noted that beta-blockers actually block the conversion of the enzymes necessary for efficient thyroid function.

15. **Smoking cigarettes** increases the risk of developing hypothyroidism. One study from Japan showed **a 42% increase in hypothyroidism in smokers versus non-smokers** (*Overcoming Thyroid Disorders*, David Brownstein, 2002, p. 69).

Smoking also contributes to the depletion of vitamins B_1, B_6, B_{12}, C, and D, as well as the mineral potassium, all of which are necessary for healthy thyroid function.

16. **Alcohol. The presence of alcohol in the bloodstream inhibits thyroid function.** Alcohol has also been found to elevate estrogen levels in women (another contributor to suppressed thyroid), as well as **depleting FOURTEEN of the 16 (NEARLY ALL) nutrients necessary for healthy thyroid function!** Not only that, but alcohol and antidepressants are a dangerous combination. And don't forget, the candida yeast infection ferments sugar into alcohol.

17. **Environmental Toxins.** There are many **thyroid "poisons"** in your environment, which greatly contribute to the suppression of the thyroid, such as chloride (or chlorine), fluoride, lead, mercury, bromine, and even certain perfumes, as well as some fluorescent lighting.

18. **Sucralose (Splenda™) – The Chlorine Connection.** There is a fairly new artificial sweetener on the market called sucralose, sold under the name Splenda™. It is a white crystalline powder substitute for sugar, has zero calories, and is about 600 times sweeter than sucrose, resulting in intense sweetness. However, sucralose is produced by chlorinating sugar. This involves chemically changing the structure of the sugar molecules by substituting three chlorine atoms for three hydroxyl groups (http://www.sucralose.org/facts.html).

Very few studies of safety for human consumption of this product have ever been published. And despite the manufacturer's claims to the contrary, **sucralose most definitely is significantly absorbed and metabolized by the body.** According to the FDA's *"Final Rule"* report, 11% to 27% of sucralose is absorbed in humans, and the rest is excreted **unchanged** in feces (Federal Register, Vol. 63, No. 64, Rules and Regulations 16417-16433, Friday. April 3, 1998, page 16426, paragraph two). **However, according to the Japanese Food Sanitation Council, as much as forty percent of ingested sucralose is absorbed**, (http://www.splendaexposed.com/articles/2005/02/weird_science_h.html), which is likely less biased and more accurate. Furthermore, **the absorbed sucralose has been found to concentrate in the liver, kidney, and gastrointestinal tract.**

Incidentally, if you are looking for a safe alternative to sugar, **Xylitol actually looks, tastes and pours just like regular sugar.** Discovered simultaneously by French and German chemists in 1891, Xylitol has been safely used since the 1970s as an ingredient in gums and candies. You can use it on your morning breakfast cereal or on anything you'd like to sweeten naturally, as well baking. For an all-around sugar replacement, Xylitol is my favorite. It comes in convenient packets, or can be purchased in bulk as well.

What Is "Normal" Thyroid Function?

Considering the statistics, let's see what one of the foremost authorities on thyroid dysfunction, has to say on the subject. According to the late Dr. Broda Barnes, M.D., Ph.D., in his book *Hypothyroidism – the Unsuspected Illness* (1976), ***"Forty percent of the American people today are suffering needlessly and many dying for lack of an ingredient vital for health"*** (p. VII). The vital ingredient Dr. Barnes was referring to is a natural glandular extract, called Armour™ thyroid, which we will soon be discussing.

It is important to point out that Dr. Barnes' book was actually published in 1976, making his statistical information more than thirty years old. Today we should expect to see statistics that would reflect a considerably larger portion of the population experiencing hypothyroidism, and thus thyroid related problems, resulting from many of the changes that have taken place the past thirty years, (such as replacing iodine with bromine, and the introduction of drugs such as the SSRI antidepressants), which are known to contribute to reduced thyroid function.

The **appropriate** dosage of thyroid hormone in my opinion, is the one at which you feel your best. That amount often varies between individuals, and there are actually many different factors involved. According to Dr. Broda Barnes, (*Hypothyroidism: The Unsuspected Illness*, 1976), quite simply ***"The proper dosage for any individual is the minimum needed to relieve symptoms"*** (p. 285). For example, he suggests that additional thyroid hormone may be necessary when consuming a high-protein diet (up to 4 additional grains daily).

Dr. David Brownstein, M.D., author of the book *Overcoming Thyroid Disorders* (2002), has found that some people simply require a higher dosage of thyroid to overcome the problem of cellular resistance (regarding the iodine receptors throughout the body and brain, which incidentally is **discussed in detail at the end of this book, in the chapter on Additional Technical Information**). Once the problem of hormone resistance is eliminated (if possible), the dosage may be reduced accordingly. Incidentally, one of the many problems associated with the fluoride in Prozac™ is "damaging receptors", which would contribute to hormone resistance at the cellular level.

Another influencing factor, according to retired professor Dr. Ray Peat, Ph.D., is that people quite often require more thyroid hormone (again, up to four grains more) in the winter months than during the summer (http://www.thyroid-info.com/articles/ray-peat.htm). It makes perfect sense that when the ambient (surrounding) temperature is colder during the winter months, the body would be required to produce more heat (the thyroid's responsibility), in order to maintain our normal body temperature of 98.6 degrees.

Dr. Neal Rouzier, M.D. FACEP, author of *Natural Hormone Replacement* (2001), tells of one professor, Dr. Lavene, who found that most of his brightest students actually tended to be slightly hyp**er**thyroid ("above" what is considered as normal). Thus, he claims to have taken 3 grains of Armour™ thyroid daily for the past 30 years. Teaching students who are brighter than you can be quite a challenge. Although we can't change our genetics, there are things we can control, as Dr. Lavene apparently discovered. Just keep in mind that excessively elevated thyroid can be a risk factor as well. I believe that our current evaluation process is likely flawed.

What is actually subclinical (marginally low), although still considered as being in the normal range, in my opinion is still not optimal, and should thus be addressed. It's rather like accepting a low (although "normal") IQ, when it could be easily increased without any drastic measures. Your metabolism seems to have an influence on both your energy level and your mental capacity, which Dr. Lavene recognized.

We will now learn how you can do a self-test at home to determine if you likely have a low thyroid condition. We will then be looking at ways you can bring your thyroid function back to normal (if it's too low). Having normal thyroid function has a major influence on your entire overall health and energy levels. So we will now look at some potential solutions.

Do The Self Test (Evaluate Your Own Thyroid Function)

This can be accomplished by placing a normal glass thermometer underarm, first thing in the morning before arising. Just lie still and leave it there for ten minutes and record your temperature. Repeat the process for five consecutive days, and then average your temperature. If your average temperature is 97.4° or less, you should consider some of the options provided later in this chapter.

Comparing Thyroid Hormones

If either you or your doctor discovered that you are hypothyroid (low thyroid), getting the very best form of thyroid hormone is critical. Many doctors absolutely insist on prescribing what I consider the "very worst" form of thyroid hormone. I will provide you with the facts that you can take to your doctor if necessary. The late Dr. Broda Barnes was considered to be one of the foremost authorities on thyroid conditions and hormones, and I believe you will soon learn why he chose Armour™ thyroid over Synthroid™. Once you learn the whole unbiased story, you will be in a better position to make an intelligent decision regarding which form of thyroid hormone would be the safest and most effective for you.

What Do We Know About The Prescription Thyroid (Synthroid™)

1. Synthroid™ is a chemical form of the T_4 thyroid hormone.

2. In his book *Natural Hormone Replacement* (2001), Dr. Rouzier states that most of his new patients were still experiencing typical thyroid symptoms, although they had been taking the thyroid medication known as Synthroid™, (thus it was obviously not as effective as it should have been).

3. The basic problem is, many people have difficulty converting the T_4 thyroid, to the much more active T_3 form. Many different factors can easily undermine the efficient thyroid conversion process in the liver. One good example is Insulin resistance, associated with type II diabetes.

4. As with drugs in general, Synthroid™ not only has its share of associated side effects, but also some troubling potential risks, which should make any doctor think twice before prescribing it over a much safer, and proven effective alternative.

5. It has been reported in the *Journal of the American Medical Association*, that **Synthroid™ depletes calcium** (http://www.vitaminevi.com/Index/Drug_Index-F.htm).

6. Some **common side effects** associated with Synthroid™ include:

* Diarrhea
* **Irritability**
* Headache
* Hand Tremors
* Leg cramps
* Insomnia
* Vomiting
* **Nervousness**
* Changes in menstrual periods

7. Then, some of the **symptoms from possible overstimulation** are:

* Abdominal cramps
* **Emotional instability**
* **Heart attack or failure**
* Increased heart rate
* Shortness of breath
* Sleeplessness
* **Anxiety**
* Hair loss
* Irregular heartbeat
* **Irritability**
* Nervousness
* Muscle weakness
* Chest pain
* Headache
* **Hyperactivity**
* Tremors
* Palpitation

8. We are also warned that **Synthroid™ can interact with a wide variety of medications,** which just happen to include some widely used medications, such as:

* Oral Contraceptives
* Blood pressure medications
* **Diabetes drugs**
* **Antidepressants**
* Asthma medication
* Blood thinning drugs
* Antacids
* Diuretics
* Aspirin

9. A surprising number of women are placed on Synthroid™, (and **normally left on the drug**), yet we also find the warning that: ***"Postmenopausal women on long-term Synthroid™ therapy may suffer a loss of bone density, increasing the danger of osteoporosis* [brittle bones]"** (http://www.healthsquare.com/newrx/syn1421.htm).

10. Most importantly, **the majority of diabetics are hypothyroid (requiring thyroid medication).** They would thus be taking "diabetic drugs", which as you can see, can interact with Synthroid™! There are very few seniors today that at least one of the following risk factors would not apply to, (that is, unless they are high school seniors). Seriously though, if they continue placing children on Ritalin™ and Prozac™ at a very young age, some of the following conditions could very well apply to high school seniors as well! So let's take a look at our risky list, as one source warns us that:

> ***If you have diabetes,*** *or if your body makes insufficient adrenal corticosteroid hormone,* ***Synthroid® will tend to make your symptoms worse. Synthroid® has profound effects on the body.*** *Make sure your doctor is aware of all your medical problems, especially heart disease, clotting disorders, diabetes, and disorders of the adrenal or pituitary glands* (http://www.healthsquare.com/newrx/syn1421.htm).

While another source additionally warns:

> ***Tell your doctor if you have or have ever had diabetes;*** *hardening of the arteries (atherosclerosis); kidney disease; hepatitis; cardiovascular disease such as high blood pressure, chest pain (angina), arrhythmias, or heart attack; or an underactive adrenal or pituitary gland.*
> (http://www.nlm.nih.gov/medlineplus/druginfo/medmaster/a682461.html)

As you can easily see, we have some obvious concerns regarding the use of the Synthroid™, which most doctors insist on prescribing for a thyroid disorder that is intimately connected with both diabetes, and cardiovascular disease.

Then there is the concern of possibly experiencing some of the more serious side effects associated with overstimulation (drug overdose), such as **emotional instability** or possibly even **heart attack or failure.** That risk is greatly increased, when combined with any of the many commonly prescribed medications that Synthroid™ can interact with. I would assume that by far, the majority would also be taking at least one of the medications on the list. For instance, women are already ten times as likely to experience a low thyroid condition as men, however many women are likely taking oral contraceptives, which is not only on the list of potentially interacting drugs, but is also a known thyroid suppressant.

Also, as mentioned earlier, depression is one of the most common symptoms associated with a hypothyroid condition, and even though **"Synthroid™ seldom resolves the condition",** patients are normally placed and then left on Synthroid™. Thus another serious medication on our list of potentially interacting drugs, (an antidepressant), is often added, greatly increasing potential risks! If you recall, Mary Lou was even placed on "two antidepressants," along with Synthroid™, (which is a very risky combination). Then, as she also developed diabetes, (a common side effect of Prozac™), she was also placed on diabetes medication, which is another drug that Synthroid™ can interact with. Drugs, in combination, can become very risky, and it's difficult to find an adult on medications that is taking only one, unless they just got started on the typical drug regimen.

Many in the nation are also taking at least one over-the-counter medication such as antacids or aspirin, which also increases the potential for drug interaction. The more potentially interacting medications you find on that list, that you might possibly be taking while on Synthroid™, the greater your risk will be. Then as usual, there is a much safer alternative, known as Armour™ Thyroid, which we will now examine.

Some of the Many Benefits of Armour™ Thyroid

1. Armour™ thyroid is a natural product, and not a chemical compound, thus your liver will not attempt to remove it, as it would with Synthroid™. Consequently, your effective dosage can be more easily controlled and maintained.

2. In Armour™ thyroid we find a combination of both T_4 and T_3, in the same proportion our body normally produces. Although T_3 is approximately four times as fast acting as T_4, both actually work well together, as the T_4 helps moderate the action of T_3. Sometimes the T_3 thyroid, (if not combined with T_4), can result in overstimulation unless slowly released, as only the body can efficiently do. Although a time-release form of T_3 is available, it can only be obtained through a compounding pharmacy, and there appears to be a concern. It is very difficult (if not

impossible) to accurately achieve even distribution of the time-release agent with the T_3 thyroid hormone. Our thyroid normally produces an adequate level of T_4 thyroid, thus that is seldom the cause of the majority of hypothyroid conditions. It is instead an inefficient conversion process, and thus an insufficient level of free T_3 thyroid.

3. Companies such as *Standard Process™, Inc.*, which produce quality supplements from natural sources only, include glandulars in their formulas that they refer to as protomorphogens. They contain extracts of organs such as heart, adrenals, kidneys, liver, thymus, or thyroid, etc. The extracts are normally from either bovine (beef) or pork organs. We find they are not species specific, but instead organ specific. Thus, in our body they are not broken down as other proteins to individual amino acids, but instead go directly to the specific target organ, and are beneficial for maintaining or regenerating the specific organ intended.

As Armour™ thyroid is a glandular extract, it would likely strengthen the thyroid as well. Then, according to Dr. David Brownstein, M.D., it also contains T_1 and T_2 thyroid, as well as the beneficial cofactors calcitonin and selenium. Most importantly, although Synthroid™ seldom works, Armour™ thyroid seldom fails. The importance of proper metabolism cannot be over stressed, so getting the most effective form of thyroid hormone is essential.

4. We can only begin to appreciate the value of Armour™ thyroid, if we consider that many in the nation are needlessly placed on potentially dangerous antidepressants, when Armour™ thyroid would often resolve the depression (as well as many other conditions). And by taking a thyroid hormone that truly works, the action of all 3,000 enzymes in the body will also begin working more efficiently. Then, many who were unable to lose weight, due to insufficient metabolism, would finally be much more successful.

5. And last but definitely not least, I believe we are all aware of the tremendous deterioration to the overall body, especially the cardiovascular system, the eyes, and kidneys, associated with diabetes. And then we have **the amazing discovery of both Dr. C. D. Eaton and Dr. Broda Barnes, that thyroid therapy (using Armour™ thyroid) prevented the typical complications normally associated with their patients' diabetes!** We also find that many of the conditions we normally attribute to diabetes, are actually influenced by a hypothyroid condition, which can only be truly resolved by Armour™ thyroid (not Synthroid™).

We will next evaluate exactly how Armour™ thyroid is both formulated and regulated.

The Natural Armour™ Thyroid Versus Synthroid™

A typical response by many doctors upon a patient's request for Armour™ thyroid, seems to be that it is not as well regulated as Synthroid™. In reality, quite the opposite is actually true. Incidentally, if you have trouble getting your doctor to prescribe Armour™ thyroid, you can go to http://www.armourthyroid.com to locate doctors nearest you who prescribes Armour™ thyroid for their patients.

The problem with Synthroid™ is, like other medications, it is a chemical compound, which is treated as a toxin by the liver. Then it also interacts with many other commonly prescribed medications, as we just learned. Especially when taking multiple medications, drinking alcohol, or even eating grapefruit (which suppresses the P450 enzyme in the liver responsible for detoxification), how can anyone accurately predict the effective dosage they might get on any particular day? So, even if the amount of T_4 thyroid in Synthroid™ was closely regulated, your effective dosage can still vary considerably.

Now, let's compare that with the Armour™ thyroid. First we'll evaluate the process for producing Armour™ thyroid, in order to assure that an accurate level, and ratio of both natural T_4 and T_3 are properly maintained. We find that:

> *Armour™ Thyroid is made from desiccated (dried) pork thyroid glands. The amount of thyroid hormone present in the thyroid gland may vary from animal to animal. To ensure that Armour™ Thyroid tablets are consistently potent from tablet to tablet and lot to lot, analytical tests are performed on the thyroid powder (raw material) and on the actual tablets (finished product) to measure actual T_4 and T_3 activity.*
>
> ***Different lots of thyroid powder are mixed together and analyzed to achieve the desired ratio of T_4 to T_3 in each lot of tablets. This method ensures that each strength of Armour™ Thyroid will be consistent with the United States Pharmacopoeia (USP) official standards and specifications for desiccated thyroid lot-to-lot consistency.*** *The ratio of T_4 to T_3 equals 4.22:1 (4.22 parts of T_4 to one part of T_3)* (http://www.armourthyroid.com/faq.html#q3).

We then find that **Armour™ thyroid meets all the USP standards for accuracy and safety**, as follows:

> *Armour™ Thyroid Tablets, USP contain the labeled amounts of levothyroxin* [T_4] *and liothyronine* [T_3], *as established by the United States Pharmacopeia (USP). To meet quality standards* ***it must also pass bacteriological testing and must meet other product quality tests.*** *The ratio of Armour ™ Thyroid T_4 to T_3 is 4.22:1 (4.22 parts of T_4 to one part of T_3)* (http://www.armourthyroid.com/faq.html#q7).

If you want even more proof that should convince any doctor with an open mind, we just happen to have another opinion from a very credible source, **(The New England Journal of Medicine)!**

NEJM STUDY PROVES ARMOUR THYROID BETTER THAN SYNTHROID

> ***Patients with hypothyroidism show greater improvements in mood and brain function if they receive treatment*** **[with]** ***Armour thyroid rather than Synthroid*** *(thyroxine). Hypothyroidism, where the gland has ceased to function or been removed, is usually treated with daily doses of Synthroid. But the researchers found that substituting* ***Armour thyroid led to improvements in mood and in neuropsychological functioning.***
>
> *Not all tissues that need thyroid hormone are equally able to convert thyroxine to triiodothyronine* [T_4 to T_3], *the active form of the hormone. But most patients with hypothyroidism (reduced thyroid function) are treated only with thyroxine* [T_4]. *On 6 of 17 measures of mood and cognition -- a catchall term that refers to language, learning and memory --* ***the patients scored better after receiving Armour***

thyroid than after receiving Synthroid. *No score was better after Synthroid than after combination treatment.* ***The authors also detected biochemical evidence that thyroid hormone action was greater after treatment with Armour thyroid.*** *The patients who were on Armour thyroid had significantly higher serum concentrations of sex hormone-binding globulin.*
The New England Journal of Medicine 1999;340:424-429, 469-470
(http://internationalhealth.net/NewsArticles.htm#armour)

So the question is: Where did most doctors learn that Armour™ thyroid is not adequately regulated? Likely from the Abbott Laboratories representative who was promoting his company's product (Synthroid™). If the doctor had done his own research, he obviously would have known better.

Another thing to consider is that although **Armour™ thyroid** is standardized for its T_3 and T_4 content, it **also contains calcitonin, and selenium. Calcitonin stimulates the movement of calcium into the bones, (helping prevent osteoporosis), yet Synthroid™ actually increases the risk for osteoporosis! Selenium is a trace mineral that is not only an antioxidant, but is also necessary for the action of the enzyme 5'deiodinase, which converts T_4 thyroid hormone into the much more active T_3 thyroid hormone.**

Thus, although the Synthroid™ contains the "less active T_4 thyroid only", Armour™ also contains the more active T_3, plus the calcitonin that would help prevent osteoporosis, and even the trace mineral selenium, necessary for converting the T_4 thyroid when necessary! Yet most doctors still insist on prescribing Synthroid™ for their patients, who incidentally are mostly women, (concerned about getting osteoporosis), or are unnecessarily dealing with depression. Not only that, but many resort to taking antidepressants, as the Synthroid™ they were placed on is often ineffective in resolving their hypothyroid condition. If you consider that our thyroid normally produces the very same hormones and cofactors found in Armour™ thyroid, and that antidepressants are one of the drugs on the list of contraindications, then why in the world do doctors still insist on prescribing the "incomplete chemical T_4 form" with all its associated side effects?

Dr. Neal Rouzier discovered that many of his new patients were still suffering from typical thyroid symptoms, although they had been placed and often left on Synthroid™ (T_4) for years. The problem is, far too many don't efficiently convert the T_4 thyroid to the much more active T_3 form. However, Dr. Rouzier found that **his new patients immediately noticed a major improvement when placed on Armour™ thyroid. Yet, in spite of the noted improvement, their own personal doctor normally insisted on placing them back on Synthroid™** (artificial T_4 thyroid), and absolutely refused to prescribe Armour™ thyroid! Is there something drastically wrong with this picture?

The fact that many doctors will only prescribe Synthroid™, and absolutely refuse to prescribe Armour™ thyroid, is inexcusable. Armed with the above information, your doctor will have a difficult time justifying his or her position, if that's the case. And if your doctor still refuses to prescribe Armour™ thyroid, in my opinion a change of doctors is likely in order. Some doctors have a hard time admitting their patient might be better informed than they are, but it's your body, and thus your ultimate decision, (and not your doctor's)! Although a prescription is necessary for Armour™ thyroid, it can be obtained through *Women's International Pharmacy* by calling (800) 699-8143, or visiting http://www.womensinternational.com. Or to locate a doctor nearest you, who prescribes Armour™ thyroid, visit http://armourthyroid.com.

Natural Solutions for Promoting Healthy Thyroid Function

Remember, resolving any health issue involves first eliminating as many contributors to the condition as possible, and then adding nutrients important for restoring good health.

Following are some do-it-yourself approaches you might try first that wouldn't require finding a doctor willing to prescribe Armour™ thyroid. It is important to remember that the recommended dosage of all supplements is normally the average suggested dosage. The most beneficial dosage for a particular individual can sometimes vary considerably between individuals. A knowledgeable nutritionist should be helpful in determining which dosage of each might be appropriate for you, if you don't seem to be getting the results you were looking for. Just keep in mind that nutrients don't suppress symptoms as drugs do. Thus you shouldn't expect "immediate results", but you will achieve real results by using the proper approach.

1. **Drug withdrawal (if necessary)** should be your first priority in order to restore your health to optimum levels. Unfortunately, taking supplements will have little value, as long as you also continue taking medications that are known to deplete them. Also, as drugs only suppress symptoms, and do so in an unnatural way, you have absolutely no way of determining if a condition has been truly resolved, as long as you continue taking the medication. Drugs would only suppress symptoms and undermine any effort you might be making to truly identify the underlying issue, or effectively evaluate your progress. For instance, if you are taking pain medications, how will you possibly know when (or if) the cause of pain has been truly resolved? Suppressing symptoms is a life-long project, thus you will often be required to take medications for the remainder of your life, (very profitable for the pharmaceutical companies). Drugs are not only "not resolving the underlying condition" that is creating the symptom in the first place, but they instead allow the condition to worsen, and create others as well, (which is obvious from their side effects). Your health is in a downhill spiral as long as you remain on drugs, and most importantly, it's seldom (if ever) necessary!

If you recall, **nearly 87% of the 200 most prescribed drugs, evaluated for their nutrient depletion, were found to deplete nutrients important for healthy thyroid function.**

2. **Iodine** is critical to supporting healthy thyroid gland function, and Iodoral™ appears to be an excellent option. It's a natural iodine formula, consisting of both iodine and potassium iodide.

Dr. David Brownstein, M.D. found in a study, that **91.7% of the patients that were tested for low iodine levels, actually had an iodine deficiency.** According to Dr. Brownstein, this appears to be a huge public health problem, stating that ***"All individuals with a thyroid disorder should be screened for an iodine deficiency"*** (*Iodine: Why You Need It, Why You Can't Live Without It,* 2004, p. 99). He also notes that *"My clinical experience has proven, beyond a doubt, that a combination of iodine/iodide* [or Iodoral™] *is much more effective than an iodide only supplement"* (p. 50).

Dr. Brownstein points out that although other tissues and organs can concentrate either form, the obvious objective would be to provide both iodine and iodide, allowing the body to manage the details, (something it was designed to do). Contrary to drugs' typical "side effects", natural supplements instead have many "side benefits", which also applies to Iodoral™ (two forms of organic iodine). For example, **once you ingest the Iodoral™, it immediately gets busy eliminating "the iodine impersonators", such as chorine, fluoride, and bromine, as**

well as the heavy metal mercury, which disrupts the trace mineral selenium, responsible for thyroid enzyme conversion in the liver. You can easily see the wisdom of anyone who has been exposed to high levels of fluoride, (found in Prozac™ for instance), to begin phasing it out and ingesting Iodoral™, to start the fluoride detoxification process. Remember, fluoride is a well-known environmental toxin that somehow ended up in your antidepressant, (how depressing that would be!). Then if you consider that every single molecule of Prozac™ actually contains "three molecules of fluoride", we're talking about an unbelievably high dose of an "environmental toxin" accumulating in both the body and brain!

Then according to Dr. Brownstein, women who have low levels of iodine are much more prone to acquire breast cancer, and with men it's prostate cancer. Interestingly, over 60 years ago a man named Harry Hoxsey was curing tens of thousands of cancer patients that were sent home by their doctors to die, as they were considered as incurable, (referred to as Stage IV cancer). **Other than herbs, his cancer formula known as the Hoxsey formula, just happened to contain "potassium iodide", (one ingredient in Iodoral™)!**

3. **Celtic sea salt**, from the *Grain & Salt Society*, is an excellent source of iodine, as well as many other minerals important for supporting thyroid function, and in their natural easily absorbable ionic form. Celtic sea salt is available at most health food stores, or directly through the *Grain & Salt Society* by calling (800) TOP-SALT, or by visiting http://www.celtic-seasalt.com/.

4. **Water.** Adequate water greatly influences every part of the body, and is necessary in all areas of health. It is especially important regarding the thyroid, as dehydration is considered a stressor, contributing to thyroid suppression. According to Dr. Batmanghelidj, M.D., dehydration also causes cells to become more insulin resistant, which reduces the liver's ability to efficiently convert the thyroid hormones. I recommend ten 8-ounce glasses of water, along with 1 teaspoon of the Celtic sea salt daily.

5. **Thyromin™** is one natural option that doesn't require a prescription. It is a fairly new product used to nourish the thyroid, balance metabolism, and reduce fatigue. It was developed by Dr. N. Gary Young, N.D., and sold only through his company *Young Living™ Essential Oils*. Thyromin™ contains a combination of specially selected glandular nutrients, herbs, amino acids, minerals, and essential oils. All the oils are therapeutic-grade and perfectly balanced to bring about the most beneficial and nutritional support to the thyroid. Thyromin™ contains vitamin E, Iodine, Potassium, CoQ_{10}, L-cysteine, and adrenal/pituitary extracts from bovine sources. It also contains the essential oils peppermint, spearmint, myrtle, and myrrh.

It is best taken at bedtime, starting with 2 capsules immediately before going to sleep. Then check your temperature first thing in the following morning, and if your basal temperature indicates no improvement, add 1 additional capsule that morning. If there is still no significant improvement by the next morning, then increase the dosage to 2 capsules in the morning and 2 at night, as Dr. Young notes it is best to take half of the total amount at night and half in the morning. Continue using this stepped approach until your temperature reaches the correct range (97.8° - 98.6°). According to Dr. Young, another product called VitaGreen™ (also sold only through *Young Living™ Essential Oils*) will also enhance the effect of the Thyromin™. For a *Young Living™* distributor nearest you, call (800) 371-2928 or visit http://www.youngliving.com.

6. **Selenium.** As previously mentioned, Dr. David Brownstein, M.D. has observed that **selenium-deficient individuals are almost always hypothyroid**. Selenium has also been shown to elevate mood and decrease anxiety, with the recommended daily dosage being 200 mcg of selenium yeast (the most absorbable form). Selenium is important for the enzyme in the liver that converts the T_4 thyroid hormone to the more active T_3 form.

7. **Vitamin A.** Insufficient vitamin A can cause a deterioration of the pituitary gland's basophil cells where the thyroid-stimulating hormone is synthesized, limiting the amount of iodine that the thyroid gland can absorb, and reducing the amount of thyroid hormone it produces. Vitamin A can be depleted by substances such as cholesterol-lowering drugs, antibiotics, caffeine, alcohol, and bad fats. One tablespoon of cod liver oil naturally contains approximately 4,500 IU. Normally 25,000 IU of supplemental vitamin A (in soft gels) daily should be sufficient, unless you have liver disease, in which case it is recommended that you not exceed 10,000 IU daily.

8. **Vitamin B-complex.** Vitamin B_2 (riboflavin) strongly influences how well the thyroid gland synthesizes its hormones. Sufficient vitamin B_3 (niacin) is essential to the good health of all glands, especially the thyroid, by assisting in the respiration of cells and the efficient metabolism of carbohydrates, fats and protein. A thyroid gland deficient in vitamin B_6 (pyridoxine) has difficulty converting iodine into thyroid hormone. In fact, in one study, when cattle were fed a diet resulting in a vitamin B_{12} deficiency, there was a significant reduction in the conversion of T_4 to T_3. At the same time, low thyroid function decreases our ability to absorb vitamin B_{12}. As you can see, vitamins are codependent. Thus, the best solution is to take a good 100 mg B-complex vitamin daily, which includes all the B-vitamins. It's not recommended that you take individual B vitamins without also taking the entire B complex as well. Keep in mind that microwave cooking can destroy the majority of B vitamins (60 to 90 percent) in your food.

9. **Vitamin D** is necessary for healthy thyroid function. Vitamin D is commonly depleted by such things as alcohol, antidepressants, antibiotics, aspirin, smoking, stress, and all cholesterol-lowering drugs, just to name a few. 1,000 IU daily should be adequate. Although, during the winter months, when you are not getting as much exposure to the sun, you would be more inclined to be deficient in vitamin D.

10. **Tyrosine.** For the thyroid hormone to form, a biochemical union of the amino acid tyrosine and iodine must occur. **Tyrosine is commonly depleted by estrogen and oral contraceptives.** It's easy to see why women are ten times as likely to experience a low thyroid condition than men are. Although meat, fish, and eggs contain tyrosine, some may benefit from 1,000 mg of supplemental tyrosine daily.

11. **Zinc** levels appear to be directly correlated with levels of the active thyroid hormone T3. According to David Brownstein, M.D. (*Overcoming Thyroid Disorders*, 2002), ***"My experience has clearly shown a decrease in the conversion of T4 into T3 in zinc deficient individuals"*** (p. 67). The suggested dosage is 50 mg daily, (do not exceed 100 mg total daily). If you recall, selenium is also involved in that process.

12. **DHEA** (**D**e**h**ydro**e**pi**a**ndrosterone) increases sensitivity to thyroid production, or conversion in the liver. 25 mg daily is normally recommended for women, and 50 mg for men.

13. **Relora™** is an herbal formula containing magnolia and philodendron, and is available at most health food stores. **It has two important functions: Reducing the stress hormone cortisol (which suppresses the thyroid), while increasing the level of DHEA.** Elevated cortisol, (caused by stress and SSRI antidepressants), actually lowers the level of DHEA, (which assists in thyroid hormone production). The recommended dosage is 150 mg, three times daily.

14. Iron deficiency has been reported to impair the body's ability to make its own thyroid hormones. In my opinion, the best source of organic iron is blackstrap molasses, which is also a good source of organic sulfur. One tablespoon daily should normally be sufficient.

15. Foods that enhance the production of thyroid hormones are: Sea vegetables (kelp, dulse), garlic, radishes, egg yolk, wheat germ and brewer's yeast.

16. **Valerian root.** As we have learned, stress hormones are a major contributor to thyroid suppression, and Valerian is a very effective herb for relieving stress. It is fast acting, perfectly safe, and doesn't cause drowsiness. I would recommend taking two capsules (450 mg each) anytime you experience stress. Valerian is an inexpensive herb, and should be available at your local health food store.

17. TG100 is a non-prescription item that contains 40 mg of thyroid tissue, along with 5 mg each of adrenal, pancreas, thymus, and spleen tissue, plus 120 mg of vitamin C (ascorbic acid). The other glandulars are important for supporting the thyroid function.

I found that the combination of Iodoral™ (potassium iodide / iodine) and TG100™ was effective in maintaining my wife's metabolism, without the necessity of using thyroid hormones. I have her take 1 capsule of TG100™, along with 1 tablet of Iodoral™, twice daily, (once in the morning and again in the evening). The best dosage might vary with individuals, which is true with all supplements. It will obviously be more effective if you can also avoid as many thyroid suppressants as possible. TG100™ can be purchased through *Women's International Pharmacy* by calling (800) 699-8143, or by visiting http://www.womensinternational.com.

18. **Armour™ Thyroid**. One last thought: If all else fails, you can always attempt to find a doctor who would be willing to prescribe Armour™ thyroid. As previously mentioned, one solution to that problem is to call a pharmacy such as the *Women's International Pharmacy* at (800) 699-8143, which handles Armour™ thyroid, as well as other bio-identical (natural to the body) hormones, and ask for a list of doctors who prescribe Armour™ thyroid in your area. You can also find a complete list of doctors in your zip code area that are familiar with Armour™ thyroid, and can prescribe it for their patients, by visiting their Website http://www.armourthyroid.com.

A Summary On the Importance Of Adequate Thyroid Function

The importance of maintaining adequate thyroid function (or metabolism), for efficient detoxification, and maintaining optimum energy levels, as well as maintaining a healthy weight, can't be overstressed. It's also important for avoiding depression, edema (fluid retention), and fibroid tumors, as well as many other undesirable conditions. Just remember, the efficient action of all 3,000 enzymes in the body and brain depend upon your body temperature, and just one degree can make a major difference. That is especially a concern for women, who are "ten times" as likely as men, to experience a hypothyroid (low thyroid) condition.

As you are now likely aware, the thyroid system in general is very sensitive to both thyroid suppressants, and proper nutrition, (and at times the proper thyroid hormone). Once your thyroid function is normalized, many undesirable conditions will soon begin disappearing.

A Word Of Caution – And An Observation

Just don't ever allow yourself to get caught in the web (of the madness in medicine), as Mary Lou and many others unknowingly did. It all began with an undiagnosed and untreated hypothyroid condition (which was the underlying cause of her depression) that eventually led to prescriptions for nine "totally unnecessary medications". So, sixteen years after Mary Lou received the original prescription for the new wonder-drug Prozac™, which was eventually followed by the other eight, I discovered that she still seemed to be dealing with a hypothyroid condition, because she had been taking the wrong form of thyroid (Synthroid™) that seldom works, although it is the thyroid hormone that **most doctors insist on prescribing!**

Far too many adults (such as Mary Lou) have been unnecessarily placed on more and more medications, due to what I refer to as the typical domino effect. Basically, drugs are often prescribed just to treat the side effects of your other drugs. Unfortunately, the pharmaceutical industry is now turning to our innocent children as another financial resource, and we can't possibly allow that to continue any longer!

Dr. Matthias Rath, M.D. states the problem rather well, in his own words, as follows: ***"We live in an era in which 98% of pharmaceutical preparations have no proven beneficial effects, in which the pharmaceutical industry has created the fourth largest cause of death herself, the side effects of medication, with the sole purpose of creating new markets for its products"*** (http://www.rath-eduserv.com/English/index/html).

It is beyond belief that after decades of research and trillions of dollars invested, the obvious continues to be overlooked. The basic problem is: The true solutions, (as well as disease prevention), are not profitable. Unless we change our priorities in medicine, and place our health before profit, we will continue to experience an increase in our rate of disease, along with the constant escalation of the cost of our healthcare, in the nation.

We must finally take a stand and say: I will now take more responsibility for my own health, and my very first step will be to no longer be held hostage by my medications, and begin phasing them out of my life forever. And as I mentioned, those who chose to do so found it was perfectly safe, and surprisingly easy, as they normally never needed them all those years to begin with. They are quite often just an inappropriate response, (some symptom-suppressing drug), for some condition that was not properly addressed. And as we discovered, resorting to those drugs just leads to more drugs, due to the nutrient depletion and side effects associated with drugs in general. Remember to play it safe, and monitor your levels (such as your blood pressure and blood sugar). It's important that you listen to your body, and use caution during your withdrawal. It will definitely be worth your effort. If you would be more comfortable having a doctor's assistance, that's perfectly OK. Just make sure that your doctor's goals are the same as yours. If not, I suggest you find a doctor who is familiar with nutrition, and willing to assist you with your withdrawal. Best of luck in your effort!

CHAPTER FOURTEEN

Hypoglycemia – A Very Controllable Condition Often Confused With Hypothyroidism

The Symptoms All Too Often Lead To A Prescription For An Antidepressant, Which Just Makes Matters Worse!

The various symptoms associated with hypoglycemia are typical of the very symptoms that so many children (and adults) are being placed on medications for. Depression is one common symptom associated with hypoglycemia, and as a result, many are being placed on Prozac™, or some other SSRI antidepressant, for typical hypoglycemic (low blood sugar) symptoms. The primary reason is, most doctors were never trained in nutrition. Thus, their response is normally some drug for suppressing a condition. Prozac™ stimulates the release of glucose from the liver, due to the major increase in the stress hormone cortisol, resulting in the daily elevation of glucose and insulin, thus Prozac™ would not only worsen the hypoglycemia, but it would also precipitate the progression from hypoglycemia to type II diabetes as well.

Hypoglycemia is often a precursor that eventually leads to diabetes. They are both blood sugar related disorders, meaning that they both affect the body's ability to use sugar effectively, thus the same basic therapy actually applies to both. Unfortunately, drugs such as Prozac™ increase the progression of hypoglycemia to diabetes, when just a simple diet modification along with a few nutritional supplements should instead reverse the process, as you are about to learn. I don't know about you, but that certainly makes a lot more sense to me. In his book *How to Eat Your Way Out of Fatigue* (1969), Dr. Clement G. Martin, M.D. does an excellent job of describing the symptoms of hypoglycemia, as follows:

> ***Profound brain damage is, unfortunately, an anticipated result when the disease had progressed long enough.***
>
> *The outstanding symptom is fatigue.* ***Most commonly both mental and physical,*** *though it can be only one or the other. Sudden sweating, varying from mild to an absolute drench, is a not too infrequent sign. These may be accompanied by chills, and usually the feeling of weakness grows greatest because the blood sugar is dropping rapidly in these sessions. This is the point where there is a real craving for food – some high energy food most likely. It might be candy, coffee and a sweet roll or some other pastry.* ***Marked obesity is apt to be the eventual result of this disease if it is allowed to persist.***
>
> *Fortunately, the treatment is simple and largely dietary* (pp. 13, 21, 31).

Although hypoglycemia is occasionally influenced by heredity, Dr. Martin claims that **ninety-five percent of hypoglycemia is considered to be self-caused by diet.** However, Dr. Martin's book was written in 1969, which was before we were blessed with Prozac™ and the other SSRI antidepressants that soon followed, (as well as the ADHD drugs such as the stimulants Ritalin™ and Adderall™) that many are currently taking. Their effects on blood sugar levels are well known, and explained below by Dr. Diana Schwarzbein, M.D., as follows:

> ***Stimulants cause insulin levels to rise too high, which stimulates an excessive rush of stored serotonin – a temporary rush – which is quickly used up. Then, because serotonin levels drop rapidly, you begin to feel down again. This depletion sets up a vicious cycle:*** *You experience the symptoms of low serotonin, and in response you eat an excess of carbohydrates or use stimulants to obtain the rush of serotonin again* (*The Schwarzbein Principal*, 1999, p. 42).

According to a list of the 200 most prescribed drugs, a total of 102 prescription medications (51%) actually list diabetes, hypoglycemia or blood sugar fluctuations as a potential side effect, or note that taking that drug will worsen the condition or interfere with its treatment. And on that same list, more than 91% of the medications that had been tested were found to deplete nutrients that either assist in treating diabetes, controlling blood sugar, (or contribute to diabetes or hypoglycemia when deficient).

Interestingly, **the symptoms of hypoglycemia (low blood sugar) and hypothyroidism (low thyroid) are almost identical, and in many cases they actually are identical!** That is an important issue that many doctors fail to recognize. If you stop to think about it, the brain requires both adequate thyroid hormone, and glucose, in order to provide energy, and both are equally important. So you would expect the brain to react in a similar way, if there was a deficiency of either. It's basically attempting to get your attention, and hoping you will respond appropriately, (and not with some drug)!

Typical symptoms associated with hypoglycemia, as well as a low thyroid condition, are depression, mood swings, difficulty with concentration, poor memory, fatigue, irritability, anxiety, and insomnia. Other symptoms of hypoglycemia may include cravings for sweets and constant hunger, as well as **becoming very aggressive at times, losing their tempers easily,** most commonly occurring a few hours after eating sweets or fats. This is the type of behavior that many children are placed on various medications for, (which medication often depends on which pharmaceutical rep was the most convincing, or sometimes even the most attractive). This is an issue that pharmaceutical companies are very aware of.

Resolving Hypoglycemia Without Drugs

The first plan of action is to assure the brain receives a steady supply of energy; not just an excess one minute, stimulating an inappropriate elevation of insulin in the process, and soon a deficiency of glucose to follow. This normally results from consuming too much simple sugars, or drinking alcoholic beverages, which are rapidly absorbed, and deficient in nutrients necessary for their own metabolism, or for producing "quality insulin", (as not all insulin is created equal). It also contributes to insulin resistance, which is the very same principal as mind-altering drugs (stimulating an excess of a hormone, followed by a deficiency). Both lead to hormone receptors becoming resistant, whether it's insulin or serotonin, the same basic principle applies.

Rather than the typical solution of resorting to the use of diabetic medications, in an attempt to reduce the blood sugar (often causing or worsening hypoglycemia), as usual there is a much better solution, as you are about to discover. I might mention that diabetic medications actually deplete some nutrients necessary for producing insulin!

Supplying Adequate Energy For Your Brain

Although glucose is sometimes considered the only source of energy for the brain, another excellent source is **Celtic sea salt (from the *Grain & Salt Society*), with all its minerals still intact, along with water (free of chlorine and fluoride).** This is a potential resource that even many natural practitioners are still unaware of, although something I learned from Dr. Batmanghelidj several years ago.

Water is essential for healthy receptors, and dehydration causes insulin receptors to become resistant. An adequate intake of water should resolve the problem. Water is also necessary for preventing acidosis (low pH) in the body, as well as maintaining all aspects of good health. Water is an excellent solvent, and important for the effective removal of toxins.

Celtic sea salt contains 84 trace minerals, all in their natural ionic, easily assimilatable form. Two of those trace minerals are chromium and vanadium, both beneficial for maintaining stable blood sugar and improving insulin utilization. Celtic sea salt also contains both sodium and potassium, necessary for maintaining a proper pH balance, thus avoiding acidosis (which also reduces insulin sensitivity). They also function as a team in the transfer of nutrients into cells, as well as the removal of toxins.

According to Dr. Batmanghelidj, ***"A low salt diet is not conductive to the correction of a diabetic's high blood sugar."*** He also notes that: *"The brain is designed to resuscitate itself,* ***when there is water and salt shortage in the body. It raises the levels of sugar in circulation. If the blood sugar is to come down, a slight upward adjustment of daily salt intake may become unavoidable****"* (*Your Body's Many Cries For Water*, 1992/1998, pp. 125–127).

I would suggest taking one teaspoon of sea salt, along with ten 8-ounce glasses of non-chlorinated, non-fluoridated water daily. Celtic sea salt is available at most health food stores, or directly through the *Grain & Salt Society* by calling (800) TOP-SALT, or by visiting http://www.celtic-seasalt.com/.

The amino acid L-glutamine is another source of energy for the brain, which also reduces carbohydrate cravings, and helps prevent hypoglycemia. According to a study at Louisiana State University Medical College, 2 grams of glutamine were given to nine healthy athletes 45 minutes after a light breakfast in the morning, and it was reported that ***"Blood levels of growth hormone rose 430 percent above initial levels 90 minutes after glutamine supplementation"*** (*American Journal of Clinical Nutrition*, 1995, Vol. 61, pp. 1058-1061).

Glutamine is quickly depleted by prolonged exercise and other stressors, and the more stress you're under, the sooner your glutamine supply is depleted. This was proven when the health status of more than 150 runners were compared in a study at Oxford University, as follows: *"Half of the test subjects were given 5 grams of glutamine after a strenuous bout of exercise, while the other half took a placebo.* ***Almost twice as many in the group with glutamine stayed healthy during the next 7 days compared to the placebo"*** (*Sports Medicine*, 1996, Vol. 21, pp. 80-97).

L-glutamine comes in both powder and capsules, with the recommended dosage between 2 to 5 grams daily. Remember that 1 gram = 1,000 mg. Sometimes body builders take five grams following a workout!

Maintaining a healthy pH (7 to 7.4) helps provide the brain with the necessary oxygen it requires for the energy to metabolize nutrients. The best way to **deplete** oxygen is to produce an acidic environment in the body, as more oxygen is required to neutralize the pH. Although oxygen helps increase the pH (or reduce acidity), it is depleted in the process. Thus, in order to preserve oxygen, we should maintain a healthy pH. The more high alkaline (low acid) foods we eat, the healthier the pH level will normally be. Keep in mind that, although common table salt is acidic, Celtic sea salt is instead alkaline!

You should be able to purchase pH-testing paper in a roll, at most pharmacies and health food stores. On the back of the dispenser you will find a chart with colors identifying your pH level. One common tape, which comes in a roll, is called Phydron™. It can evaluate a pH ranging from 5.5 (yellow, very acidic) to 8.0 (blue, very alkaline), and in between (varying shades of green). The healthy saliva range falls somewhere between 7.0 and 7.4. **Most people are too acidic**, (although too alkaline is not considered healthy either). It's very similar to maintaining a healthy pH or acid/alkaline balance in your swimming pool.

You can find an excellent list of foods that are alkaline, and those more acidic, as well as their pH ratings, at http://www.thewolfeclinic.com/acidalkfoods.html. Just keep in mind that drugs (legal or illegal, prescription or over-the-counter) are acidic, as is sugar, alcohol and soft drinks. Water (free of chlorine and fluoride) is instead alkaline. Incidentally, cancer thrives in an acidic (oxygen deficient) environment. Cancer patients often have a pH ranging from 4.5 to 5, which is very acidic. An acidic condition also causes cravings for sugar, alcohol, soft drinks, and caffeine, (which are all very acidic). Just remember, the more acidic the body is (the lower the pH), the more oxygen will be depleted.

Dietary Suggestions For The Hypoglycemic - What To Eat and Why To Eat It

Just as the **cause** of this disease is often due to eating the wrong diet, the **solution** is often in eating the correct diet. It is important to remember that everything you put into your mouth will affect your blood sugar and insulin levels in some way, and that all carbohydrates are definitely **not** created equal. Generally, it is the combination of fiber, proteins, and fats consumed during a meal, as well as the amount of each that will help control blood sugar levels and the production of insulin.

✓ **In general, hypoglycemics should eat as many low glycemic foods in their diet as possible.** The glycemic index is a classification of carbohydrates and their blood glucose-raising potential, determined by measuring their rate of entry into the bloodstream. An extensive list of foods and their glycemic indexes can be found at http://www.mendosa.com/gilists.htm.

✓ **Fiber,** (also known as roughage), is the indigestible remnants of plant cells. Consuming small amounts of fiber with everything you eat is an extremely effective way to manage insulin levels. According to researchers at UCLA, obese men were allowed to eat as much high-fiber, low-fat food as they wanted, combined with daily exercise, for **three weeks.** At the end of that time, they were still overweight, but ***"their high blood pressure was reversed; cholesterol dropped 20%, insulin levels dropped 46%. No drug in the world can do this"*** (*Fearless Health*, Dr. Julian Whitaker, M.D., pp. 29-30).

Although very few foods in the typical American diet provide two or more grams of soluble fiber per serving, it is possible to boost fiber levels slightly with certain raw vegetables (especially lima beans, Brussels sprouts, zucchini, and squash), fruits (especially cantaloupe, dried prunes, raisins, and papaya), seeds (especially flax), and oatmeal or oat bran. Unfortunately, the refining process removes much of the natural fiber from our foods, as well as their protective coating of fiber (as in the case of white rice). Fiber supplements are also available, such as Glucomannan, guar gum, lignin, or pectin.

Be sure not to take any fiber with fat-soluble vitamins (such as vitamins A, D, E, and K), as the fiber can absorb and remove them, and thus reduce their effectiveness. Excessive amounts of fiber may also decrease the absorption of zinc, iron, and calcium, thus it's best to take fiber separately from your supplements.

✓ **Protein**, in moderate amounts, can slow digestion and sugar absorption (as does fat and fiber), preventing insulin spikes after a meal. In fact, eating a small amount of protein with everything you eat can be very beneficial in maintaining stable blood sugar levels. Eggs are an excellent source of protein! In case you're the least bit concerned, although eggs do contain cholesterol, they will not increase your cholesterol level. Cholesterol is involved in many important functions, in both the body and brain. Some other good protein sources are nuts, fish, and poultry.

However, too much protein (especially meat) can cause your body to become highly acidic (promoting the release of insulin), as well as increasing the need for additional thyroid hormone. But most importantly regarding blood sugar, in his book *The Rosedale Diet* (2004), Dr. Ron Rosedale, M.D. warns us:

> ***Protein that the body doesn't quickly use to repair or make new cells is largely broken down into simple sugars, which increases blood sugar and promotes insulin resistance.*** *Furthermore, protein itself triggers insulin production, which can worsen insulin resistance. (That is why* ***diabetics should never go on a very high protein diet.****)*
>
> *The more protein you eat, the more proficient you become at making glucose from the protein in your diet, and from the protein in your muscle and bone. As I tell my diabetic patients, this is something that you don't want to be good at!* (pp. 13, 23).

✓ **Good fats** not only prevent insulin receptors from becoming insulin resistant, but fat also slows digestion (just like fiber and protein), which reduces the absorption rate of sugar into the bloodstream, preventing insulin spikes after a meal.

"Good fats" are found in the omega-3 Essential Fatty Acids (EFAs), which include Docosahexaenoic acid (DHA), eicosapentaenoic acid (EPA), gamma linolenic acid (GLA), and conjugated linoleic acid (CLA), and are also known as "good" polyunsaturated fats. CLA is also beneficial for weight loss, and is normally found in soft gels, at your local health food store.

Although the body cannot produce these fats, they can be found in cold water fatty fish, fish oil, flax seed oil, deep green vegetables, algae, and some nuts. You can also purchase fish oil or flax seed oil in liquid or soft gel form, also normally available at your local health food store.

It is important to be aware that there are numerous dietary and lifestyle factors that can decrease and even eliminate any potential benefits that may be obtained through consuming EFAs. Some examples are the consumption of sugar, alcohol, and trans (bad) fats, as well as a lack of vitamins and minerals (often depleted by medications).

Other good fats are monounsaturated (omega-9) fatty acids, primarily found in cold-pressed extra virgin olive oil, extra virgin coconut oil, avocado, and nuts. Other healthy saturated fats are also found in salmon, walnuts, olives, lamb and goat meat, goat's and sheep's milk and cheese, and other properly prepared dairy products, such as butter produced from the milk of grass-fed animals free from growth hormones.

Unfortunately, the typical non-organic pasteurized milk that most people normally drink today comes from cows that have been fed hormones and antibiotics. Once milk has been pasteurized, it no longer contains the good bacteria, or the good enzymes, vitamins, minerals, and good fats that raw fresh unpasteurized milk contains. Keep in mind that non-fat products (especially dairy) are naturally a bit higher on the glycemic index because they have had the fat removed (the fat is what slows the rate of digestion, and sugar absorption into the bloodstream).

Saturated fats tend to be solid at room temperature, and are normally found in tropical oils such as **processed** coconut, palm and palm kernel oils. When fats are heated, their bonds change and they soon become trans fatty acids. Regardless of whether they started out good or not, they are irrevocably changed for the worse when heated or hydrogenated, thus they should obviously not be used for cooking.

✓ **Eat plenty of flax**. Flax seeds are both a rich source of omega-3 fatty acids (as they contain flax seed oil), as well as a good source of fiber. You can get as much as 20 grams of fiber from ¼ cup of ground flax seeds! Flax seed is an easy, effective, and inexpensive way to bring more balance to blood sugar levels. Flax seeds in bulk are very inexpensive. You can normally purchase a grinder for approximately $20. Just grind and take a couple tablespoons with 8 ounces of water prior to a meal. Another option might be adding a tablespoon or two of flax seeds ground into your soups, salads, or cereal. Flax seeds oxidize fairly rapidly when exposed to light or oxygen, once the seed is ground and the oil is released. Thus either grind it just before you use it, or store the ground seeds in a dark container in the refrigerator.

Flax seed oil is another option. The oil must be kept refrigerated and will stay fresh for up to 8 weeks after it is opened, or it can safely be kept frozen for at least a year. Never expose flax oil to direct heat, as it contains EFAs and will become trans fatty acids. However, flax oil works well as a salad dressing base, or added to hot cereal, soup, sauces, or dips as well. It can also be taken as a supplement in the soft gel form, if you prefer.

✓ **Raw vegetables** are an excellent source of fiber, however it is important to remember that cooking changes everything! Heat breaks down the fiber, changing the quality of the vegetable to a more readily available form of carbohydrate, causing a more rapid release of blood sugar. Some examples of vegetables with the very lowest glycemic index are: asparagus, artichoke, cucumber, fennel, lettuce, bell peppers, tomatoes, avocados, green beans, broccoli, cabbage, kale, collards, parsley, cilantro and cauliflower.

✓ **Fresh fruit.** The body can more efficiently utilize fruit in its natural state: FRESH. There is considerably less nutritional benefit from eating processed fruit, or fruit that has been altered by heat in any way. This includes canned fruit, cooked applesauce, baked apples, etc. Remember, heat breaks down the fiber in foods, necessary for controlling blood sugar levels, thus raising the glycemic index. Cooking also alters the fruit's pH balance, leaving them more acidic, which increases insulin production.

✓ **Ezekiel 4:9™ bread** is made of sprouted organically grown grains and legumes, sea salt, water and yeast, with no added flour, and should thus not cause a sudden spike in blood sugar. This bread is often found in the freezer section of your local grocery store or health food store. If not, you can call the makers, *Food For Life Baking Company*, at (800) 797-5090 for a location nearest you, or visit their Website at http://www.food-for-life.com/. Ezekiel 4:9™ Flourless Organic Sprouted Grain bread is the only bread I am aware of that is a complete protein, which by itself should assist in maintaining blood sugar levels. It contains 18 amino acids, including all nine essential amino acids, as well as fiber. In order to maintain freshness, it should remain frozen until eaten.

Things You Should Avoid To Maintain Healthy Blood Sugar

✓ **Sugar (which also includes fructose, glucose, corn sweeteners, corn syrup, fruit sugar, table sugar, and brown sugar), and simple carbohydrates.** As stated by Dr. Ron Rosedale, M.D. (*The Rosedale Diet*, 2004), ***"A bowl of cereal is a bowl of sugar, a slice of bread (with few exceptions) is a slice of sugar, and a potato is a big lump of sugar.*** *Unfortunately, these are the foods that have become the mainstay of the American diet"* (p. 77).

✓ **Simple carbohydrates (starchy foods), such as corn, noodles, pasta, white rice, white potatoes, and white bread.** According to an article in *The McAlvany Health Alert* (January 2004 issue), **eighty-five percent of the grains we consume are refined (meaning the healthy fiber and nutrients have been removed) before they ever reach our plate.** The *"enriched grains"* that most people consume in processed food, not only contribute to insulin resistance, but they also deplete vitamins, especially the B vitamins.

✓ **Bad fats (trans-fatty acids) and fried foods. This includes bacon, cold cuts, gravies, ham, and sausage.**

✓ **Overcooking your food.** Heat changes everything, and not for the better.

- When food is overcooked, fiber is lost, changing the quality of the food and allowing it to be more quickly absorbed into the bloodstream. Thus, the glycemic index of the food rises, (sometimes dramatically). Hog farmers discovered years ago that, although pigs would not put on weight when fed raw vegetables, that soon changed once they were fed cooked vegetables. It proved to be worth the added expense of cooking their food.
- The following important nutrients are depleted by heat and cooking: Vitamin B_1 (thiamine), vitamin B_5, vitamin B_6, folic acid, vitamin C, vitamin D, vitamin E, and bioflavonoids.
- Overcooked food can become acidic, which in turn promotes insulin production.
- And, overcooking food destroys the natural digestive enzymes, making digestion more difficult. Digestive enzymes with a meal could be helpful in this case.

✓ **An acid pH.** A diet of acidic foods, causing an acid pH, contributes to insulin insensitivity (or resistance), which causes too much insulin to be produced, (one contributor to hypoglycemia).

✓ **Microwave cooking**. The very worst form of cooking for nutrient depletion, as well as changing the natural structure of not only foods, but also water (which is also important). For details, read about the nutrients depleted by Microwave Cooking, in the next chapter (regarding Other Possible Contributors to Depression).

✓ **Alcohol**. It is a carbohydrate, derived from grain or fruit or both, which are all forms of sugar. After the initial sugar rush (which rapidly raises insulin levels), extremely low blood sugar levels soon follow, resulting in hypoglycemia, as well as depleting many important nutrients.

✓ **Stress, caffeine, nicotine, and other stimulants (i.e. Ritalin™)**. When the body is stressed for any reason, it stimulates the secretion of insulin, as well as stress hormones, which results in a surge of glucose into a system that is often already burdened with excess sugar. **This can contribute to the destruction of the beta cells in the pancreas, as well as the**

suppression of insulin receptors, leading to insulin resistance and type II diabetes. Prozac™ also stimulates the release of the stress hormone cortisol.

✓ **Artificial sweeteners**. Did you ever wonder why so many of the obese actually drink diet beverages, yet are still overweight? It obviously doesn't work. NutraSweet™ (aspartame) is by far the most popular artificial sweetener. When anything sweet enters our mouth, the body assumes it is sugar, and thus secretes insulin to deal with it. When no sugar follows, and the two stimulating amino acids in aspartame (phenylalanine and aspartic acid) also kick in, you are basically creating hypoglycemia, and thus a craving for carbohydrates to feed the brain, (a perfect way to create the many undesirable symptoms associated with hypoglycemia, and contribute to weight gain as well). Most people assume that, as NutraSweet™ contains no calories, they can drink all they want, (and they often do). Another ingredient in NutraSweet™, which is of particular concern, is ethyl alcohol, which converts to the brain toxin formaldehyde, in the body. You should stop trying to trick Mother Nature – it just won't work!

Additional Supplements Helpful For Regulating Blood Sugar

As I've mentioned before, the recommended dosage of all supplements is normally the average suggested dosage. The most beneficial dosage for a particular individual can sometimes vary considerably between individuals. A knowledgeable nutritionist should be helpful in determining which dosage of each might be the most appropriate for you or your child, if you are not getting the desired results.

Vitamins

✓ **Vitamin B-complex.** I would recommend that everyone take a good vitamin B-100 complex. A vitamin B_6 deficiency is more common in those with diabetes or hypoglycemia, thus I would recommend they also take an additional 100 mg of vitamin B_6. It is involved in more important actions than any other B vitamin, and vitamin B_6 levels tend to decrease as we age.

✓ **Vitamin C** is something we all need, although diabetics need it most. If you smoke, you need it even more, as smoking is well known for depleting vitamin C. Vitamin C reduces the cravings for both sugar and alcohol, and is calming to the nervous system. It is especially important for repairing damage to the epitheal (smooth muscle) cells in the vascular system (blood vessels), caused by both elevated blood sugar and insulin.

Although the ascorbic acid form of vitamin C is acidic, ester-C is not, and the body also utilizes ester-C more efficiently. The best form of ester-C also includes bioflavonoids, which help strengthen the arteries and capillaries.

If you are a non-smoker, and a non-diabetic, 1,000 mg twice daily should normally be adequate. Although, if you are coming down with a virus, or just had an injury or surgery, I would recommend 10,000 mg in divided doses daily. I would recommend 5,000 mg in divided daily doses for a diabetic or smoker.

✓ **Biotin, a member of the B vitamin family,** enhances glucose utilization and is beneficial in diabetic neuropathy. **A deficiency can produce high blood sugar.** Although 100 mcg – 200 mcg of biotin is usually included in most B-complex formulas, according to *The Life Extension Foundation's Disease Prevention and Treatment, Expanded Fourth Edition* (1997/2003), the recommended diabetic dosage is considerably higher, at 8,000 mcg – 16,000 mcg daily. That is equal to 8 mg – 16 mg (1,000 mcg = 1 mg).

✓ **Vitamin D** reduces insulin resistance, just as a deficiency of vitamin D increases insulin resistance. Vitamin D also enhances the immune system. I would recommend 400 IU in the summer, and 800 IU in the winter, as our body produces vitamin D when we are exposed to the sunlight.

✓ **Vitamin E** improves insulin sensitivity, and reduces blood glucose levels. I would recommend 800 IU daily.

✓ **Vitamin K** assists in converting glucose to glycogen for storage in the liver, and enhances the immune system. In fact, vitamin K may actually protect the body from both abnormal insulin response to sugar, and insulin resistance. It also helps escort calcium to the bones, where it belongs. **A deficiency interferes with insulin release and glucose regulation.** I would recommend 10 mg daily.

Minerals

✓ **Chromium** is necessary for maintaining stable blood sugar levels through proper insulin utilization, and assists in the treatment of diabetes and hypoglycemia. A deficiency can produce anxiety, fatigue, glucose intolerance (especially in diabetics), and increased risk of arteriosclerosis. **Deficiency symptoms parallel those of diabetes, yet it's one of the minerals depleted by diabetic medications!** Refined carbohydrates and sugar also deplete chromium. I know of several people who were able to eliminate their diabetic medications, just by reducing their intake of sugar and taking 800 mcg of chromium picolinate daily (400 mcg, twice daily). Sometimes, just replacing soft drinks and fruit juices, (often sweetened with high fructose corn syrup), with water, was all that was necessary to stabilize their blood sugar and eliminate hypoglycemia.

✓ **Magnesium** is necessary for maintaining the body's proper pH balance, as well as **maintaining stable blood sugar levels. A magnesium deficiency is often mistaken as diabetes.** Magnesium is a very important mineral, involved in 300 different enzyme actions in the body. I would recommend approximately 750 mg daily.

✓ **Manganese is necessary for blood sugar regulation,** and enhances the immune system. **A deficiency can produce abnormalities in insulin secretion and impaired glucose metabolism.** 10 mg daily should normally be adequate.

✓ **Potassium** is necessary for maintaining the body's proper pH balance. **One symptom of a potassium deficiency is diabetes.** 100 mg daily should be beneficial.

✓ **Zinc improves insulin action, and is actually one element of insulin.** Some symptoms of zinc deficiency include diabetes, obesity, and thyroid disorders. I would recommend taking 50 mg daily, (just don't exceed 100 mg).

Coenzyme Q_{10}

✓ **CoQ_{10} has proven beneficial in the treatment of diabetes, as it stabilizes blood sugar and improves circulation. A deficiency has been linked to diabetes.** I would recommend 100 mg daily. However, if you have been taking statin (cholesterol lowering) drugs or any other medications known to deplete this important nutrient, I would suggest taking 200 mg daily, at least for a few months. CoQ_{10} also has tremendous cardiovascular benefits, and is especially beneficial for the heart.

MSM (Methyl sulfonyl methane)

✓ **MSM is a special type of dietary sulfur** produced from DMSO, and is beneficial for promoting the flexibility of our cells. **Sulfur is especially important for diabetics and hypoglycemics, as it is also a necessary component involved in the production of insulin.** As with many other nutrients, MSM levels normally decline with age.

NOTE: You may be surprised to learn that **raw garlic cloves** also contain a high amount of sulfur.

Cinnamon

✓ **Cinnamon helps regulate the amount of sugars extracted from carbohydrates in the bloodstream.** Not only does cinnamon activate essential enzymes in the body thus stimulating the receptors in the cells so they will respond more efficiently to insulin, but it also inhibits the enzymes responsible for deactivating the insulin receptors, causing insulin resistance. Cinnamon bark actually contains calcium, chromium, copper, iodine, iron, manganese, phosphorus, potassium, zinc, and vitamins A, B_1, B_2, and C, many of which are important for the prevention or treatment of diabetes. Cinnamon in capsules is also available.

Researchers from the U.S. Department of Agriculture found that less than one-teaspoon (one gram) of cinnamon worked just as well as higher doses, in reducing blood glucose levels 20 percent on some 60 volunteers. They also found that blood sugar levels started rising when the volunteers stopped eating cinnamon (http://care.diabetesjournals.org/cgi/content/abstract/26/12/3215).

Is It Really Hypoglycemia? Or Could It Actually Be Hypothyroidism?

Anyone with hypoglycemia would likely experience an even worse low thyroid condition, as hypoglycemia means you have less sugar (glucose) available, which is necessary to assist in the process that must take place in the liver for a efficient thyroid function. In fact, according to Dr. Broda Barnes, M.D., *"Treatment usually recommended for hypoglycemia is usually a diet high in protein and low in carbohydrate, with frequent feedings. **I have seen many patients with hypoglycemia who have responded to thyroid therapy.** Their symptoms have been ended and they have been able to eat normal diets"* (*Hypothyroidism – The Unsuspected Illness,* 1976, p. 238).

If you suspect you may be suffering from hypoglycemia, it is important to stop and think: When did this all start? Was it perhaps shortly after experiencing an emotionally stressful situation, such as divorce, death, birth, or surgery? If so, **you might consider the possibility that it might instead be hypothyroidism,** which is often brought on by a sudden stressful situation, with extremely similar symptoms. Hypothyroidism can only be identified and resolved with the proper diagnosis, and treatment of the problem early on. Rather than resorting to the typical solution of medications for diabetes, in an attempt to reduce the blood sugar (often causing or worsening hypoglycemia), as you can see, there are much better solutions available.

However, if you have ruled out hypoglycemia, and hypothyroidism, and even Candidiasis, there are still many other possible contributors to depression, as well as natural solutions, as you will learn in the following chapter.

CHAPTER FIFTEEN

Further Possible Contributors To Depression, And Natural Solutions

Are Your Medications Possibly Making You Depressed?

Your medications could quite easily be a major contributing factor to your depression in several ways.

First, on our list of the 200 most commonly prescribed drugs, we encountered a total of 109 prescription medications (54.5%) that actually listed "depression" as a potential side effect.

Then, **on that same list, although there are 20 medications that have not been evaluated to determine their nutrient depletion, (which does not guarantee that none were actually depleted), of the 180 remaining prescribed medications, we found that every single medication depleted nutrients that, when deficient, contributes to depression!**

The depletion (or a deficiency) of any of the following **18 nutrients** can result in depression. In addition to the nutrients listed, are the drugs, class of drugs, substances, or conditions such as stress that can contribute to their depletion. Anyone suffering from depression will likely be able to identify multiple risk factors:

1. **Vitamin B_3 (niacin)** – depleted by sulfa drugs, **SSRI antidepressants,** steroids and corticosteroids, sleeping pills, **estrogen (and oral contraceptives),** caffeine, antibiotics, alcohol, sugar, and physical and mental stress.

2. **Vitamin B_5 (pantothenic acid)** – depleted by sulfa drugs, sleeping pills, **estrogen (and oral contraceptives),** caffeine, alcohol, sugar, cooking, and physical and mental stress.

3. **Vitamin B_6 (pyridoxine)** – depleted by vasodilators (i.e. nitroglycerin), sulfa drugs, steroids and corticosteroids, smoking, sleeping pills, **estrogen (and oral contraceptives),** diuretics, diabetic medication, caffeine, asthma medications, **antidepressants and MAO inhibitors**, antibiotics, alcohol, sugar, heat (canning & roasting), and physical and mental stresses.

4. **Vitamin B_{12}** – depleted by sulfa drugs, **SSRI antidepressants**, smoking, sleeping pills, proton pump inhibitors (i.e. Nexium™), muscle relaxants, mineral oil and laxatives, Histamine H_2 blockers (i.e. Tagamet™, Pepcid™, Zantac™), **estrogen (and oral contraceptives),** diuretics, diabetic medications, all cholesterol-lowering drugs, including statins and bile acid sequestrants (i.e. Questran™, Colestid™), calcium deficiency, caffeine, antiseizure medication (i.e. barbiturates), amphetamines and diet pills, antibiotics, and alcohol.

5. **Biotin** – depleted by sulfa drugs, **estrogen and oral contraceptives,** caffeine, antiseizure medication (i.e. barbiturates, phenytoin), antibiotics, alcohol, and saccharin.

6. **Folic Acid (folate)** – depleted by sulfa drugs, **SSRI antidepressants**, steroids and corticosteroids, smoking, NSAIDs (i.e. ibuprofen), mineral oil and laxatives, Histamine H_2 blockers (i.e. Tagamet™, Pepcid™, Zantac™), **estrogen (and oral contraceptives),** diabetic medication (especially Metformin), diuretics, decongestants (i.e. pseudoephedrine), caffeine, all cholesterol-lowering drugs, including statins and bile acid sequestrants (i.e. Questran™, Colestid™), aspirin, antiseizure medication (i.e. barbiturates), antibiotics, antacids, alcohol, food processing, heat and boiling, and physical and mental stress.

7. **Inositol** – depleted by sulfa drugs, lithium, food processing**, estrogen (and oral contraceptives),** caffeine, antiseizure medication, antibiotics, and alcohol.

8. **PABA (Para-Amino benzoic Acid)** – depleted by sulfa drugs, **estrogen (and oral contraceptives),** food processing, and alcohol.

9. **Vitamin C** – depleted by amphetamines (i.e. Ritalin™) and diet pills, analgesics, antiarrhythmics (i.e. digoxin), anticoagulants (blood thinners), antiseizure medication (i.e. barbiturates, phenytoin), **antidepressants (most)**, aspirin, asthma medications, antihistamines, caffeine, alcohol, diabetic medication, diuretics, **estrogen (and oral contraceptives)**, muscle relaxants, NSAIDs (i.e. ibuprofen), steroids and corticosteroids, high fever, smoking, physical and mental stress.

10. **Vitamin D** – depleted by alcohol, analgesics, antacids, antiarrhythmics, (i.e. digoxin), **antidepressants,** antibiotics, antiseizure medication (i.e. barbiturates, phenytoin), aspirin, asthma medications, all cholesterol-lowering drugs, including statins and bile acid sequestrants (i.e. Questran™, Colestid™), diabetic medication, diuretics, **estrogen (and oral contraceptives)**, Histamine H_2 blockers (i.e. Tagamet™, Pepcid™, Zantac™), mineral oil (laxatives), NSAIDs (i.e. ibuprofen), smoking, steroids and corticosteroids, high fever, and physical and mental stress.

11. **Calcium** – depleted by sulfa drugs, steroids and corticosteroids, **SSRI antidepressants,** NSAIDs (i.e. ibuprofen), mineral oil (laxatives), Histamine H_2 blockers (i.e. Tagamet™, Pepcid™, Zantac™), high fluoride intake (Prozac™), **estrogen (and oral contraceptives),** diuretics, caffeine, all cholesterol-lowering drugs, including statins and bile acid sequestrants (i.e. Questran™, Colestid™), aspirin, antiseizure medication (i.e. barbiturates), antifungals, antibiotics, antiarrhythmic agents (i.e. digoxin), antacids, alcohol, high protein diet, high sugar diet, high saturated fat diet, soft drinks, excess salt or white flour, excess sweating, smoking and emotional and physical stress.

12. **Copper** – depleted by Histamine H_2 blockers (i.e. Tagamet™, Pepcid™, Zantac™), penicillamine™ (chelating agent for copper removal), excess zinc, ethambutol™ (tuberculosis treatment), bile acid sequestrants (Questran™), antiviral HIV medication, and antacids.

13. **Iron** – depleted by NSAIDs (i.e. ibuprofen), mineral oil and laxatives, narcotics, histamine H_2 blockers (i.e. Tagamet™, Pepcid™, Zantac™), choline magnesium trisalicylate (an

anti-inflammatory), all cholesterol-lowering drugs, including statins and bile acid sequestrants (i.e. Questran™, Colestid™), Carisoprodol™ (pain reliever), caffeine (especially the tannic acid in coffee and tea), aspirin, antibiotics, antacids, high phosphorus diet (bran), excess sweating, heavy bleeding (i.e. menstruating women, bleeding ulcers), candida yeast infection, phosphate food additives and EDTA (**e**thylene**d**iamine **t**etraacetic **a**cid – a food preservative).

14. **Magnesium** – depleted by steroids and corticosteroids, **SSRI antidepressants,** NSAIDs (i.e. ibuprofen), Immunosuppressants, high levels of zinc, **estrogen and oral contraceptives,** diuretics, diabetic medication, all cholesterol-lowering drugs, including statins and bile acid sequestrants (i.e. Questran™, Colestid™), antiseizure medication (i.e. barbiturates, phenytoin), antifungal medication, antibiotics, antiarrhythmic agents (i.e. digoxin), antacids, alcohol, antihypertensive (blood pressure lowering) drugs (including ACE inhibitors, beta-blockers and calcium channel blockers), large amounts of fats, sugar, refined flour, fluoride, soft water consumption, and physical and emotional stress.

15. **Potassium** – depleted by steroids and corticosteroids, sodium bicarbonate (Alka Seltzer™), smoking, Parkinson's disease medication, NSAIDs (i.e. ibuprofen), muscle relaxants, laxatives, immunosuppressants, diuretics, caffeine, antiarrhythmic agents (i.e. digoxin), asthma medication, aspirin, antifungal medication, antibiotics, amphetamines and diet pills, alcohol, Acetazolamide™ (a carbonic anhydrase inhibitor), ACE inhibitors and other blood pressure lowering drugs (including beta-blockers), excess sugar and refined foods, large amounts of licorice, and physical and mental stress.

16. **Sodium** – depleted by narcotics, muscle relaxants, laxatives, diuretics, beta-blockers (blood pressure lowering drugs), aspirin, antigout medication, antifungal medication, **antidepressants (especially SSRI antidepressants),** Acetazolamide™ (a carbonic anhydrase inhibitor), ACE inhibitors and other blood pressure lowering drugs, dehydration (fever, heat, diarrhea, vomiting).

17. **Tyrosine – depleted by estrogen and oral contraceptives.**

18. **Essential Fatty Acids (EFAs)** – depleted by NSAIDs (i.e. ibuprofen), **estrogen (and oral contraceptives),** antiseizure medication (i.e. barbiturates, phenytoin), high saturated fat diet, bronchodilators, aspirin, and food processing.

If you recall, Prozac™ depletes a total of 16 nutrients, (nine of which just happen to be on the above list), that are known to contribute to depression when deficient. That is just one of several reasons why a worsening of depression is one potential side effect associated with Prozac™. And once again, does it look like something we would want our children taking?

Microwave Cooking – Another Source of Major Nutrient Depletion

An adequate level of B vitamins is especially important for healthy brain function, and those most often depleted by drugs. Although food preparation in general is important, the greatest concern is in regard to **microwave cooking**. In Dr. Lita Lee's book, *Health Effects of*

Microwave Radiation – Microwave Ovens, she stated that every microwave oven converts substances cooked in it to dangerous organ-toxic and carcinogenic products, and goes on to quote portions of the Russian investigations published by the *Atlantis Raising Educational Center* in Portland, Oregon, as follows:

> ***DECREASE IN NUTRITIONAL VALUE -*** *Russian researchers reported a marked acceleration of structural degradation leading to* ***a decreased food value of 60 to 90% in all foods tested****. Among the changes observed were:* ***Decreased bio-availability of vitamin B complex, vitamin C, vitamin E, essential minerals and lipotropic factors in all food tested;*** *various kinds of damage to many plant substances, such as alkaloids, glucosides, galactosides and nitrilosides;* ***the degradation of nucleo-proteins in meats*** (http://www.vaccinetruth.org/microwave.htm).

This is a very serious concern, regarding "major nutritional depletion", that very few are even aware of. Especially if you consider that microwave cooking destroys the majority of some of the most important nutrients we all need. Even heating water in a microwave is not advisable, as the structure of water is also changed, and water structure is important to the body as well. I would guess that by far, the majority of people in the nation use their microwave on a regular basis, and just for the sake of convenience. If they only knew, (now you know!)

Sugar Robs The Body Of Nutrients For Its Own Digestion

One thing that sugar and medications appear to have in common is their ability to deplete nutrients. Although Prozac™ and Paxil™ are two of the most efficient drugs for nutrient depletion that I'm aware of, (depleting 16 nutrients each), sugar definitely comes in a close second, at twelve. Even worse, according to Dr. Tracy, **Prozac™ causes cravings for both sugar and alcohol.** So anyone taking Prozac™ would be inclined to consume more sugar than normal, potentially creating an even more serious nutritional deficiency.

The following nutrients are those that sugar is responsible for depleting, and those **7 that are bolded** are actually some of the nutrients also depleted by Prozac™ and Paxil™:

1. **Vitamin B_1**
2. **Vitamin B_2**
3. **Vitamin B_3**
4. Vitamin B_5
5. **Vitamin B_6**
6. Choline
7. **Calcium**
8. Chromium
9. Copper
10. **Magnesium**
11. **Manganese**
12. Potassium

Prozac™ combined with sugar is a deadly duo. Together, "all the B vitamins will be depleted", as well as both vitamins C and D. Most of the minerals will also be depleted, (even magnesium used in over 300 different functions). Then we also have the critical combination of the sodium, depleted by Prozac™, combined with the potassium, depleted by sugar. Both are necessary for getting nutrients into each cell, (including the brain), as well as the removal of toxins. The combination also supplies an alternate source of energy for the brain, (when combined with water). **That is, unless they were depleted!**

We then find that Prozac™ depletes the major energy molecule, CoQ_{10}, as well as the most important detoxifier in the liver, glutathione.

Then of course, if a person just happens to have the candida yeast infection, as we discussed, the Prozac™ would greatly potentiate (increase by ten times) the level of alcohol fermented from sugar by the candida yeast infection. And vitamin C, CoQ_{10}, and Zinc, (all depleted by Prozac™), are effective in strengthening the immune system, which is important for controlling or resolving the candida yeast infection.

Only by delving more deeply than traditional medicine tends to, can you fully appreciate just how extensive the potential influence of a drug such as Prozac™ can truly have, on both the body and brain, (either directly or indirectly), due to its critical nutrient depletion. Especially considering the many important functions that each nutrient is responsible for.

Now let's take a moment and evaluate what we just learned, so we can better understand why depression, (due to nutrient depletion), is such a widespread problem in the nation today. **Of the eighteen nutrients important for preventing depression, we find that:**

1. **Nine (half) are actually depleted by antidepressants.** We also find that **one of the potential side effects of antidepressants is depression.**

2. Also, **eight (nearly half) are depleted by the cholesterol-lowering medications** (basically for a non-disease).

3. And, **six (one third) are depleted by sugar consumption, (and made worse by the addition of SSRI antidepressants).**

4. If we look closely, we can also see why **far more women than men suffer from depression. Estrogen and oral contraceptives actually top our list by far, at thirteen of seventeen contributing to the problem!**

5. If we then consider that many are also taking NSAIDs for pain, or H_2 blockers for acid reflux, or possibly various medications for lowering cholesterol or blood pressure, we can better understand why anyone on prescription and over-the-counter medications is a prime candidate for depression, due to nutrient depletion

6. Many eat fast food quite often, as well as frozen TV dinners heated in a microwave oven, which depletes nutrients (by 60% to 90%). It is quite easy to see how both depression and disease in general are not only possible, but also quite likely.

There is always an underlying cause of poor health or depression, and as we just discovered, even prescription medications can be a major factor contributing to depression. Although a nutritional deficiency or a mineral or hormonal imbalance in the brain is the most likely suspect, there are other possibilities, which we will now address.

Additional Contributors To Depression

✓ **Elevated estrogen.** One common side effect associated with elevated estrogen is depression. And as we just pointed out, **estrogen and oral contraceptives (another form of estrogen) contributes to the depletion of FOURTEEN of the 18 nutrients previously listed as being necessary for the prevention of depression!** Estrogen is also a thyroid suppressant.

✓ **Fluoride** not only disrupts the binding of iodine in the thyroid (reducing the metabolism and suppressing the thyroid), but is also a known enzyme inhibitor (reducing the liver's enzyme action), as well as a contributor to elevated estrogen.

Incidentally, every single molecule of Prozac™ (as well as Luvox™) actually contains three molecules of fluoride. And, according to one study conducted at the University of Western Ontario (2002): ***"Most of the symptoms of Fluoride toxicity point towards some kind of profound metabolic dysfunction, and are strikingly similar to the symptoms of Hypothyroidism"*** (http://www.nccn.net/~wwithin/fluoride.htm). This particular website, devoted to the dangers of fluoride, firmly states: ***"We are convinced that all fluoride toxicity is related to disturbances caused in thyroid hormone activity."*** And as we have learned, **one of the most common conditions associated with hypothyroidism (which fluoride obviously contributes to) is depression.**

✓ **Bromine** is another concern. It is yet another toxic halogen (like fluoride and chlorine), which disrupts the binding of iodine in the thyroid (reducing the metabolism and suppressing the thyroid).

As we discussed earlier, it is often used as a dough conditioner in baked goods, as well as a clouding agent in many popular drinks. Toxicity of bromine has been reported from ingestion of some carbonated drinks (i.e. Mountain Dew™, AMP™ Energy Drink, some Gatorade™ products), which contain brominated vegetable oils (*Clinical Toxicology*, 1997, pp. 315-320). Bromine is also still used today in many prescription medications (i.e. asthma treatment). Dr. David Brownstein, M.D. notes the following:

> ***Bromine intoxication*** *(i.e. bromism) has been shown to cause delirium, psychomotor retardation,* ***schizophrenia, and hallucination. Subjects who ingest enough bromide feel dull land apathetic*** *and have difficulty concentrating.* ***Bromide can also cause severe depression,*** *headache, and* ***irritability.***
>
> ***Recent research has demonstrated that some symptoms of bromide toxicity can be present with low levels of bromide in the diet*** (*Iodine: Why You Need – Why You Can't Live Without It,* 2004, p. 78).

✓ **Candidiasis Yeast Infection**. Some of the common symptoms of Candidiasis are **depression, mood swings**, yearning for isolation, **insomnia,** and in some cases **manic depression or suicidal tendencies.** Candidiasis and its treatment are covered in detail in an earlier chapter in this book.

✓ **Suppressed dopamine** levels also contribute to depression. According to Dr. Glenmullen, SSRI antidepressants can actually promote depression, as they are known to suppress another important feel-good hormone, dopamine, by approximately 50%. It's quite amazing how many different ways antidepressants can actually contribute to depression, (even one of the potential side effects), and we can easily see why.

✓ **Stress,** which most of us experience all too often, creates an elevation of the hormone cortisol, which is not only known to suppress the thyroid, but also contributes to brain damage. This then often leads to either one or both of the most common side effects associated with suppressed thyroid function, (depression and mood swings). And as you have just seen, **physical and mental stress contributes to the depletion of NINE (half) of the 18 nutrients previously mentioned as necessary for preventing depression.**

✓ **SSRI antidepressants such as Prozac™**, cause stress. And as we have learned, just one single 30 mg dose of Prozac™ increases the level of the stress hormone cortisol by an amazing 200%! And, it has been proven that excess cortisol is a marker for depression, a fact that was established by studies published three years before Prozac™ was approved. In her book *Prozac: Panacea or Pandora?* (1991/1994), Dr. Ann Blake Tracy poses the question: ***"If one single dose causes such a significant increase in cortisol, then what kind of increase in cortisol levels can be expected when someone is taking Prozac on a daily basis?"*** (p. 84). A very thought-provoking question, I would say.

Not only that, but as we pointed out, **NINE of the 18 nutrients listed as necessary for the prevention of depression, are actually depleted by antidepressants!**

✓ **Statin (cholesterol lowering) drugs / Low Cholesterol Levels.** Following is a portion of an article by Sally Fallon and Mary G. Enig, Ph.D., originally posted on The Weston A Price Website, (http://www.westonaprice.org/moderndiseases/statin.html), regarding statin drugs and the importance of cholesterol:

The Dangers of Statin Drugs:
What You Haven't Been Told About Cholesterol-Lowering Medication

> ***Hypercholesterolemia* [high cholesterol] *is the health issue of the 21st century. It is actually an invented disease, a "problem" that emerged when health professionals learned how to measure cholesterol levels in the blood.***
>
> ***Many people who feel perfectly healthy suffer from high cholesterol--in fact, feeling good is actually a symptom of high cholesterol!***
>
> ***Cholesterol is vital to proper neurological function. It plays a key role in the formation of memory and the uptake of hormones in the brain, including serotonin, the body's feel-good chemical. When cholesterol levels drop too low, the serotonin receptors cannot work.***
>
> ***Numerous studies have linked low cholesterol with depression. One of the most recent found that women with low cholesterol are twice as likely to suffer from depression and anxiety.***
>
> ***Dr. Edward Suarez found that men who lower their cholesterol levels with medication have increased rates of suicide and violent death,*** *leading the*

*researchers to theorize **"that low cholesterol levels were causing mood disturbances."***

✓ **Combining different prescription medications, and possibly even mixing over-the-counter medications,** considerably increases the risk for depression. The more medications you are taking, the greater the risk will be.

✓ **Drinking grapefruit juice** can actually suppress the major detoxifier in the liver, the P450 enzyme, for up to 24 hours. That alone could easily complicate matters even further, by increasing the potential for side effects, as well as potentially leading to a serious overdose of both alcohol and drugs. Also keep in mind that the P450 enzyme in the liver is responsible for detoxifying both alcohol and Prozac™, as well as other toxins.

✓ **Alcohol is a depressant!** Drinking alcohol also requires the exact same enzyme in the liver that most drugs, (including SSRI antidepressants), require for detoxification, greatly increasing the potential for a drug overdose. The importance of avoiding alcohol becomes especially apparent when you consider that **alcohol depletes THIRTEEN of the 19 nutrients previously mentioned as necessary for preventing depression.**

✓ **Elevated Histamine (or Histadelia) can cause a person to experience depression, obsession, thoughts of suicide, misperceptions, and thought disorder.** According to the late Dr. Carl C. Pfeiffer, Ph.D., M.D., histadelia is most often hereditary, and he suggests that ***"The easily elicited history of suicide, depression, and allergies among near and distant relatives is a strong indication of possible histadelia"*** (*Nutrition and Mental Illness*, 1987, p. 28). Other common symptoms of histadelia may include a history of allergies or periodic headache, a very low threshold to pain, oversensitive and crying easily, and severe insomnia.

Histamine is actually considered a neurotransmitter, and has several important functions in the body and brain. The late Dr. Batmanghelidj, M.D. has pointed out that **there is a *"direct connection between histamine and serotonin"*,** has noted that ***"the higher the blood histamine, the lower the serotonin level"*** (*Water – Rx For A Healthier Pain-free Life*, 1997, cassette recording). High histamine levels can be the direct result of dehydration, or a copper deficiency. For more detailed information, refer to the "Histamine" section of the Bipolar Disorder chapter.

✓ **Elevated Copper (Zinc deficiency), also known as Pyroluria.** Although a copper **deficiency** can contribute to histadelia, (as we just mentioned), **elevated** copper levels have their own set of problems! The most common cause of elevated copper is drinking water that comes from copper pipes, although zinc offsets copper, thus a zinc deficiency can result in elevated copper levels. Another contributor to excess copper is contraceptive pills, (which causes elevated estrogen).

According to local author Eva Edelman, (*Naturally Healing Schizophrenia*, 1996/1998), another concern is that **excess copper *"may foster right brain dominance"*** (p. 38). And **there is a direct relationship between right-brain dominance and depression,** as explained in this portion of *MegaBrain Report* (Vol. 2, No. 3), edited by Michael Hutchison, titled ***"The Cry-Baby Biomarker & Depression in the Brain"*,** as follows:

> ***There is also evidence that these brainwave asymmetries may be linked to depression.*** *The researchers tested the EEGs of a group of normal subjects who had never been treated for depression, and a group of subjects who had been previously depressed and later successfully treated for depression. They found that* ***the previously depressed subjects had far less left-frontal activity, and far more right-frontal activity,*** *than those who had never been depressed.*
>
> *A recent* ***brainmapping study of depressive patients*** *by C. Norman Shealy, M.D., Ph.D. at the Shealy Institute in Springfield, Missouri, revealed that* ***100 percent of the patients had abnormal brainwave activity, with the most common finding being "Asymmetry of the two hemispheres with right hemisphere dominance."***
>
> *Another study revealed that* ***patients who had just been diagnosed with depression and were about to begin treatment had less left-frontal activity than non-depressed subjects.*** *"You find similar brain patterns in people who are depressed, or who have recovered from depression, and in normal people who are prone to bad moods," said one of the researchers, Dr. John Davidson, of the University of Wisconsin, Madison.* ***"We suspect that people with this brain activity pattern are at high risk for depression."***
>
> *Davidson has studied the behavior and the EEG patterns of 10-month old infants during a brief period (one minute) of separation from their mothers, and found that* ***"those infants who cried in response to maternal separation showed greater right-frontal activation during the preceding baseline period compared with infants who did not cry."*** *Observed Davidson,* ***"Every single infant who cried had more right-frontal activation. Every one who did not had more activity on the left."*** *He concluded that* ***"Frontal activation asymmetry may be a state-independent marker for individual differences in threshold of reactivity to stressful events and vulnerability to particular emotions"*** (http://beyond-the-illusion.com/files/Altered-States/Brain-Programming/bwave.txt).

So as you can see, the right-brain dominance Eva Edelman referred to could be a significant factor in regards to the predisposition towards depression, often the result of a high copper-to-zinc ratio. Also, according to Dr. Carl C. Pfeiffer, Ph.D., M.D., **a deficiency of either vitamin C or B_3 can also cause copper levels to rise. NOTE: Further information on Pyroluria can be found in the back of this book, in the chapter on Additional Technical Information.**

✓ **Vitamin D deficiency** appears to be an *"increasingly prevalent, but largely unrecognized, problem,"* as reported in an editorial by Alan R. Gaby, M.D., in *the Townsend Letter for Doctors & Patients* (July 2004). Dr. Gaby points out that ***"Vitamin D deficiency might be a contributing factor to depression, particularly seasonal affective disorder (winter depression),"*** and goes on to note that *"**even a mild deficiency may cause depression**."* **Note: Both Prozac™ and Ritalin™ deplete vitamin D.**

✓ **Vitamin C deficiency.** According to *Life Extension Disease Prevention and Treatment, Expanded Third Edition,* (1997/2002), ***"depression is the first clinical symptoms detected when humans are deliberately deprived of vitamin C for purposes of study"*** (p. 231). In fact, one study compared the diets of 12 women who attempted suicide, compared with 12 women who were not depressed and had not attempted suicide, and found the diets very similar, *"except that* ***the 'suicide' group was taking in much less vitamin C.****"*
Note: Both Prozac™ and Ritalin™ deplete vitamin C.

✓ **Essential Fatty Acid (EFA) deficiency.** According to an article in the December 1998 issue of *Psychiatric Times* (Vol. XVI, Issue 12), previous investigation by Drs. Hibbeln and Norman Salem Jr., Ph.D. confirmed that ***"the depletion of certain EFAs had been indicated as a probable factor for major depression."*** In fact, one study, reported in the German journal *Fortschritte der Neurologie-Psychiatrie*, states that ***"decreased consumption of omega-3 fatty acids could be a risk factor for human depression and suicide"*** (*Life Extension* magazine, July 2006, p. 48). And as pointed out in an article in *Preventative Medicine* (January 2006), ***"Supplementation with fish oil could potentially prevent many of the 765,000 suicide attempts and 30,000 suicides committed each year in the U.S."*** (pp. 4-14).

If those promoting TeenScreen were truly concerned about suicide prevention, they might want to take a look at the benefits of EFAs, as well as the previously mentioned vitamin C, regarding suicide prevention, (obviously inexpensive solutions, with multiple benefits).

✓ **Sleep deprivation**. According to a recent study published in the journal *Sleep* (January 2007 issue), ***"Sleep-disturbed children are more severely depressed and have more depressive symptoms compared with children without sleep disturbance"*** (http://www.sciencedaily.com/releases/2007/01/070101104155.htm). And although sleep deprivation contributes to depression, this same study confirmed that depression contributes to sleep deprivation, especially in children. This is particularly important if you consider the number of children now being placed on the stimulant Ritalin™, known to cause insomnia and interrupt REM sleep, (further contributing to depression). For more on this subject, see the chapter on "ADHD".

✓ **Chronic back pain** may seem unrelated to depression, however **a chiropractic adjustment might possibly be in order,** as we find that back pain may actually alter brain chemistry.

> *Back pain doesn't just affect patients' backs – it also influences their brains, say scientists. According to a recently published report in the journal* Pain, ***chronic back pain (CBP) alters patients' brain chemistry.***
>
> *Researchers at SUNY Upstate Medical University in Syracuse, New York used a magnetic resonance spectroscopy to measure the relative concentrations of several brain chemicals (N-acetyl aspartate, creatine, choline, glutamate, glutamine, gamma aminobutyric acid, inositol, glucose and lactate) in 9 CBP sufferers and 11 pain-free volunteers. Measurements were conducted in six different brain regions. Patients with CBP also underwent evaluations for pain and anxiety.*

Findings revealed that, "in chronic back pain, the interrelationship between chemicals within and across brain regions was abnormal, and there was a specific relationship between regional chemicals and perceptual measures of pain and anxiety. These findings provide direct evidence of abnormal brain chemistry in chronic back pain."

The Chiropractic Health Research Information Service (CHRIS) February 9, 2001
(*Pain* – December 2000, 15;89:7-18)
(http://hub.elsevier.com/pii/S0304395900003407)

Are You In The Dark?
Seasonal Affective Disorder (SAD)

The National Association for Mental Illness (NAMI) defines Seasonal Affective Disorder (SAD) as a condition *"characterized by recurrent episodes of depression – usually in late fall and winter - alternating with periods of normal or high mood the rest of the year"* (http://www.nami.org/Template.cfm?Section=By_Illness&Template=/TaggedPage/TaggedPageDisplay.cfm&TPLID=54&ContentID=23051). **For many people, SAD is a seriously disabling illness, and is often misdiagnosed as hypothyroidism, hypoglycemia,** infectious mononucleosis, and other viral infections. For others, it is subsyndromal (a mild but debilitating condition), often referred to as the "Winter Blues".

According to the Seasonal Affective Disorder Association (SADA) in England, this disorder is *"caused by **a biochemical imbalance in the hypothalamus** due to the shortening of daylight hours and the lack of sunlight in winter,"* (http://www.sada.org.uk/index.htm).

Years ago, I took a course on Interior Decoration (one of my interests), taught by a prominent decorator in San Jose, with many years experience. She mentioned that psychiatrists would often have her consult with many of their patients who were depressed. She noticed that their homes were often very drab with dark colors and insufficient light, and that normally a few decorating changes would dramatically improve their overall mood. Sunlight stimulates the production of serotonin, so we want to let as much light in as we possibly can, and use light colors to reflect as much light as possible.

On the other hand, when it's time to go to sleep, we should eliminate as much light from our bedrooms as we possibly can. Doing so would stimulate the production of melatonin necessary for the quality REM sleep to promote the restoration of our mind and body. Sleep deprivation is just one contributor to depression. Prozac™ and other SSRI antidepressants cause an elevation of the stress hormone cortisol, which among other things disrupts the REM sleep cycle.

Let There Be Light – Lots of Light

Light therapy has proven to reverse the winter depressive symptoms of Seasonal Affective Disorder (SAD). The *Psychiatric Times* claims that **light therapy is now being recommended as "first-line defense for SAD", as well as non-seasonal depression, post-partum depression, and prepartum depression** (http://www.psychiatrictimes.com/p041068.html).

In fact, the *American Journal of Psychiatry* reports: *"Systematic review of studies on the effectiveness of light therapy conducted between 1975 and 2003 has concluded that* ***bright***

light therapy is as effective for non-seasonal depression as most pharmaceutical treatments (prescription drugs)," (2005 April, pp. 656-662), but bright full-spectrum fluorescent lights (not ordinary light bulbs), are necessary. Even the average household or office lighting, which emits an intensity of 200-500 LUX, is not enough. The minimum dose necessary to be beneficial is 2500 LUX, although more is often required. The intensity of a bright summer day can be as much as 100,000 LUX! **In the winter months, using a 10,000-LUX Full Spectrum Light Box for 30 minutes each morning is normally enough to help produce serotonin and reduce depression.** This is especially beneficial during the winter months in the northern latitudes, when sufficient natural sunlight is often not available. Keep in mind though, that using the light box in the evening can cause overstimulation, and thus insomnia, as serotonin is stimulating. Taking 3 mg of melatonin approximately ½ hour before bedtime is one way to help promote deep sleep.

Light therapy consists of sitting two to three feet away from a specially designed light box, usually placed on a table, allowing the light to shine directly through the eyes. Tinted lenses, or any device that blocks the light to the retina of the eye, should not be worn. It is not necessary to stare at the light, although it has been proven safe. You can carry out your normal activities such as reading, working, or eating, while sitting in front of the box. After a week or two, either reducing or increasing the daily duration may be necessary. Improvement is normally noticed within three to four days, and should continue as long as necessary. There are several companies that sell light boxes in the 10,000-LUX range.

Because Light Therapy (phototherapy) is no longer considered experimental, and is a mainstream type of psychiatric treatment for SAD or depressive/anxiety conditions, **many insurance companies will cover the cost of a therapeutic light box.** The recent discovery that several forms of depression respond to daily exposure to bright light has called attention to the popular notion that **sunlight is one effective therapy for depression.**

In her un-dated booklet titled *"The Miracle of Simple,"* Susan M. Lark, M.D. sheds some light (pun intended):

> ***Take us out of the sunlight for any length of time and we become depressed.*** *A blue light will make your pulse rate slow, your breathing relax, and your adrenal glands and immune system respond magically.*
>
> ***A red light*** *heightens your sense of smell and taste, and awakens your libido by* ***stimulating all the endocrine glands****. Energy levels soar, blood flow increases, and* ***metabolic rates pick up****.*
>
> *My dad, who was a medical doctor and research scientist himself, built* ***a simple light box*** *for my mom, and fitted it* ***with a red light filter****. She loved it – and said* ***it was as effective as a cup of coffee, but without the jitters*** (p. 30).

Our body responds to different frequencies, and different colors have varying frequencies, and thus our brain also responds accordingly. Light therapy, utilizing a whole spectrum of colors, is one method proven beneficial for various conditions.

Of all the stimulants the human brain responds to, one of the most powerful is light. **The body has hundreds of biochemical and hormonal rhythms, all of which are governed by light and dark**. In a study done by a Harvard medical team, volunteers were taken through a series of light-exposure tests, experimenting with intensities ranging from 7,000 LUX to 12,000 LUX. Scientists measured the change in brain-wave patterns immediately following this exposure and were able to establish the link between the retina and an area of the brain known as the suprachiasmatic nuclei. According to professors Richard Kronauer, Ph.D., and Charles Czeisler, M.D., the two scientists who headed the three-year Harvard study, this confirms that **there is a direct connection between light exposure and the part of the brain that is thought to play a key role in attention focus and energy production** (*Low Fat Living*, Dr. Robert Cooper, 1996, p. 71). Therefore, **if you have a hard time getting going in the morning**, try turning on every light in the house and see if that helps get you moving! The most benefit can be achieved when using full-spectrum lighting.

Let There Be Lots of the *Right Kind* of Light

Another concern is regular fluorescent lighting, which was discussed earlier (in the chapter on "ADHD"). Much research has been done regarding the negative, harmful effects of **artificial fluorescent lighting**, and research has proven that it **not only produces increased levels of stress producing hormones, but it can also promote depression.** According to a study performed by elementary school principal, William Titoff, **depression actually increased in fourth-graders studying under standard fluorescent lights, compared to those students studying under full-spectrum lighting.** His controlled study verified that ***"depression was lowered among those students who experienced learning under full-spectrum lighting"*** (http://www.fullspectrumsolutions.com/lighting_for_schools.shtml).

I replaced all the fluorescent lights in our home and my office, with full spectrum bulbs. We actually have twelve in our kitchen, and it is the most cheerful room in our home. I also replaced all reading lamps with full spectrum incandescent bulbs. When purchased by the case, full spectrum fluorescent bulbs are fairly inexpensive, and are well worth the price. In my opinion, due to the above findings, all schools should replace any cool fluorescent lighting with full-spectrum fluorescent lighting. It's a simple change that could easily reduce or eliminate depression in hundreds of students. I would even work at home!

Now that we've discovered how to brighten our future, and better light the way, we will take a look at many other options to choose from. When it comes to natural solutions, it's quite amazing how many natural options Our Creator has provided for our benefit. We just need to stop ignoring them, and begin taking advantage of them. Just keep in mind that all our options actually provide many different benefits, (versus drugs' many side effects), thus the choice should be obvious. So let's take a look at several additional options to choose from.

Helpful Suggestions For Resolving Depression Without Drugs

Although some people just seem to cope more effectively than others, there is normally a good explanation. The late Dr. Carl C. Pfeiffer, Ph.D., M.D., author of the book *Nutrition and Mental Illness* (1987), discovered that a nutritional deficiency or hormone imbalance in the brain is often the underlying factor that can potentially influence how we might possibly respond to various events in life. **Some of the most important neurotransmitters, critical for our brain's functioning, are dopamine, norepinephrine, and serotonin, and doctors have concluded that depression occurs when these levels become too low, or out of balance.**

It was once believed that the brain could somehow protect itself from nutritional deficiencies, but we now know that is not really true, and that the brain actually requires certain nutrients. A sufficient supply, as well as the proper balance, of vitamins, minerals, and amino acids, is important for healthy mental function, and it's your responsibility to assure it's provided with the necessary nutrients. If this supply is not met, biochemistry changes take place, resulting in symptoms such as fatigue, depression, and irritability, just to name a few.

One potential problem arises when people choose to rely solely on their doctor's advice for their healthcare. Most traditionally trained doctors are all too quick to prescribe medications for any symptom, while failing to consider the importance of nutritional deficiencies. At times, doctors even discourage taking vitamins, suggesting that they are just a waste of money. In some cases, doctors also warn of the potential for some supplements interacting with their medications. Interestingly, those at the greatest risk of taking the most medications are patients unfamiliar with nutrition (the majority of people), who are also the most concerned about their health. Unfortunately, **although few doctors have any training in nutrition, they still tend to discredit its potential benefits.** The problem lies in many people's total confidence in their doctor's opinion, which they seldom, if ever question. Thus, we must all become better informed, and then take a more active part regarding our healthcare, which is our ultimate responsibility.

For instance, a friend of mine was unfamiliar with nutrition, although very conscientious regarding his health, and previously had a great deal of confidence in his doctor. He took taking his medications very seriously, especially due to his doctor's warning that his life depended upon them. This is a good way to motivate your patient, (although based on a false premise). Incidentally, after becoming better informed, he decided that a change of doctors was in order, and I believe that under the circumstances, that was a wise decision.

Sometimes, openly discussing your symptoms, or various health concerns with your doctor could very well be detrimental to your health. Due to most doctors' restricted training in medical school, as well as the limited time normally allotted for each patient, another drug is often the most likely solution (just one more quick fix). It is rather difficult for a doctor to justify charging for an office visit unless he either writes, or renews a prescription, or recommends some surgery. Unfortunately, the only solutions available to most traditionally trained M.D.s are those approved by the American Medical Association (AMA).

Our Emotions Can Be Controlled

We all normally experience various episodes in our lifetime that can contribute to either stress or depression. These events are normally transient, and should soon resolve. It is how we deal with the adverse incidents, such as the death of a loved one, divorce, or possibly a financial reversal, in the interim that makes the difference.

If a loved one passes on, we must remember that death is beyond our control, and something no one can escape. Only God can make that decision, and although we obviously will miss them, life must go on until our time comes. Making the most of the remainder of our lives is the very best thing we can do for them, as well as ourselves. You might begin by making a list of your goals and blessings, and then review them the first thing every morning. You can continually expand your list, whenever new ones come to mind.

Learn to focus on positive uplifting thoughts only. Negative thoughts tend to lead to stress or depression, two conditions that far too many are unnecessarily taking medications for. Whenever a thought comes to mind that is not uplifting, remove it immediately, and replace it with another that is. Remind yourself to review your list each morning, and it will soon become a habit. Abraham Lincoln summed it up pretty well when he said***: "Most folks are about as***

happy as they make their minds up to be," so make up your mind to be happy every single day. Happiness is basically a state of mind that seems to come naturally for some, although something others might need to work on at times. Parents' attitudes and moods are often reflected in their children. If your parents tended to be pessimistic, rather than optimistic toward life, you might have to work a little harder at developing a positive attitude than others, (and make sure that you are "not" one of those pessimistic parents).

Actually, service to others can be very rewarding. It allows us to focus on others who are less fortunate, which not only brings a great deal of satisfaction, but also reminds us just how fortunate we really are. By focusing on the problems of others, we also tend to forget our own. Service to others was an important principle Jesus taught by example during His lifetime.

If your depression is possibly the result of an unwanted divorce, keep in mind that it was likely for our own good. No matter how much you might love someone, if that person does not share that love, whatever the reason, you can never be truly happy. You must give them their freedom, and avoid any hostile feelings, even though it may seem justifiable. Harboring negative feelings is basically self-destructive, and can negatively influence your personality. It will just make your chances of finding another spouse (or happiness) much more difficult. For example, if a man meets a divorced woman with a bad attitude toward men, possibly due to a bad experience from her previous marriage, he will likely assume that she was the problem, although that might not necessarily have been true.

A cheerful optimistic personality is a characteristic that both women and men are drawn to, not only in the opposite sex, but also as a choice of friends. In order to attract a mate, or just develop good friendships, we should begin developing those positive attributes that we admire the most in others. Nothing can be more depressing than being around someone with a negative attitude. On the other hand, a cheerful person with a positive attitude is rather like a ray of sunshine, or a breath of fresh air (something we all can use more of). So let's see if we can begin developing the characteristics that we so much admire in others.

It is not necessarily our experiences in life that dictates our happiness, but rather how we react to them. We can't always control the events we encounter throughout our lifetime, although how we respond to each is our choice. We must learn to adapt to our environment, and look for the good in every situation, no matter what our initial response might possibly be. We must remember that it is difficult to retract something inappropriately said in haste, and an apology might not always undo the damage. It is rather like the judge during a trial, instructing the jury to disregard a statement made by a witness (believe me - they won't forget!) We must learn to control our emotions when appropriate. It is much easier than damage control after the fact. Just by developing good social skills, we can often avoid the depression we might possibly experience from dwelling on foolish mistakes, by preventing them in the first place.

While conducting research on addictions, I discovered that many alcoholics tend to suffer from personality disorders, which often leads to depression, thus influencing their interactions with others. Depression then leads to excessive drinking, which then results in worse behavior. It is basically a vicious cycle that often repeats itself over and over. Our interaction with others (not only who we interact with, but also how we interact with them) can have a major influence on our quality of life in general. Serious introspection might be helpful, and remember to be objective. Recognizing that a problem exists is the very first step in the recovery process. Motivation is important, and input from others might be helpful, as we might tend to rationalize at times, in an attempt to justify our actions.

Drink Sufficient Water

An adequate supply of water (preferably ten 8-ounce glasses a day) is essential for effective neuron transmission of critical hormones in the brain. The body basically responds to dehydration as a stressor, and any stress will suppress the thyroid function. Then, a typical symptom of suppressed thyroid is depression. When we are dehydrated, the viscosity (thickness) of our blood also increases. When the blood thickens, the amino acid L-tryptophan, (which is a relatively large molecule), finds it difficult to cross the blood-brain barrier. Tryptophan is the basic building block of serotonin, which is important for avoiding depression. Incidentally, vitamin B_6 (depleted by many medications, including Prozac™) is necessary for the conversion process to take place.

When you are dehydrated, your brain is in need of an energy source, and unless you provide it with the proper nutrients (or hydration), it will crave a quick source of energy (i.e. carbohydrates, sugar, alcohol, etc.). Thus, another reason to assure you drink plenty of water, along with Celtic sea with all its minerals still intact, is that it can provide an alternate source of energy for the brain. It's an excellent way to provide energy without stimulating the release of insulin, which is one contributor to hypoglycemia.

No other drink can replace water, and some beverages such as coffee, caffeinated soft drinks, and alcohol are actually very dehydrating. Most fruit drinks are basically loaded with sugar, often in the form of high fructose corn syrup, which contributes to elevated insulin, and then hypoglycemia. One of the many symptoms associated with hypoglycemia is depression. As previously discussed, the symptoms of hypothyroidism (low thyroid) and hypoglycemia (low blood sugar) are surprisingly similar, with depression being a common denominator. So as we can easily see, water is also helpful in avoiding depression, and basically something we can all afford. Just make sure there is no chlorine or fluoride in the water you drink, as both can suppress the thyroid function, which would just reduce the benefit of drinking water.

Get Moving!

Exercise is also beneficial, as it balances the nerve chemicals and hormones, increases endorphins, curbs hunger, relaxes the body, and improves the quality of sleep. Exercising outdoors, whenever possible, is the best way to get more natural light exposure, which causes the body to naturally produce vitamin D, thus increasing levels of serotonin in the brain. When walking, get away from traffic as much as possible. The carbon monoxide fumes from vehicles can considerably reduce your oxygen level.

Dr. Hyla Cass explains, in her book *Natural Highs* (2002), that exercise stimulates the release of powerful, mood-elevating endorphins. She also states that *"regular exercise can actually reduce the amount of adrenal hormones the body releases in response to stress. In addition, it raises the levels of the mood-elevating hormones, or endorphins, in the brain"* (p. 193).

According to researcher James Blumenthal, professor of medical psychology at Duke University in Durham, North Carolina, **when compared to antidepressants, *"after sixteen weeks of treatment exercise was equally effective in reducing depression among patients with MDD*** [Major Depressive Disorder]."
(http://www.ncbi.nlm.nih.gov/entrez/query.fcgi?cmd=Retrieve&db=PubMed&list_uids=10547175)

Check Your Thyroid!

Although depression can eventually lead to other conditions, depression can only be effectively treated and resolved by addressing the underlying problem. One seemingly unrelated contributor to depression might be the thyroid, and if you have a hypothyroid condition, that should be your very first focus (explained in detail in earlier, in the Hypothyroidism chapter of this book). Just remember to use the natural hormone Armour™ thyroid, (not Synthroid™).

Nutritional Supplements for Resolving Depression

1. **Goji and/or Mangosteen Juice.** For thousands of years, goji has been known in Asia as "the happy berry". One to two ounces, one to two times daily, has been historically used to "uplift and elevate" mood. With 19 amino acids (including the 8 essential amino acids) and 21 trace minerals (as well as other important nutrients), goji also enhances energy and eliminates fatigue.

Drinking two ounces of mangosteen juice, three times daily is also very effective, and often all that is necessary for resolving depression. Although we are each unique, and results may vary based on many different factors, mangosteen has in many cases elevated the mood and eliminated depression. It also seems to be very effective in relieving chronic (long-term) pain. As told in his book *Tame the Flame* (2004), Dr. Sam Walters, N.MD. discovered that mangosteen had effectively resolved the long-term pain that he had been taking medications for, due to a serious parachute accident over twenty years ago. In his book, Dr. Walters states that ***"Often chronic pain will lead to psychological responses such as anxiety, fear, sleeplessness, and even suicidal thoughts."***

Although we have yet to discover exactly how the these fruits resolve so many different conditions, I can see a few ways it could possibly help eliminate depression. First, according to Dr. Sherry Rodgers, M.D., 95% of the feel-good hormone serotonin that antidepressants are attempting to increase, is actually produced in the intestinal tract. Dr. Tracy makes the same claim, although she claims it's 90%. Both the mangosteen and goji have been proven beneficial for resolving common intestinal disorders. They are also effective in eliminating a condition in the small intestine known as leaky gut syndrome, as well as acid reflux disease. Both conditions make the digestion and assimilation of proteins less effective, (especially when antacids are used). These proteins are important for producing amino acids required for building both the important neurotransmitters such as serotonin and dopamine, and the enzymes critical for our sense of well being.

As both the mangosteen and goji juices are adaptogens with multiple benefits, another beneficial influence they both appear to have is on the thyroid gland. Dr. Sam Walters discovered that mangosteen is sometimes effective in eliminating the need for thyroid medication. And Dr. Victor Marcial-Vega claims that goji helps stabilize the body temperature. That can be an important factor, as a low thyroid condition, referred to as hypothyroidism, is one common cause of depression. Insufficient metabolism is also often the underlying cause of inappropriate weight gain, and the inability to effectively lose weight on any diet, and just being overweight can be very depressing. So, a low thyroid condition (insufficient metabolism) is often a potential contributor to depression in more ways than one. This condition is covered in considerable detail earlier in the chapter on Hypothyroidism. It is an absolute must-read for anyone suffering with depression (especially for women, who are ten times as likely as men to become hypothyroid). This condition is, in my opinion, the greatest contributor to depression. If it is a problem, it must be resolved in order to truly eliminate your depression.

Mary Lou soon experienced both an elevated mood and increased energy from using mangosteen. And if you recall, Mary Lou was able to eliminate a 16-year dependency on Prozac™, and do so in only two months, by using the mangosteen juice, along with a good vitamin B-complex and essential fatty acids (flax seed oil). Following her withdrawal, she not only experienced an elevated mood, but also an increased level of energy. Although Mary Lou used XanGo™, similar results would likely occur with (undiluted) mangosteen, or goji juice, in lower dosage, as well.

2. **SAMe. S**-**a**denosyl**m**ethionin**e** (SAMe) is a natural substance, normally produced by the liver when an adequate supply of nutrients is available. Due to their nutrient depletion, prescription medications (especially the SSRI antidepressants) can quite easily reduce the liver's ability to effectively produce SAMe. It is especially beneficial for anyone attempting to phase out any of the SSRI antidepressants such as Prozac™, Paxil™, or Zoloft™, as it elevates the mood in a natural way, and is safe to take until the antidepressants are phased out. As some people on SSRI antidepressants such as Prozac™, Paxil™ or Zoloft™ for several years (or on multiple antidepressants) risk accumulating toxic levels of serotonin, (a condition called Serotonin Syndrome), which can be potentially dangerous, it's best, (at least initially), to avoid anything like 5HTP that can increase your serotonin level.

According to Teodoro Bottiglieri, Ph.D., senior research scientist and director of neuropharmacology at Baylor University Medical Center, Institute of Metabolic Disease in Dallas, ***"SAMe posses a rapid onset of action (five to 10 days) in seven clinical trials vs. standard antidepressant medication, which can take 14 to 20 days to become effective."*** He goes on to note that:

> *It is a fact that about 50 percent of patients stop their antidepressant medication within three months, primarily due to its side effects. Patient compliance is better with SAMe because it is a natural substance with a low side-effect profile. Furthermore,* ***SAMe may be used in combination with other*** **[supplements]** ***to enhance their effect*** (http://www.hsrmagazine.com/articles/161feat2.html).

SAMe has also been proven beneficial in repairing damage to the liver (a potential with prescription drug use), and reducing elevated homocysteine, as well as resolving depression in most people. In a double-blind study, SAMe was found to have even **less** side effects than a sugar pill, (as we know, sugar is not good for us!). Just contrast that with Prozac's extensive list of potential side effects. It seems that 400 mg of SAMe, twice daily is normally effective in resolving depression.

3. **TMG (tri methyl glycine).** Although TMG can do some of the same things in the body that SAMe can, (such as controlling homocysteine levels), SAMe is more beneficial in resolving depression, and SAMe is considerably more expensive than TMG. Thus, in order to use SAMe to its full depression-fighting potential, for financial reasons, I would suggest taking also TMG, a natural extract from the sugar beet, along with folic acid, and vitamins B_6 and B_{12},, to help control homocysteine, in addition to SAMe. Thus more SAMe would be available for doing what it does best, (fight depression). This is actually explained in extensive detail in the back of this book in

the chapter on "Additional Technical Information", under "The Connection Between Elevated Homocysteine and Depression").

If cost is an issue, you might first try 200 mg of SAMe, twice daily, along with two capsules of TMG, which will as I mentioned, make the SAMe go further. If that's not sufficient, I would suggest you work your way up to 400 mg of SAMe, twice daily, instead of 200 mg.

4. **B Vitamins.** The B vitamins are critical to normal brain function, and are unfortunately depleted by many prescription medications, (especially antidepressants). The B vitamins are also necessary in assisting the brain in creating neurotransmitters that enable brain cells to communicate with each other. For example, vitamin B_6 is necessary for the conversion of the amino acid tryptophan to serotonin. And, all three vitamin B_6, B_{12}, and folic acid help control homocysteine, which can damage the neurons in the brain when elevated. Another thing is, most people suffering with dementia were found to be deficient in folic acid and B_{12}. Unfortunately, most physicians seldom recommend B vitamins to treat depression, (or any vitamins, for that matter).

Just taking a good "coenzyme vitamin B complex," along with flax oil, was sufficient for eliminating my granddaughter's depression. Incidentally, regular B-complex vitamins made her nauseated, (a problem some people experience). As a result, I suggested she try the coenzyme form, which didn't cause her any nausea. It's also the best form for anyone with a liver disorder, or liver damage. The coenzyme formula actually contains the B-complex vitamins in the form used by the body, and the conversion by the liver is not necessary. (I suggested she take two daily, produced by *Country Life™*, although there are others available.)

Normally, I would recommend taking a high-potency vitamin B-complex, such as B-100 (100 mg of each B vitamin) daily, although if you happen to experience the problem that my granddaughter did, you might consider taking a coenzyme form of B-complex vitamins instead.

5. **Essential Fatty Acids (EFAs).** The essential fatty acids (EFAs) in both fish oil and flax oil are very beneficial for resolving depression, (as well as the bipolar disorder). They are essential for creating and maintaining healthy cell walls and receptors for important neurotransmitters such as serotonin and dopamine. Numerous studies have been done to prove the benefits of EFAs on mood and the mind. According to an article in *Preventative Medicine*, *"Growing evidence likewise suggests a role for omega-3 fatty acids in helping to relieve disabling depression.* ***Fatty acids may provide relief for people of all ages and genders who are afflicted by depression"*** (2006 January, pp. 4-13). In fact, one specific study reported in the *American Journal of Psychiatry* (June 1, 2006, pp. 1098-1100), reported that ***"children with depression benefit from omega-3 supplementation."***

Dr. Bruce West, in *A Special Report from Health Alert* (2001), states that flax seed and flax oil are *"Probably the most remarkable source of nutrition in our entire food chain…* ***flax oil is the supreme source of essential fatty acids****"* (p. 1). He goes on to point out that our bodies cannot manufacture EFAs, which is why they are called essential fatty acids. They cannot be manufactured in the body, and thus must be consumed in our daily diet. Not only do they help control cholesterol and prevent cardiovascular disease, but **in a matter of just a few hours,** ***"your mood can be improved and a feeling of calm can be experienced, along with initial relief from depression"*** (p. 2).

It is important to note that EFAs are most commonly depleted by a diet high in saturated fatty foods, aspirin, **estrogen (and oral contraceptives)**, NSAIDS (i.e. ibuprofen), and bronchodilators (commonly used to treat asthma or bronchitis).

I would recommend taking four 1,000 mg gel caps of either fish oil or flax seed oil daily, or two capsules of each.

6. **Minerals.** A good multi-mineral that includes calcium, magnesium, zinc, and copper is most beneficial, as they are often depleted by medications, thus you could quite easily be deficient in minerals if you have been taking medications. According to the late well-known and respected psychiatrist Dr. Carl C. Pfeiffer, Ph.D., M.D., **a vitamin or mineral deficiency can result in various brain disorders, including depression.** We just need to provide the resources and allow our brain to take care of the details (something it can do very efficiently). It's when we attempt to use drugs to force it to do what we think it should, that we begin encountering problems.

7. **Amino acids**. As some amino acids act as either neurotransmitters or precursors of neurotransmitters, they are thus critical for the brain to effectively receive and send messages.

Even if vitamins and minerals are absorbed and assimilated by the body, they cannot be effective unless the necessary amino acids are present, no matter how well balanced your diet. Impaired absorption, infection, trauma, stress, drug use, age, and imbalances of other nutrients can all affect the availability of essential amino acids in the body.

While a good multi-amino acid complex containing all essential amino acids should be beneficial, it is also suggested that you take the following additional individual amino acids, (but at a separate time). Each amino acid has its own unique benefit. Some are more calming, while others are more stimulating. If an individual amino acid, such as Taurine for example, was taken along with the complex containing all essential amino acids (those that the body can't produce), you might not realize the same benefit. The Taurine could possibly be combined with other amino acids and used for some other purpose. When combined, they have multiple uses in the body, such as producing enzymes, red blood cells, tissue repairs, etc. We can more effectively regulate how they will be used, when taking some separately from others.

It is normally wise to take the more stimulating amino acids such as tyrosine in the morning for most people, or when anyone suffering from a bipolar condition is experiencing depression. In contrast, the more calming amino acid would ordinarily be best if taken in the evening, or when experiencing a manic episode by those with the bipolar or manic-depressive disorder.

Following are some of the more beneficial amino acids for depression:

✓ **Glutamine** – an energizer, memory booster, and stress reliever. It is an alternate source of fuel for the brain and helps build and balance the neurotransmitters. It improves mental energy and promotes relaxation, as well as stabilizing blood sugar, thus reducing cravings for sugar and alcohol.

✓ **Taurine** –helps reduce anxiety, irritability, insomnia, migraine, alcoholism, obsessions, and depression. It also enhances the activity of the calming neurotransmitter Gama-Aminobutric Acid (GABA).

✓ **Tyrosine** – acts as an energizer and mood enhancer, and is a precursor to the neurotransmitters dopamine, adrenaline, and noradrenaline, as well as the thyroid hormone.

✓ **L-theanine** – last but certainly not least, this is another fairly new amino acid, discussed in the January 2002 issue of the *Health Sciences Institute* newsletter. One article explains how research has revealed that **L-theanine effectively crosses the blood-brain barrier** and induces several distinct chemical changes in the brain that reduce feelings of stress:

> ***Approximately 30 minutes after it is ingested, L-theanine stimulates the production of alpha waves. Such brain waves leave a person feeling alert but deeply relaxed.*** *Theanine also stimulated production of gamma aminobutyric acid. GABA, our most widespread neurotransmitter, limits nerve cell activity in those areas of the brain associated with anxiety, and consequently* ***induces a state of relaxation, calmness, and serenity in stressed or agitated individuals*** (pp. 1-2).

It was mentioned **that L-Theanine also "significantly increased" tryptophan, an amino acid that is the basis of serotonin, a mood-altering brain chemical that is essential to the feeling of well-being and relaxation and may help alleviate symptoms of clinical depression**. Apparently, in addition to providing the foundation for substances essential to good neuron function, **L-theanine may also prevent brain cell death.**

8. **5HTP** (5-hydroxytryptophan**).** An alternate solution that might work for you is 5HTP, an amino acid derived from a West African herb, *Griffonia simplicifolia*. 5HTP is easily absorbed and is highly effective at raising serotonin levels, with up to 300 mg per day often being effective. As a serotonin enhancer, 5HTP has proven in studies to be a mood elevator for people who suffer from depression, anxiety, and stress. However, **while attempting to withdraw from Prozac™, or any SSRI antidepressant for that matter, 5HTP is not a good choice.** It could help contribute to a condition called serotonin syndrome, which is caused from excessively elevated serotonin, and something you should be aware of. Instead, SAMe would likely be a better option.

9. **Licorice Root.** While scientists believe that most forms of depression are caused either by neurotransmitter uptake, increased MAO levels, or both, they have just begun to realize that **licorice root (*Glycyrrhiza glabra*) can be extremely beneficial when battling depression. High levels of the enzyme monoamine oxidase (MAO) can destroy dopamine, norepinephrine, and serotonin, leading to depression**. Unfortunately, MAO is concentrated primarily in the brain, where it causes the most damage.

Studies in Japan suggest that **the most benefit comes from licorice's ability to inhibit MAO. Licorice has been shown to inhibit 44-64% of MAO, which is comparable to synthetic treatments, but without the side effects, thus making licorice nature's form of an MAO inhibitor.** And you don't have to avoid all those healthy foods that must be avoided when taking MAO inhibitor antidepressants. Keep in mind that licorice root can sometimes worsen hypertension, so if you have elevated blood pressure, licorice root might not be the best option.

The best form is deglycyrrhizinated licorice root (DGL), and should be available in your local health food store.

10.**Rhodiola Rosea** is another herbal supplement that proves to be highly beneficial. In the book *Arctic Root (Rhodiola Rosea) – The Powerful New Ginseng Alternative*, written by Carl Germano, R.D., C.N.S., L.D.N. and Zakir Ramazanov, Ph.D. (1999), it is stated that ***"Rhodiola rosea not only decreases the levels of stress hormones in the body****… but evidence also suggests that* ***Rhodiola rosea may help those people, buried by feelings of depression, climb out of their psychological hole"*** (pp. 46, 139).

And, an article in *Life Extension* magazine (2004/2005 winter special edition), explains: *"Rhodiola works primarily on the mitochondria in the central and parasympathetic nervous system. In small doses,* **Rhodiola increases the bioelectric activity of the brain and stimulates norepinephrine, dopamine, and serotonin, all major neurotransmitters***"* (p. 39). The article goes on to explain that, although 17 varieties of Rhodiola rosea are available, positive effects were achieved using the **Russian Rhodiola**, standardized to 3% rosavins and 1% salidrosides.

11. **DHEA** (**de**h**y**dro**e**pi**a**ndrosterone). In a major study conducted in the UK, **as many as 67% of men and 82% of women reported a noticeable decrease in their depressive symptoms while taking only 25 mg/day of DHEA**. In the March 2003 issue of *Life Extension Magazine*, it was reported that researchers at the University of Newcastle Upon Tyne, UK tested DHEA to see if it offered any protection against the stress hormone cortisol, known to be elevated in patients with depression. In their study, cortisol and DHEA were measured in saliva taken from 39 patients with unipolar depression who had been medication free for at least six weeks. These samples were then compared with those of 41 non-depressed subjects. The results showed that **the level of cortisol was significantly higher than that of DHEA in the depressed patients, when compared with healthy subjects** (pp. 27-28). The article concludes:

> ***This indicates that reduced DHEA levels may be a marker for depressive illness and a contributing factor to the associated deficits in learning and memory.*** *These results also suggest that* ***the administration of DHEA or other anti-glucocorticoid treatments may reduce neurocognitive deficits in major depression.*** *(Am J Psychiatry 2002 Jul;159(7):1237-9)*

According to the book *DHEA – Unlocking the Secrets to the Fountain of Youth*, written by Beth M. Ley (1996): ***"DHEA regulates diabetes, obesity,*** *carcinogenesis, tumor growth, virus and bacterial infection,* ***stress,*** *pregnancy,* ***hypertension****, collagen and skin integrity,* ***fatigue, depression, memory*** *and immune responses"* (p. 32). Beth goes on to point out that:

> ***Stressful events depress DHEA production. The Cortisol/DHEA ratio in individuals with panic disorder is depressed by about 50 percent.***

A number of drugs, not only pharmaceuticals, but also alcohol and tobacco, lower levels of DHEA, probably due to the increased stress on the body. Birth control pills especially have a detrimental effect. Alcohol puts an added stress on the body*. Alcohol has numerous and various effects on hormone production in the body* (p. 35).

It was also found that *"**people taking DHEA simply claim that they feel better; less stressed, less depressed, more energetic. DHEA has shown to improve memory by increasing formation of brain cells. DHEA has also shown to decrease aggressive behavior and decrease depression"*** (pp. 81-82).

As we can see, **both stress and the stress hormone Cortisol (increased 200% by Prozac™) can reduce DHEA and thus contribute to depression!** Just one of many ways Prozac™ can eventually contribute to depression, **(as well as having a negative influence on the memory!)**

12. **Relora™,** which contains extracts from the two herbs Philodendron and Magnolia, is yet another safe and effective supplement, found to **increase DHEA levels, while also lowering cortisol**, **both associated with depression.** It is available at most health food stores and through mail order.

The cover story of the June 18, 2002 edition of *Woman's World* magazine, featured Dr. Jim LaValle explaining how Relora™ was tested in a human study and found to be a **safe, effective, rapidly acting, non-sedating dietary supplement that helps control stress and its associated symptoms: irritability, emotional ups and downs, restlessness, tense muscles, poor sleep and concentration difficulties.** The study was conducted in Dr. LaValle's clinic to measure cortisol and DHEA levels in patients with mild to moderate stress. **Elevated cortisol levels and depressed DHEA levels are associated with chronic stress.** A two-week regimen of **Relora™ caused a significant increase in salivary DHEA (227 percent) and a significant decrease in morning salivary cortisol levels (37 percent)**. These significant findings support **Relora's ability to relieve stress and its potential role in depression (a major issue).**

13. NADH is basically an **energizer that stimulates the production of the neurotransmitters serotonin, dopamine, and noradrenaline.** It is also an antioxidant, and **improves mental clarity, memory, alertness, and concentration.**

14. Noni has been used in the Hawaiian Islands for years, for all types of ailments. In her audiotape titled *Help! I Can't Get Off My Anti-Depressants!* (1999), Dr. Tracy suggests that, ***"Noni juice will help you to get rid of the disassociative state that comes from these drugs* [Prozac™, etc.]*. That 'almost being in a dream state' that you feel in the withdrawal."*** She goes on to say that ***"It will help prevent mania. I have been amazed at what I have seen Noni do with those who have gone manic because of these drugs."***

In her book *Understanding the Nature and Cause of Addictions*, Dr. Mary L. Reed, CNHP, MH, ND also encourages the use of Noni, indicating that *"Tahitian Noni seems to be a lifesaver for many who have an addictive personality"* and goes on to say that, ***"It has been used successfully by those with drug addictions, cigarettes, alcohol and sugar. It is also helpful for depression** and vitality"* (p. 4).

15. **Pregnenolone** is a hormone that appears to be an excellent resource to assist in **reducing stress and maintaining emotional health.** Just be aware that pregnenolone is produced from cholesterol, (one of its many benefits). Because it is a precursor for all steroid hormones, pregnenolone helps regulate proper hormone balance. It is also **involved in emotional health, assists with proper sleep, and reduces stress, and is known for its ability to promote feelings of balance and harmony.** Clinical studies have examined its role in **relieving depression, improving memory, reducing stress,** treating arthritis, and increasing longevity. Pregnenolone has been used for many years in high doses, and most importantly with no reported side effects. It can normally be found at your local health food store. I personally take one 30 mg capsule daily.

16.**Protein-Rich Diet.** Not only serotonin, but also another neurotransmitter, dopamine, is also suspected to decrease with reduced exposure to light. **Dopamine is the brain activator, and it has been proven that people are more alert and think more clearly when dopamine levels are high.** If you consider that according to Dr. Glenmullen, M.D., author or *Prozac Backlash*, SSRI antidepressants such as Prozac™, Paxil™, and Zoloft™ actually suppress dopamine by more than 50%, you can see the concern of placing children on these drugs in increasing numbers. If they would be more alert and think more clearly when dopamine levels are higher, does it make any sense to be placing our children on drugs known to lower dopamine? Especially due to their many serious side effects, and very poor performance record, in studies, compared to a placebo.

A dietary approach to combat low dopamine levels is a protein-rich diet. Foods such as cheese, extra-lean meat, chicken or turkey, fish and salmon, and eggs raise dopamine levels and help boost energy and mood. In addition, protein does not trigger a high insulin response, allowing the blood sugar to remain steadier.

17. **Vitamin D Supplementation.** Another level that drops during the winter months due to less sun exposure is vitamin D. Canadian researchers, at Mt. Sinai Hospital in Toronto, report that vitamin D levels have been found to drop in the winter months, compared to summer months. Additionally, it has been found that ***"Vitamin D deficiency also might be a contributing factor to depression,*** *particularly seasonal affective disorder (winter depression)"* (http://www.townsendletter.com/July2004/gabyeditorial0704.htm).

Canadian Dr. Reinhold Vieth, Ph.D., lead vitamin D researcher in Toronto, advises: *"If I were to provide advice, I would say that anyone in North America should be able to walk into any drug store and buy 1,000 IU vitamin D supplements. And if you consume those supplements every day, you should feel better"* (http://www.webmd.com/content/Article/91/101374.htm). In my opinion, a health food store might be a better place to find quality vitamins, rather than a drug store.

As Dr. John Cannell, M.D. explains on *WebMD*, ***"Basically, what vitamin D does is increase levels of the serotonin in the brain. About 90% of patients in my hospital are vitamin D deficient, and I put them on a vitamin D regimen, and it does improve their mood disorders,"*** (http://www.lightupthenet.com/news_studies/index.html).

Although the best source of vitamin D is exposure to the sunlight, the only food sources that provide more than trace amounts are cod-liver oil and fish oil. One-thousand milligrams daily of vitamin D_3 (the natural form) is normally adequate, although recent evidence has suggested that doses up to 4,000 IU per day are safe (*Mayo Clinic Proceedings*, Rochester MN, 2003, pp. 1463-1470).

18.Vitamin C. According to *Life Extension Disease Prevention and Treatment, Expanded Third Edition*, (1997/2002), ***"Supplemental doses of vitamin C have helped depressed patients of all ages,"*** and recommend the following: *"Start with 1 gram (1000 mg) of vitamin C twice a day. Then gradually increase the dosage until you are taking at least 3000 mg twice a day"* (p. 231).

19.**Celtic sea salt.** Replace common table salt, which is acidic and missing the mineral potassium, (as well as many important trace minerals), with Celtic sea salt. Celtic sea salt is instead alkaline, and contains both sodium and potassium, as well as 84 trace minerals in the ionic form, which is important for effective assimilation and utilization by the cells.

According to Dr. Balch (in regards to the mineral potassium), **the secretion of stress hormones (caused by Prozac™) causes a decrease in the potassium-to-sodium ratio both inside and outside of the cells.** This is just one more reason to get off Prozac™, which stimulates the stress hormone cortisol. Adding Celtic sea salt to your diet, during and after withdrawal, will help restore proper mineral ratios. This is an important issue, as the sodium-potassium pump is responsible for the transfer of nutrients into the cell, as well as the removal of toxins from the cell. Although common table salt contains only sodium, (which contributes to fluid retention or edema), Celtic sea salt also contains the important mineral potassium.

Celtic sea salt is available at most health food stores, or directly through the *Grain & Salt Society* by calling (800) TOP-SALT, or by visiting http://www.celtic-seasalt.com/

20. Then Last, But Definitely Not Least, The Herb "Ashwagandha" - Instead of the Dangerous SSRI Antidepressants

We will now take a moment and compare a safe and effective herb from India, called Ashwagandha, (easily accessible in the U.S.), with SSRI antidepressants. The following was taken from an article in the June 2006 issue of *Life Extension* magazine:

> ***Ashwagandha,*** *an exotic Indian herb,* ***has remarkable stress-relieving properties comparable to those of powerful drugs used to treat depression and anxiety.*** *In addition to its excellent protective effects on the nervous system,* ***Ashwagandha may be a promising alternative treatment for a variety of degenerative diseases such as Alzheimer's disease and Parkinson's disease.***
>
> *Even more remarkable,* ***emerging evidence suggests that Ashwagandha has anti-cancer benefits as well.***
>
> *In validated models of anxiety and depression,* ***Ashwagandha has been demonstrated to be as effective as some tranquilizers and antidepressant drugs.*** *Bhattacharya SK, Bhattacharya A, Sairam K, Ghosal S. Phytomedicine. 2000 Dec;7(6):463-9).*

Studies of chronic stress support these findings. For example, in a remarkable animal study, ***examination of the brains of sacrificed animals showed that 85% of the brain cells observed in the animals exposed to chronic stress showed signs of degeneration.*** *It is this type of cellular degeneration that can lead to long-term cognitive difficulties. Amazingly,* ***when Ashwagandha was administered to chronically stressed animals, the number of degenerating brain cells was reduced by 80%!*** *(Jain S, Shukla SD, Sharma K, Bhatnager M. Phytother Res. 2001 Sep;15(6):544-8).*

In one of the most complete human clinical trials to date, researchers studied the effects of a standardized extract of Ashwagandha on the negative effects of stress, including elevated levels of the stress hormone cortisol. ***Many of the adverse effects of stress are thought to be related to elevated levels of cortisol. The results were impressive. The participants subjectively reported increased energy, reduced fatigue, better sleep, and an enhanced sense of well-being.***

The participants showed several measurable improvements, including a reduction of cortisol levels up to 26%, ***a decline in fasting blood sugar levels,*** *and improved lipid profiles. It would appear from this study that* ***Ashwagandha can address many of the health and psychological issues that plague today's society.*** *(Unpublished study, 2005, NutrGeneisis. LLC.)*

Ashwagandha also shows promise as a treatment for Parkinson's and Alzheimer's diseases, chronic neurodegenerative conditions for which there currently are no cures. *(Choudhary MI, Yousuf S, Nawaz SA, Ahmed S, Atta uR. Chem Pharm Bull (Tokyo). 2004 Nov;52(11):1358-61).*

In addition to ashwagandha's documented neuroprotective effects, exciting recent evidence suggests that it also has the potential to stop cancer cells in their tracks. *(Altern Med Rev. 2004 Jun;9(2):211-4).*

Scientists in India recently conducted cell studies showing that Ashwagandha extract disrupts cancer cells' ability to reproduce – a key stop in fighting cancer. Additionally, laboratory analysis indicates that Ashwagandha extract possesses anti-angiogenic activity, also known as the ability to prevent cancer from forming new blood vessels to support its unbridled growth. (Mathur R, Gapta SK, Singh N, J Ethnopharmacol. 2006 Jan 9).

A recent experiment demonstrated that Ashwagandha extract produced a marked increase in life span *and a decrease in tumor weight in animals with experimentally induced cancer of the lymphatic system. (Christina AJ, Joseph DG, Packialakshmi M. J Ethnopharmacol. 2004 Aug;93(2-3):359-61).*

One of the consequences of chemotherapy is neutropenia, a decrease in white blood cells called neutrophils that can leave patients dangerously vulnerable to infection. A study of animals demonstrated that orally administered Ashwagandha

extract protected against this decline in infection-fighting neutrophils. (Gupta YK, Sharma SS, Rai K, Katiyar CK. Indian J Physiol Pharmacol. 2001 Apr;45(2):253-7).
Another animal study investigated Ashwagandha extract's effects in normalizing the immune-suppressing effects of chemotherapy.

Chronic stress exacts a high price from our bodies as well as our minds. *Many degenerative diseases, as well as premature aging, are associated with chronic nervous tension. There is great need for safe and effective prevention strategies to combat the ravages of stress on our nervous system.*

Of primary importance is the fact that **Ashwagandha has been demonstrated to be as effective as some tranquilizers and antidepressants**. Then, **instead of having "many troubling side effects," which Prozac™ is so well known for, just the opposite is actually true with Ashwagandha.**

If a pharmaceutical company could create a drug with that kind of potential, the whole world would soon hear about it, and you could rest assured that the price would not be cheap. The cost of most medication normally reflects what it might be worth to someone, rather than the cost to produce it.

For instance, **Prozac™ is well known for greatly increasing the stress hormone cortisol, and raising the blood sugar, eventually resulting in diabetes. Yet, Ashwagandha appears to instead lower both cortisol and blood sugar.** And as we discussed earlier, the elevated cortisol caused by Prozac™ contributes to neuron damage in the area of the brain responsible for long-term memory, and regulating hormones. It was also discovered that many with Alzheimer's disease have elevated cortisol in the brain. Although, Ashwagandha was instead found to be neuro-protective, and that it might even be effective in the treatment of both Alzheimer's disease and Parkinson's disease.

Then we come to cancer. As we learned, every molecule of Prozac™ actually contains three molecules of the toxin fluoride, which among many things, is thought to contribute to cancer, as it tends to cause cell mutilation. And once more we find that Ashwagandha not only has documented neuroprotective effects, but it might very well be a resource in stopping cancer's progression as well. And that it also helps restore some of the damage to the immune system caused by chemotherapy.

In every single instance, Prozac™ is busy creating problems, while Ashwagandha is instead resolving them, and is proven effective in resolving depression as well. And as we just learned, Ashwagandha is just one of many natural alternatives we have to choose from. And some of the others have proven every bit as effective as Prozac™ in resolving depression.

Due to the preponderance of evidence presented, do you see any possible reason to justify allowing such a potentially dangerous drug to remain on the market, and to be continually promoted and prescribed (especially to our innocent children)? As adults, it's our ultimate responsibility to look out for our children's best interest. Someone should be held accountable for such an obvious deception! The question is: How can the FDA possibly justify approving such a dangerous drug as Prozac™ with its hundreds of potential side effects, and thousands of official complaints regarding serious reactions, for children's use? One can't help but wonder if the FDA hasn't somehow lost sight of whose interest they were originally established to protect!

Next: Phase Out Your Medications

Although this step is important, I would recommend you begin re-building your body with sufficient nutrition initially. You might consider first taking supplements such as goji, noni, and/or mangosteen juices, as well as SAMe, vitamins, minerals, amino acids, and essential fatty acids, for a couple of weeks. You could then try slowly reducing the dosage of your medications, (in an attempt to phase them out), while carefully monitoring your blood pressure and blood sugar levels (when appropriate, if necessary). Although it is helpful to maintain healthy levels of both blood pressure and blood sugar, on a temporary basis neither should be life threatening, (unless extremely elevated).

One medication you should, in my opinion, stop taking immediately is any statin drug for lowering cholesterol. Everyone I know that did, son began feeling much better. Elevated cholesterol is not a disease! If you are on several medications, or are at all concerned, you might ask your doctor if he or she can assist you in the drug withdrawal process.

As I have always stressed, you better than anyone else, can more effectively evaluate your pain and depression level, if that is what you are taking medication for. Keep in mind that one side effect associated with many medications is depression, thus just eliminating some medications might be sufficient to resolve your depression.

In most cases, (if not all of them), the supplements we discussed are more effective than medications such as Prozac™ and Paxil™ in truly resolving depression. In addition, they have many "side benefits", versus the antidepressants' many "troubling side effects", thus the choice should be obvious!

Then, Phase Out Antidepressants

If you are currently taking any antidepressant, this is the most important step in your recovery process. It is critical for restoring the natural balance of neurotransmitters in the brain (something only the body can accomplish). It would be most beneficial if you could phase out **all other** prescription medications, **BEFORE** attempting to phase out any antidepressant (especially the SSRI antidepressants). This will help strengthen your body for the withdrawal process. And, regarding the SSRI antidepressants, such as Prozac™, Paxil™, or Zoloft™, there are many different benefits from phasing them out of your life once and for all. One thing people soon discover after withdrawal, is a return of their emotions, and often claim that it feels as though a fog is lifting. Just avoiding the potential long-term side effects, such as diabetes, cancer, adrenal fatigue, and possibly brain damage, along with any of the 575 potential side effects associated with the drug Prozac™, definitely makes it well worth the effort. Any drug such as Prozac™ that can increase your level of the stress hormone cortisol by 200% is obviously a major concern, as cortisol is a major contributor to many of the side effects associated with Prozac™, (thus worsening the condition). And we certainly can't forget the potential damage associated with the fluoride found in Prozac™.

Dr. Ann Blake Tracy, in her book *Prozac: Panacea or Pandora?* (1991/1994), recommends improving the diet, and reducing the dosage of your antidepressant very slowly. She said that at times it might take as long as two years, and would require slowly shaving the pill in the process. Although reducing your dosage of the antidepressant slowly is sometimes advisable, in my opinion that would be extremely difficult to accomplish over that long a period of time, especially as some are in capsule rather than pill form. And personally, I couldn't visualize reducing the dosage for two years! How could you possibly keep track of how much you shaved off your pill the day before? However, as far as I know, at the time Dr. Tracy wrote her book, neither the mangosteen nor goji juices were widely available in the U.S. yet, (and possibly she wasn't familiar with some of the supplements we covered as well).

Although I have actually seen some people go off their antidepressants cold turkey and do so without any problem, there are multiple factors involved, and thus is not normally advisable. It typically depends upon the particular antidepressant, how long you have been taking the antidepressant, your overall health, nutrient intake, and daily stress levels. In my opinion, it's usually best to begin by reducing the dosage by ¼ for two weeks, and then go on a half-dose for another two more weeks, and finally reduce the dosage by ¾, to ¼ for dose the last two weeks. Although, if you have only been on the antidepressant for a few months, that is normally not really necessary.

People often tend to have difficulty dealing with stress following the use of SSRI antidepressants, especially for an extended period of time. The continuous stimulation of cortisol caused by Prozac™ (200% increase from one 30 mg dose) for example, in time can result in adrenal fatigue, as well as **a hair-trigger response to any stress.** One of Dr. Tracy's patients discovered that when attempting to stop her antidepressants, after an unusually stressful day at work (she didn't deal well with stress). She found that drinking a cup of chamomile tea along with several hours of rest helped her recover.

There are many helpful herbs for dealing with stress (possibly even better than the chamomile tea), without causing drowsiness. One I find very effective is called Valerian root. It is fast acting, very effective, and yet quite inexpensive. If you try to avoid stressful situations, (especially during the withdrawal process), and take Valerian root when necessary, you should likely be more successful, and experience less symptoms during the withdrawal process.

Remove / Eliminate Fluoride

It's interesting that even thousands of years ago, the Egyptians were fully aware of the dangers associated with Fluoride in their water. And the Chinese were also concerned about fluoride found in their well water in some provinces, yet we continue "adding" it to our water systems! The aluminum industry just found a convenient way to dispose of a well-known environmental toxin, and have gotten away with it for years, and at our expense.

The Egyptians discovered long ago that gold was effective in the removal of fluoride in the body, although I'm not sure exactly how they accomplished it. It's amazing that, thousands of years ago, they were fully aware that fluoride is a serious toxin, (something that many scientists today still seem to be ignoring).

There just happens to be a product containing gold that I am aware of. It's a colloidal gold liquid, containing a concentration of approximately 50 parts per million. It's a super small molecule that is rapidly absorbed. According to David Hinkson, the founder of the company *Water Oz*™, some symptoms of a gold deficiency appear to be brain dysfunction, depression, gland dysfunction, and insomnia

Interestingly, those symptoms just happen to be very similar to the side effects associated with Prozac™. And it appears that the Egyptians were right all along, although we just happen to have technology now to produce a colloidal form that readily absorbs. According to David Hinkson, **gold *"neutralizes fluoride poisoning"*** (noted in the *Water Oz Retail/Buyer's Club Catalog*, 2004, p. 10).

It's important to incorporate a molecule small enough to penetrate the blood-brain barrier, as fluoride also can. What convinced me that their products can rapidly absorb, was regarding their liquid magnesium. At times, it can resolve a headache, (especially tension headaches). With my wife, it will normally resolve a headache in less than five minutes. Their colloidal minerals can be purchased through *Water Oz™* by calling (800) 547-2294.

As we discussed, every single molecule of Prozac™ contains "3 molecules of fluoride"! And if you recall, Dr. Cade discovered that Prozac™, (and thus fluoride), not only accumulates, but also remains in the brain for years. If you consider that fluoride damages hormone receptors, suppresses enzyme action, and disrupts the iodine receptors found throughout the brain, you can see **the wisdom in "getting the fluoride out"!**

NOTE: Further information regarding iodine receptors in the brain, and fluoride interaction, can be found in the chapter at the end of this book on Additional Technical Information.

In addition to the colloidal liquid gold, another way of accomplishing the removal of fluoride involves using the supplement Iodoral™, which contains both iodine and potassium iodide (as we previously discussed). It will help kick start the thyroid gland by removing accumulated fluoride and replacing it with the proper form of iodine necessary for producing the thyroid hormone. In his book *Iodine: Why You Need It – Why You Can't Live Without It* (2004), Dr. David Brownstein discovered that ***"after one day of supplementation* [referring to the Iodoral™]*, fluoride excretion increased 78%"*** (p. 88). However, he also goes on to note that ***"My experience has shown that in an iodine deficient state, it takes from three to six months of iodine supplementation before iodine saturation is reached"*** (p. 88).

Dr. Brownstein states that many different conditions such as thyroid disorders, chronic fatigue, fibromyalgia, and cancer of the breast and prostate are often the result of an iodine deficiency, and he goes on to note that ***"The most important facet of iodine supplementation is that it helps patients improve their health and helps them feel better"*** (p. 88).

I personally purchase Iodoral™ from the *Women's International Pharmacy*, as the owner Wally Simons, R.Ph. is a good friend whom I trust, although there are likely other sources. They can be contacted at (800) 699-8143.

It would also be helpful to take fish oil to help rebuild the hormone receptors in the brain, (which fluoride damages), and Iodoral™ (iodine/iodide), to also restore the iodine in the receptors of the thyroid and the brain, which fluoride replaces. Iodine is necessary for efficient metabolism in both the body and brain. The Iodoral™ should soon begin restoring normal balance in the brain.

Dr. Brownstein has stated that the thyroid hormone is more effective when an adequate level of iodine is available, and that most people do better on a combination of iodine and potassium iodide, (found in Iodoral™). He also indicates that in the patients he tested for iodine levels, 91% were found to be below normal. I might just mention that it's interesting that Harry Hoxsey discovered a very effective cancer therapy, over 60 years ago, that just happened to contain potassium iodide, (found in Iodoral™), along with herbs. As usual, natural supplements provide many benefits, (versus drugs' many side effects). The choice should be quite obvious.

Drugs that target the brain, (be they legal or illegal), are very damaging to the brain, and disrupt normal hormone balance. That eventually results in an unsteady and abnormal condition, such as the bipolar disorder, for which even more dangerous drugs are then prescribed to treat, as we will be discussing next.

CHAPTER SIXTEEN

The Bipolar Disorder

To begin with, I might first explain that, after completing my original version of this chapter, I soon realized that I was introducing some new concepts, as well as explaining various actions and interactions, in considerable detail. I could see that, to the average person (which this book was actually written for), it could appear rather complex, and possibly even confusing to some. That prompted me to re-write this chapter for you, and place **the expanded, more technical version, in the back of this book,** for other doctors or scientists who might be interested in details, and a more in-depth explanation. And of course, you are welcome to read it as well, if you so choose. Some are just curious, as I always have been, or possibly looking for a challenge.

How SSRI Antidepressants Actually Contribute to the Bipolar Disorder (And They Are Actually Less Effective Than A Placebo!)

Serotonin affects nearly every area of brain activity. Prozac™ actually over-stimulates serotonin receptors, by suppressing the natural reuptake of any excess serotonin secreted, as nature had intended. This is where the bipolar condition normally begins. The excessive stimulation of neurotransmitters is an abnormal condition that initiates a chain reaction resulting in an unsteady environment in the brain. Not only illegal drugs, but also legal drugs such as Prozac™ and other SSRI antidepressants, eventually contribute to very similar problems, as they are all basically stimulants. Although some are considered as legal, they can at times be every bit as dangerous, (each in its own way).

The normal serotonin reuptake's primary function in the brain is intended to prevent any over-stimulation. Another is preserving any excess serotonin for use elsewhere. Serotonin has many functions, in both the body and the brain, (and there is not an unending supply). Due to the overstimulation of the serotonin receptors in the brain, they soon begin shutting down. That is the same basic concept that results in insulin resistance in the body, from elevated insulin. That's what we refer to as insulin resistance, or type II diabetes, which results in the inefficient utilization of glucose, although in this case, it's the inefficient use of serotonin. That is especially true with long-term usage, which can eventually become potentially life threatening, often leading to the bipolar disorder, and even worse depression. That's just one of several reasons that "depression" is one potential side effect associated with Prozac™ and other SSRI antidepressants.

One big problem is, doctors often leave their patients on one or more antidepressants, contributing to the bipolar disorder for years, thus it would likely continue. Then rather than removing the problem (i.e. Prozac™), they instead add another dangerous drug to deal with the side effects (a typical, although inappropriate approach in medicine today). Not only that, but the patient would then be on both a stimulant (Prozac™), as well as a depressant (lithium), which are opposing actions that would basically be attempting to cancel the effect of the other. How "unscientific" can they possibly get? It would make more sense to phase out the contributor to the condition, which is not really that difficult, if properly withdrawn.

And most importantly, for people with the bipolar disorder, these SSRI antidepressants were proven in some studies to be no better than a placebo! As announced March 22, 2007, in the *New England Journal of Medicine*, Dr. Gary Sachs and colleagues, of Massachusetts General Hospital in Boston, studied 366 people with bipolar disorder, and reported the following:

> ***Of the 179 subjects who received an antidepressant and mood stabilizer, about 24 per cent were able to go eight weeks with no more than two depressive or manic symptoms.***
>
> ***In comparison, 27 per cent of those in the placebo group reached the same level, a difference that is not statistically significant,*** *the researchers said* (http://www.cbc.ca/health/story/2007/03/28/bipolar-medication.html).

It's interesting that the researcher claims that it's not "statistically significant", when actually it is, as **it proves that the placebo was actually more effective,** (something they obviously don't want to admit)!

Elevated Histamine (Histadelia) – One Contributor To The Bipolar Disorder

Histadelia is a term referring to a condition where the body has high levels of histamine, and in his book *Nutrition and Mental Illness* (1987), Dr. Carl C. Pfeiffer, Ph.D., M.D. states that ***"histamine causes a tendency to hyperactivity, compulsive behavior, and depression"*** (p. 26), which actually defines the bipolar disorder. Dr. Pfeiffer then warns that ***"when histamine levels are not controlled, they can lead to chronic depression and even suicide."***

Histamine is actually considered a neurotransmitter, and has several important functions in the body and brain, although both the regulation and distribution of water levels in the body appear to be two of the more critical functions that histamine is responsible for. The problem arises when the histamine level becomes excessively elevated.

Ten Natural Ways To Lower Histamine:

1. **Celtic sea salt and water.** Celtic sea salt is a natural antihistamine, and full of trace minerals. Incidentally, one of them is copper, which is necessary for regulating histamine. Dr. Batmanghelidj insists that simply increasing your salt intake will help prevent elevated histamine, and in his book *Your Body's Many Cries for Water* (1997), he points out that one of the most common causes of elevated histamine in the body is dehydration. I recommend taking one teaspoon of sea salt, and drinking eight to ten 8-ounce glasses (or more) of water daily.
2. **Copper** is necessary for regulating histamine. As I indicated, copper is one of the important trace minerals found in Celtic sea salt. As copper is a "trace" mineral, a trace amount is all that is necessary, however the natural form of copper, as found in Celtic sea salt, will not cause excessively elevated copper, which can be a concern.
3. **Limit Potassium.** Dr. Batmanghelidj also suggests: ***"Reduce orange juice intake** to one, or at the most two, glasses a day. The potassium content of orange juice is high. **High loads [levels] of potassium in the body can promote more than usual histamine production"*** (*Your Body's Many Cries For Water*, 1992/1998, p. 119).

4. Avoid stress, as stress causes dehydration, which increases histamine. Incidentally, antidepressants, diuretics, alcohol, caffeine and smoking, are all known to cause dehydration as well.

5. Vitamin C is another natural antihistamine. I would recommend a minimum of 2,000 mg of Ester C with bioflavonoids daily, in divided doses, and up to 10,000 mg daily during stress or following an injury or surgery, or during a cold or flu.

6. Essential Fatty Acids (EFAs). In her book *Natural Highs* (2002), Dr. Hyla Cass, M.D. states that *"histamine imbalances have been associated with EFA imbalances. They mediate immune function* [and] *nourish the thyroid and adrenals"* (p. 39). Two good sources of essential fatty acids are flax seed oil and fish oil, (both available in liquid or soft gel form). Both also appear to be especially beneficial for the brain. I would suggest 2,000 mg of flax seed oil, and 2,000 mg of fish oil, in soft gels, daily, or one tablespoon of each, daily.

7. Check your thyroid! As noted in his book *Wilson's Syndrome – The Miracle of Feeling Well* (1996), Dr. E. Denis Wilson, M.D. points out that **elevated histamine is common when the thyroid function is reduced (hypothyroidism).** You may want to refer to the earlier chapter on Hypothyroidism.

8. Quercetin is another possibility. As noted in an undated pamphlet by Dr. Susan Lark, M.D., titled *"The Miracle of Simple"*, ***"Knock out an allergy attack with 600 mg of 'Quercetin',*** *which is derived from onions.* ***Taken with vitamin C, it stops histamine release in its tracks."*** Incidentally, quercetin is a bioflavonoid, and included in some vitamin C formulas. As I noted earlier, I would recommend Ester C with bioflavonoids.

9. MSM has a great antihistamine effect, according to Dr. Ronald Lawrence, M.D., Ph.D., one of the speakers at the *Symposium for Health Freedom* conference in Anaheim, California, (November 16, 2002), which I attended.

10. Coenzyme Q_{10} (CoQ_{10}) is not only a natural antihistamine, but it also has proven beneficial in treating the candida yeast infection! This is due in part because it enhances the immune system, which is essential for treating Candidiasis.

Nutrient Deficiencies That Can Contribute To The Bipolar Disorder

Our brain was designed to maintain healthy levels of both calming and stimulating hormones, which it is very effective at doing, provided it is supplied with the necessary nutrients, and in the proper balance, (a very important issue). Some people are more prone genetically to experience some specific nutritional deficiencies, which can be addressed, and easily resolved. At times, a poor diet contributes to a nutritional deficiency, but by far, the greatest contributor to vitamin and mineral deficiencies is medications. And as I keep stressing, **Prozac™ and Paxil™ are two of the worst, at a total of 16 of the most critical nutrients being depleted, as well as creating an imbalance in the brain, leading to the bipolar disorder.**

Dr. William Walsh Ph.D., Senior Scientist at the Health Research Institute and Pfeiffer Treatment Center in Illinois, points out that:

> *The brain is a factory that produces serotonin, dopamine, norepinephrine, and other brain chemicals 24 hours a day.* ***The only raw materials for their syntheses are nutrients, namely, amino acids, vitamins, minerals, etc. If the brain receives improper amounts of these nutrient***

building blocks, we can expect serious problems with our neurotransmitters (http://www.healthyplace.com/communities/bipolar/treatment/alternative/nutritional_supplements.asp).

✓ **Inositol – a water-soluble cofactor of the vitamin B family.** In the *Prescription for Nutritional Healing, 3rd edition* (2000), Dr. James Balch, M.D. observes that **irritability and mood swings** are both **related to inositol deficiency,** and goes on to note that *"Research has also shown that **high doses of inositol may help in the treatment of depression, obsessive-compulsive disorder, and anxiety disorders, without the side effects of prescription medications"*** (p. 19).

Incidentally, **inositol is depleted by lithium carbonate,** as well as alcohol, caffeine, estrogen (and oral contraceptives), antibiotics, antiseizure medication, and sulfa drugs.

✓ **Choline - a water-soluble cofactor of the vitamin B family.** Both choline and inositol have many important functions, as Eva Edelman (*Natural Healing for Schizophrenia*, 1996/1998) explains:

> ***Choline and inositol nourish and strengthen nerves and brain.*** *They have been used* ***to help relieve anxiety and depression, and promote sleep. Choline is the precursor of acetylcholine, a neurotransmitter essential to memory, nerve/muscle communication, and parasympathetic activity.*** *Choline also helps maintain the myelin sheath which surrounds certain nerve axons. DMAE* [**D**i**m**ethyl**a**mino**e**thanol], *a potent form of choline, is reported to sometimes* ***benefit behavior disorders,*** *and frequently be effective in hyperactivity.*
>
> ***Choline can be depleted in histadelia*** **[elevated histamine],** *and* ***supplementation may improve mood.*** *In certain cases, choline may be helpful (once biotype imbalances are reduced)* ***in moderating the racing thoughts and hypomania*** *which can occur in paranoid schizophrenia.* ***Inositol is reported to have a mild sedative action and be useful in promoting sleep and reducing anxiety*** (p. 31).

Incidentally, **once again we find that choline is also depleted by lithium carbonate,** as well as alcohol, caffeine, sugar, estrogen (and oral contraceptives), and sulfa drugs.

✓ **Magnesium – a water-soluble essential mineral.** Magnesium is essential for a healthy nervous system. The following was obtained from Eva Edelman's *Natural Healing for Schizophrenia* (1996/1998):

> **[Magnesium is]** ***calming to the nervous system.*** *In a study of 165 boys, those with schizophrenia, depression, autism or sleep disturbances had low levels of magnesium. In other studies,* ***psychiatric patients who tried to commit suicide were also found to have depressed levels.*** *Magnesium affects cell membrane permeability, helps maintain cellular electrical potential, and supports formation of tyrosine.* ***A deficiency may produce*** *apathy,* ***agitation, irritability, personality***

> ***changes**, disorientation, bizarre movements, **sleep disturbances, depression** and, in some cases, hallucinations* (p. 35).

Actually, the "personality changes" referred to could just be another term for the bipolar disorder, which is obviously a personality change.

Also, as stressed by Dr. Balch, ***"The proper balance of magnesium, calcium, and phosphorus should be maintained at all times"*** **(*Prescription for Nutritional Healing, 3rd edition*, 2000, pp. 25-26). Dr. Balch also points out that *"a low magnesium level makes nearly every disease worse."***

Incidentally, **magnesium happens to be just one of the 16 nutrients depleted by the SSRI antidepressants such as Prozac™ and Paxil™.**

✓ **Zinc – a water-soluble trace mineral.** Again, we turn to Eva Edelman for her opinion regarding the importance of zinc, as follows:

> ***Zinc is abundant in the brain hippocampus and may function as a neurotransmitter.***
>
> ***It is needed in neuron development neurotransmitter synthesis, and copper chelation.*** *Zinc also enhances resistance to stress; and **helps maintain intellectual function, memory**, and **level moods. Deficiency can lead to** headaches, lethargy, amnesia, other **memory impairment, irritability, behavior disorders**, and **paranoia. Zinc is used in treating histamine imbalances, pyroluria, and blood sugar disorders*** (*Natural Healing for Schizophrenia*, 1996/1998, p. 34).
>
> **And again, zinc is another important mineral depleted by Prozac™ and Paxil™.**

It is important to remember, as stated by Dr. David Benton, Ph.D., of the University of Wales, Swansea, speaking at a symposium, "Mineral/Vitamin Modification of Mental Disorders and Brain Function", at the 2003 American Psychiatric Association's annual meeting, ***"the brain is arguably the most nutritionally sensitive organ in the body."***

The "Typical" Solution For The Bipolar Disorder: Lithium Carbonate - A "Very Dangerous" Drug Of Choice

The objective of prescribing lithium carbonate is to suppress the manic phase of the bipolar disorder only. It is not intended to address the depression that is also associated with this condition. Although, by reducing the manic phase (similar to being "high" on cocaine), the depressive state that eventually follows should be reduced as well. **The primary objective should be to basically level out the moods, to as close as possible to normal.** Following are just some of the dangers associated with the traditional lithium carbonate therapy.

✓ Throughout her book, *Natural Healing for Schizophrenia*, (1996/1998), Eva Edelman lists 36 potential side effects associated with lithium carbonate (although as you will discover, there are even more). Some of the side effects that she lists are:

> *Fine tremor of the hands, slurred speech…incoordination, dizziness, sedation, rigidity, central nervous system effects…**depression, goiter or Hypothyroidism (in up to 10% of patients). Lithium is known to alter adrenal cortisol levels, deplete certain neurotransmitters, and depress the thyroid.***
>
> ***Impairment of consciousness, cardiac abnormalities (20%-30%), permanently increased kidney output, bedwetting, irreversible kidney scarring, other kidney damage, liver disorders, rise in blood sugar, increased white blood cell count, blood disorders, coma, death*** (p. 155).

✓ **The suppression of the thyroid**, in this case, is at least one cause of the **depressive** phase of bipolar. **Two well-known symptoms associated with hypothyroidism are depression, and mood swings (another term for bipolar disorder), and yet these are actually the very symptoms that lithium is normally prescribed for in the first place.** As we progress, you will discover that lithium carbonate is not only a very dangerous drug, but it even **contributes to the very conditions it is prescribed for,** and does so in several ways.

✓ **The altered cortisol levels** she referred to (which is also a problem normally associated with Prozac™), contributes to the thyroid suppression, just noted.

✓ **Blood sugar disorders**. A **"rise in blood sugar"**, (as noted above), stimulates the release of insulin, which is often followed by a rapid drop in blood sugar, or **hypoglycemia.** In his book *Nutrition and Mental Illness* (1987), Dr. Carl C. Pfeiffer, Ph.D., M.D. states that ***"when the blood sugar level drops, the brain immediately suffers, resulting in fatigue and emotional chaos"*** (p. 57). Dr. Pfeiffer then lists **some conditions often associated with glucose intolerance, such as: depression, nervousness, irritability, trembling, forgetfulness, anxiety, confusion, and difficulty concentrating.**

✓ **The damage to the kidneys.** The permanently increased output would obviously affect their ability to retain an adequately regulate the level of both salt and water, contributing to dehydration and elevated histamine.

✓ **Irreversible kidney scarring,** which would then result in **elevated blood pressure**.

✓ **The kidney damage would increase the potential for dialysis,** which is a serious concern. The potential for damage to the kidneys could be even greater for anyone also placed on cholesterol lowering medication, which greatly increases the risk for kidney damage, and thus could elevate the blood pressure even further. Not only that, but kidney transplant might even be necessary.

✓ **Edema (fluid retention)** is another problem associated with both lithium, and Prozac™ use, and is also one condition associated with hypothyroidism (low thyroid). Additionally, according to studies in the *Drug-Induced Nutrient Depletion Handbook* (2001/2001, p. 483), **lithium actually *"blocks* [the] *anti-diuretic hormone effect"* in the kidneys, by decreasing its generation, which is used to regulate both salt and water.**

As strange as it might seem, you can actually be dehydrated and still experience edema. Water regulation and distribution is an important issue. For instance, when a person consumes common table salt, as most people do, they are getting sodium only. But when the accompanying potassium (found in the complete salt created by nature, such as Celtic sea salt) is present, that shouldn't happen. When the inside of the cell contains sodium, rather than potassium as it should, it causes the cell to swell, (sodium attracts water). Thus, you end up with too much water inside the cell, causing undue pressure, yet you will be deficient on water in other areas where it is needed. Possibly the greatest concern is: The sodium /potassium pump, which gets nutrients into the cell, and the toxins out, (a very important function), can't work efficiently if the accompanying potassium is missing.

What Makes Lithium Carbonate So Risky?
Even The Typical "Therapeutic" Dosage Of Lithium Can Be Life-Threatening!

First, let's see what we do know about lithium carbonate and exactly why it's so dangerous. Based on the "normal" dosage of a particular mineral, the amount is usually in either milligrams (mg) or micrograms (mcg). **Lithium is considered as a trace mineral, which is normally measured in micrograms, (not milligrams).** The problem is, the lithium carbonate that most doctors prescribe, is an **in**organic form of lithium, and thus not well absorbed. Thus, a typical dosage is thousands of times higher than the "trace minerals" normally required in order to overcome the inefficient absorption problem. In fact, a local author Eva Edelman, in her book *Natural Healing for Schizophrenia* (1996/1998), points out that, ***"Conventionally prescribed doses (starting at 900 mg Lithium Carbonate per day) approach the lethal level. Since lithium accumulates in the body****, this dosage range* ***can be particularly dangerous, so blood levels are frequently checked"*****, and then goes on to warn that:**

> ***Lithium intake at the psychiatric dose range has been associated with reduced concentration, confusion, memory defects and a blunting of emotions, thought processes and personality. Some researchers warn that lithium can cause progressive and irreversible intellectual deterioration, and should be entirely contraindicated*** (p. 155).

The question is then posed: ***"Is lithium an essential trace mineral?"*** Eva Edelman states that ***"No one knows how lithium works,*** *but these actions might contribute to its effects"* and also that, ***"Lithium influences* [the important neurotransmitters] *acetyl choline, dopamine, serotonin and GABA receptors in the limbic system and basal ganglia"*** (p. 155).

From another source, we find additional, and possibly even more critical conditions, associated with lithium use, which include the following:

> **[These side effects]** ***appear to be related to serum lithium levels, including levels within the therapeutic range:*** *muscle hyperirritability (fasciculations, twitching, clonic movements of whole limbs), hypertonicity, ataxia, choreoathetotic movements, hyperactive deep tendon reflex, extrapyramidal symptoms including acute dystonia,* ***blackout spells, epileptiform seizures, vertigo,*** *downbeat nystagmus,* ***incontinence of urine or feces,*** *somnolence, psychomotor*

> *retardation,* ***restlessness, confusion, stupor****, tongue movements, tics, tinnitus,* ***hallucinations, poor memory, slowed intellectual functioning,*** *startled response,* ***worsening of organic brain syndromes,*** *cardiac arrhythmia, hypotension,* ***peripheral circulatory collapse****, bradycardia,* ***decreased creatinine clearance and albuminuria*** **[indicating kidney damage],** *blurred vision, and* ***impotence/sexual dysfunction.***
>
> *A few reports have been received of the development of painful discoloration of fingers and toes* ***and coldness of the extremities*** **[indicating suppressed thyroid]** ***within one day of the starting of treatment with lithium.***
>
> *Cases of pseudotumor cerebri (****increased intracranial pressure*** *and papilledema)* ***have been reported with lithium use. If undetected, this condition may result in enlargement of the blind spot, constriction of visual fields and eventual blindness due to optic atrophy*** (http://www.healthyplace.com).

Could you possibly imagine anyone subjecting themselves to such serious side effects? And just to suppress the manic phase? Now that you have learned many of the serious consequences associated with taking lithium carbonate, and the nutrients it depletes, the challenge is to resolve the bipolar disorder while also protecting the brain and kidneys from potential damage in the process.

NOTE: Further information regarding the dangers of lithium carbonate therapy may be found in the chapter on Additional Technical Information, in the back of this book.

Lithium Carbonate Toxicity and Withdrawal

Toxic levels of lithium are actually very similar to the excessive buildup of serotonin caused by Prozac™, which is referred to as serotonin syndrome, and both can be life threatening. This brings us to the next important consideration: **Lithium withdrawal**. Eva Edelman quotes Drs. Pfeiffer and Richman, who both recommend increasing salt intake when withdrawing from lithium, as follows: *"For moderate excess,* ***Pfeiffer recommends withholding lithium and increasing dietary salt. Richman suggests salt water.*** *Stopping lithium may not initially reduce body storage enough to abort severe side affects.* ***In critical situations, dialysis might be indicated"*** (*Natural Healing for Schizophrenia,* Edelman, 1996/1998, p. 155). The question remains: How can we best eliminate the potentially toxic lithium carbonate, and replace it with safer alternatives?

The Therapeutic Benefits of Celtic Sea Salt

According to Dr. Batmanghelidj, **salt acts just like lithium in the body except it is excreted more rapidly.** But interestingly, **one of the contra-indications (something to avoid) listed while on the inorganic lithium carbonate therapy is "A Salt Free Diet"** (*Natural Healing for Schizophrenia,* Edelman, 1996/1998, p. 155). So, apparently lithium is not effective without salt, although I believe the Celtic sea salt (from the *Grain & Salt Society*), might possibly be effective without any additional lithium, and could possibly even eliminate the need for lithium carbonate therapy altogether. **And if salt will replace lithium during its withdrawal, as**

recommended, then why shouldn't salt be used in the first place? Although they likely used regular table salt, (sodium only), the Celtic sea salt with many trace minerals, (including organic lithium), should be much more beneficial. Celtic sea salt is available at most health food stores, or directly through the *Grain & Salt Society* by calling (800) TOP-SALT, or by visiting http://www.celtic-seasalt.com/

One major difference between lithium carbonate and Celtic sea salt is the significant damage to the kidneys caused by the lithium. The refined table salt most people consume on a daily basis is not nearly as damaging to the kidneys as the inorganic lithium carbonate is, yet according to Dr. Jacques de Langre, **excess "refined table salt" is not always adequately excreted.** As a result, regular table salt could sometimes solidify, potentially resulting in some kidney problems. Quoting Dr. de Langre (*Seasalt's Hidden Powers*, 1992), ***"Unrefined Celtic Salt has the opposite effect: its sodium drains out rapidly, keeping the kidneys at peak function,*** *as well as promoting flexibility in the articulations"* (p. 87).

Celtic sea salt seems to have some qualities similar to natural lithium (not lithium carbonate), and even contains the mineral lithium in trace amounts as nature apparently intended. In nature, trace elements are found in trace (minute) amounts, and that is why they are referred to as trace minerals. Dr. de Langre stresses this important issue when he states that *"macro-nutrients as well as* **trace elements [minerals]** ***should never be taken carelessly in any quantity. Most of them have a very narrow quantitive range between what is essential and what is toxic"*** (*Seasalt's Hidden Powers*, 1992, p. 21).

There is a major difference between **toxic doses of the inorganic lithium carbonate**, versus **trace amounts of organic lithium**. When doctors prescribe dosages of trace elements such as lithium, in an inorganic form and at toxic dosages of 900 mg or sometimes more per day, experiencing many potential serious side effects should be expected. Just the severe irreversible damage to the kidneys alone, could easily result in kidney failure, and the possibility of dialysis in the future. It is possible that many people with the bipolar disorder are just missing adequate sodium, potassium, magnesium, zinc, organic iodine, and lithium, all found in an easily assimilatable ionic form in Celtic sea salt. Even if just one important mineral were missing, some of the cellular reactions in the neurotransmitters might be influenced, as was mentioned with lithium usage. **Some neurotransmitters are stimulating, while others are calming, and still others help modulate or balance emotions.** If the lithium carbonate therapy were doing its job effectively, there would obviously not be so many serious side effects associated with its use. Its primary intended therapy is suppressing the manic phase of the bipolar disorder only, although that is obviously only half of the problem.

Although lithium is just one trace mineral found in the Celtic sea salt, it is possible that organic lithium might also play an important synergistic role along with the sodium, chloride, potassium, and magnesium, in regards to the efficient function of the neurons in the brain. According to an article in the February 2003 issue of *Life Extension* magazine, Dr. David Perlmutter, M.D., a widely known author and lecturer on brain aging and regeneration, indicates that natural lithium is neuroprotective and neurotrophic. This basically refers to the protection of the brain neurons, and stimulating the growth of neural tissue in the brain. From the article, it is obvious that Dr. Perlmutter uses natural substances in his practice, and although he did not specify the form of lithium he was referring to, under the circumstances it would obviously be the organic form. Be it lithium or hormones, there is a tremendous difference in the influence (of the natural versus the chemical form) on the body and brain.

The trace element iron, also critical to our health, is found in Celtic sea salt. Although both copper and iron can be potentially toxic at elevated levels, fortunately trace minerals in their natural ionic form do not accumulate at toxic levels in the body, as other inorganic forms sometimes can.

Dr. Balch states that calcium (also found in Celtic Sea Salt) is important for both the maintenance of a regular heartbeat and the transmission of nerve impulses. He also mentions that *"Deficiencies of calcium are also associated with* ***cognitive impairment,*** *convulsions,* ***depression,*** *delusions, and* ***hyperactivity"*** (*Prescription for Nutritional Healing, 3rd edition,* 2000, p. 28).

Another important mineral found in Celtic Sea Salt is magnesium, and Dr. Balch notes:

> *Magnesium is a vital catalyst in enzyme activity, especially the activity of those enzymes involved in energy production. It assists in calcium and potassium uptake.* ***A deficiency of magnesium interferes with the transmission of nerve and muscle impulses, causing irritability and nervousness****. Supplementing the diet with* ***magnesium can help prevent depression, and also aids in maintaining the body's proper pH balance*** (*Prescription for Nutritional Healing, 3rd edition,* 2000, p. 30).

One of the side effects associated with **in**organic lithium usage, is elevated blood sugar. Celtic Sea Salt instead contains chromium, which is an essential mineral for maintaining stable blood sugar levels through proper insulin utilization, and is especially helpful with diabetes or hypoglycemia. It has also been found that **some symptoms of a chromium deficiency are bipolar disease, depression,** obesity, **hypoglycemia**, and **diabetes**.

Vanadium is another trace mineral found in Celtic sea salt that is also beneficial for improving insulin utilization and improving glucose tolerance. It has been known for years that those with both diabetes and hypoglycemia do not properly metabolize sugar, causing them to be more prone to addictions. So, **although lithium carbonate creates a problem by elevating blood sugar levels, Celtic Sea Salt contains at least two different trace minerals that will instead help stabilize blood-glucose levels.**

The trace amounts of iodine, found in Celtic sea salt, is actually made up of two elements (lithium and tin), which benefit, rather than suppress the thyroid as lithium carbonate does. Thus, one potential problem might be resolved, rather than created. Dr. Jacques de Langre, Ph.D., explains in his book *Seasalt's Hidden Powers* (1992), that in the ocean the sea vegetation combine the two elements into organic iodine, which is then released into the ocean, and thus found in natural sea salt, along with the individual elements, tin and lithium.

In his book *Nutrition and Mental Illness* (1987), Dr. Carl C. Pfeiffer, Ph.D., M.D. mentions that **trace elements (minerals) are often the "missing link" in regards to mental illness,** and that many schizophrenics and some manic-depressives not only have high copper levels, but low levels of zinc and manganese (both found in Celtic Sea Salt). Incidentally, birth control pills can contribute to elevated copper, and a zinc deficiency.

Dr. Balch explains how organic germanium (another trace mineral also found in Celtic Sea Salt) is effective in increasing tissue oxygenation, when he states that *"like hemoglobin, germanium acts as a carrier of oxygen to the cells"* (*Prescription for Nutritional Healing, 3rd edition,* 2000, p. 28). This is just one more way the Celtic sea salt can increase the oxygen levels in the brain, which is another important issue.

Because of the diversity of the many important minerals and trace elements, and the ionic bioavailability of the organic ingredients, Celtic Sea Salt appears to have the greatest potential for stabilizing the histamine imbalances in the brain, as well as preventing dehydration, which contributes to the histamine imbalances. In fact, according to Dr. Batmanghelidj, **salt is the most effective antihistamine.** It is also interesting to note that an organic form of lithium was once used as a salt substitute!

Have You Checked Your Thyroid?

Studies have shown that our thyroid function greatly influences both our mood, and behavior. It was discovered that abnormalities of thyroid function were found in patients with depression and mania. In fact, one study found that "***approximately 25% of patients with rapid cycling bipolar disorder have evidence of hypothyroidism,*** *which contrasts with only 2-5% of depressed patients in general*" (http://www.nice.org.uk/pdf/BD_1stcons_fullguidelines.pdf).

When all else fails, whether it's depression, or the bipolar disorder, check your thyroid. Best of all, check your thyroid first, not last, especially if you're a woman, as your risk far greater than a man, (about ten times). For detailed information regarding self-testing and thyroid hormones, be sure to read the chapter earlier on Hypothyroidism.

Additional Suggestions for Lithium Withdrawal and The Bipolar Disorder

It is important to keep in mind that the most beneficial dosage for a particular individual can sometimes vary considerably. Several factors can determine what our appropriate dosage of different nutrients might be. Due to our bio-individuality, some require either a higher dosage, or possibly a specific form of vitamins or minerals, which we will also address.

1. **Supplementing Vitamins and Minerals. All the vitamins and minerals recommended for Prozac™ withdrawal should be included,** as they will benefit anyone who has been taking either Prozac™ or Lithium. They are also beneficial for anyone simply wishing to maintain their health.
2. **Essential Fatty Acids (EFAs)** are especially important. In addition to the information provided earlier in this book on depression, it is important to note that EFAs build our receptor sites and improve reception. Dr. Andrew Stoll, M.D., from the Department of Psychiatry at Harvard University, reported finding **high-dose omega-3 fatty acid supplementation to be helpful in treating patients with unstable bipolar disorder** (*Psychiatric Times*, 1998 December, Vol. XVI, Issue 12). In fact, when fish oil supplements were given to Dr. Stoll's patients, they improved so dramatically that the researchers terminated the study five months earlier than planned! Researchers reported, *"Nine of 14 patients taking the fish oil capsules responded positively, compared to only three of the 16 taking a placebo".*

And, in the book *Natural Highs* (2002), the authors Hyla Cass, M.D. and Patrick Holford discuss one study that proved that **when people with bipolar or manic depression were given 9.6 mg of omega-3 oils over a four-month period, they experienced "substantial" improvement** (pp. 148-149), although they recommend from 1,000 mg to 2,000 mg daily for anyone experiencing mental health problems, and I would as well.

3. **Withdraw from antidepressants and lithium at the same time.** If you are currently taking Prozac™, or some other SSRI antidepressant, along with lithium, it might be best to withdraw from **both** concurrently. Seldom are depression or mood swings nearly as dangerous as the antidepressants, or the inorganic lithium, can be. And, as we learned earlier, antidepressants are basically stimulants, and a major contributor to the bipolar disorder. Then, as lithium is just the opposite, (a suppressant), combining the two would appear to be opposing factors, and thus counter-productive.

4. **Lower serum lithium levels (if excessively elevated).** Two natural substances, sometimes suggested for lowering serum lithium concentration, by increasing the excretion of lithium in the urine, are urea and sodium bicarbonate. Taking one-half teaspoon of Sodium Bicarbonate (baking soda), along with urea, twice daily, is sometimes recommended. Although this might at times be necessary during withdrawal, it is only recommended if elevated lithium is suspected. Urea is normally available in the powder form through the pharmacy without a prescription.

5. **The herb Golden Seal** is also very helpful in eliminating toxins, such as the inorganic form of Lithium carbonate.

6. **Re-hydration should begin** once the lithium carbonate is discontinued. Start drinking ten 8-ounce glasses of water, along with 1 teaspoon of Celtic sea salt daily, as it contains organic iodine and lithium, as well as other important trace minerals, as we just discussed. These trace elements are much more easily absorbed and utilized by the body when in the natural organic ionized form found in the Celtic sea salt, and thus will not become toxic. The salt comes in coarse crystals and find ground salt. The coarse costs about half as much as the fine, and what I use. The fine is best to replace your common table salt for seasoning.

7. **Kelp.** Six 1,000 mg tablets of kelp, (three, twice daily), might be helpful, in addition to Celtic sea salt. Kelp has many different trace minerals, including organic iodine.

8. **Organic Lithium Orotate** is a **natural form of lithium**, which has been proven safe, and is normally sold in health food stores. Using the organic form of lithium might help reduce the manic phase in the beginning (which doctors are attempting to do with the inorganic lithium carbonate), or it might even be helpful to continue with the natural lithium orotate following withdrawal if it appears to be beneficial. Quite possibly, the organic form of lithium in the proper dosage might also prove to be a valuable resource to assist in repairing any brain damage that could have occurred from either lithium carbonate or Prozac™ use. As it absorbs much more readily than lithium carbonate, much smaller dosages of lithium orotate is sufficient. I would personally recommend Serenity™, which contains lithium orotate.

9. **"Serenity™",** a product developed by German physician, Hans A. Nieper, M.D., is another source of natural lithium. It is combined with organic orotate, which transports the natural lithium to the blood cells of our brain much more efficiently.

Apparently, *"Dr. Nieper is reported to have one of the highest cure rates for cancer in the medical world"* (http://www.healthyplace.com), and it was claimed that his **success with depression**, migraines, **and bipolar disorder**, using the organic form of lithium orotate called "Serenity™" is unsurpassed. Serenity™ is available through *Urban Nutrition* by calling (800) 515-1070, or by visiting http://www.feelserenity.com.

10. **Inositol supplementation** might possibly be another safe and effective solution for replacing lithium, as lithium instead depletes the inositol and we learned of its importance. **One safe and inexpensive source is lecithin, which contains not only inositol, but also choline, and as we learned, both are known to be very beneficial for healthy brain**

function. I personally use lecithin granules, as they are the most reasonable source. If you substitute Celtic Sea Salt for lithium, along with the minerals necessary for healthy brain function, the synergism of both choline and inositol from lecithin could also assist in their efficient absorption. I personally use two tablespoons of lecithin granules, twice daily, as it has many other health benefits, including the homogenization of fats, and the brain actually contains a great deal of lecithin.

11. **Glycine** is an amino acid, necessary for central nervous system function. It functions as an inhibitory neurotransmitter, and has been **used in the treatment of bipolar depression, as well as hyperactivity.** While a good multi-amino acid complex containing all essential amino acids should be helpful, it is also suggested to take additional glycine as an individual supplement (but at a separate time).

12. **Pregnenolone** is a hormone that modulates the neurotransmitters, and **assists in stabilizing moods.** It appears to be an excellent resource to assist in proper sleep, **reducing stress and maintaining emotional health, and is known for its ability to promote feelings of balance and harmony.** Clinical studies have examined its role in relieving depression, improving memory, reducing stress, treating arthritis, and increasing longevity. Pregnenolone can be found at your local health food store, and one 30 mg capsule daily should be adequate. Pregnenolone has actually been used for many years, even in high doses, and most importantly with no reported side effects.

13. **Goji or Mangosteen juice,** mentioned earlier in the outline for withdrawal from antidepressants, should also be beneficial when eliminating lithium, especially as neither interacts with medications. If you are on both an antidepressant, and lithium therapy, you might discover that once you have eliminated the antidepressant, your bipolar condition will likely lessen, or possibly disappear entirely. Both goji and mangosteen also help fight depression, as well as reducing stress, and without the stimulant effect, nutrient depletion, and many inherent side effects associated with antidepressant medications.

14. **L-theanine** is an amino acid made from green tea. It should be especially beneficial for anyone experiencing the manic phase of the bipolar condition. L-theanine produces the calming alpha waves in the brain, while also increasing the level of the calming hormone GABA.

15. Avoid all forms of Stress. The stress hormone cortisol is produced by emotional and mental stress, (fear, confusion, worry, anger, rage, etc.), but especially SSRI antidepressants, such as Prozac™ and Paxil™. According to an article printed in the *Eugene Register Guard* (October 29, 2004), a publication by the *Associated Press* states that **stressful situations trigger an enzyme in the brain called protein kinase C (PKC), which is also an active enzyme in bipolar disorder and schizophrenia. The active PKC enzyme not only impairs short-term memory, but it also affects the prefrontal cortex, the decision-making part of the brain as well, which researchers say *"could be a factor in the distractibility impulsiveness and impaired judgment that occurs in those illnesses."*** We can easily see the importance of eliminating all forms of stress.

If you can't always avoid stressful situations, there are a couple options. Take two capsules of the calming herb Valerian root. It helps you stay relaxed, but doesn't produce drowsiness. Another option is Relora, an herbal formula containing Philodendron and magnolia, which lowers the stress hormone cortisol and increases the calming DHEA.

16. **Many natural supplements** are known to be either calming or stimulating. The objective will be to assist your body in maintaining that delicate balance that produces both calm and peace of mind. **None of us can expect to experience an unnatural high without dealing**

with the depressing low that will ultimately follow. I am sure you are aware that **we are not only describing the bipolar condition, but also drugs such as cocaine.** Keep in mind that some of the supplements listed tend to produce more calming hormones, such as GABA or DHEA, while others are responsible for creating the more stimulating neurotransmitters, such as serotonin and dopamine.

Some Final Thoughts Regarding The Bipolar Disorder

- You now have at your disposal, more than one safe yet effective way to balance your moods. If you sense a manic phase coming on, take advantage of the more calming ones. And of course, if you are feeling a little down, use the more stimulating ones. You can experiment and find which ones work the best for you. You are basically in charge, and you better than anyone, can evaluate what works best for you. The good news is: You have several options to choose from.
- **Our bodies are each unique,** and influenced not only by our diet, but also any nutrients or medications we might be taking. **We will not all respond the same to a particular therapy or supplement,** thus some supplements might be more beneficial for you, while others might possibly be more effective for someone else.
- Although drugs can easily interact with each other, and can be potentially dangerous, that is seldom a concern with natural supplements. For example, I have taken many different vitamins, minerals, amino acids, herbs, and other plant extracts for decades, and have yet to experience a reaction or interaction from doing so. Although it is very unlikely, it might be possible, as some people may have extremely compromised immune systems and are thus allergic to many different things, including many common foods. Some may also mistake a detoxification symptom for an allergic reaction.
- Although the traditional solution of high doses of the inorganic lithium carbonate is potentially dangerous, and possibly even life threatening, the organic lithium orotate might even be beneficial to the brain. Also, if you have been taking an antidepressant, and have a bipolar condition, it is more than likely the side effect of your medication.
- As you may remember, under "Mary Lou's Story", **she was able to safely and effectively eliminate a total of <u>nine medications</u> in only two months,** and is feeling so much better since her withdrawal. Most importantly, **one was a 16-year dependence on Prozac™, (along with another antidepressant called Desyrel™), as well as lithium carbonate!** She had absolutely no problem with the withdrawal, and was totally amazed that something that many consider as impossible, was surprisingly easy to accomplish.
- If it's beginning to sound a lot like a major job of maintaining an adequate balance of the vitamins, minerals, and hormones in the body and brain, there is a very logical explanation, and a surprisingly simple solution. Get off all the drugs that are creating the unnecessary chaos by creating deficiencies (and an imbalance in nutrients and hormone levels). It's much more simple, (and more effective), to provide the body with the proper nutrients, and allow it to do the job it was designed for, by Our Creator, "managing the details." I have often wondered what our body's response might be to the continuous abuse with drugs and poor diet, if it could only talk. Actually, it can, and we call it "symptoms," which were intended for our benefit, not to induce undue suffering that must somehow be suppressed at all costs, (what drugs are designed for).

Unless you truly resolve the underlying condition, the symptoms will never go away. Thus, traditional medicine's solution is a lifetime of symptom suppression, (a very profitable approach), although obviously not a "solution" that anyone with the facts should ever consider. You now have the facts, so you can no longer be deceived, as millions of others unfortunately still are.

In Summary:

It might be helpful if we now take a moment and evaluate some important issues, **which are also discussed in further detail in the chapter in the back of this book on Additional Technical Information, (which is more in-depth, and may be more difficult to understand).**

- **Lithium can contribute to elevated calcium in the bloodstream, which could potentially result in excessive calcification of arteries, the blood-brain barrier, and neurons in the brain.**
- **Excessive calcium levels can lead to a deficiency of the minerals magnesium and zinc.**
- **A magnesium deficiency can contribute to many different potentially serious conditions. Some associated with mental and behavioral problems are: Apathy, agitation, irritability, personality changes, and depression.**
- **A low magnesium level makes nearly every disease worse.**
- **Although zinc has many important functions, and is necessary for neurotransmitter syntheses, it may also function as a neurotransmitter.**
- **Dopamine, serotonin, and acetylcholine are all very important neurotransmitters that influence our mood, which lithium is known to negatively influence.**
- **Another function of zinc is helping maintain level moods (basically preventing the highs and lows - normally referred to as bipolar disorder).**
- **A zinc deficiency can lead to irritability and behavior disorders, as well as many other conditions.**
- **Zinc also just happens to be used in treating three disorders – histamine imbalances, Pyroluria, and blood sugar disorders, (all side effects associated with lithium carbonate therapy).**

CHAPTER SEVENTEEN

Schizophrenia - Common Causes, Atypical Antipsychotics, and Natural Solutions

One Possible Cause Of Schizophrenia: Elevated Copper and/or Low Histamine

Two common contributors to schizophrenia, discovered by Dr. Carl C. Pfeiffer, Ph.D., M.D., are a low blood level of histamine, or elevated copper levels, (or both). Following are a few of the late Dr. Pfeiffer's findings, taken from his book *Nutrition and Mental Illness* (1987):

> *On a careful study of the* ***data from thousands of schizophrenic patients, we find that 50 percent have a low blood level of histamine.***
>
> ***Many cases of "schizophrenia" were really cases of copper poisoning.***
>
> *We had found that* **a sub-group of about 50 percent of our diagnosed "schizophrenic" patients were high in copper.** *These patients often experienced paranoia and hallucinations.* ***With nutritional therapy designed to reduce the copper burden of the body, the paranoia and hallucinations improved. The antidote was extra zinc, or zinc and manganese.***
>
> **[Vitamin]** ***B_3 deficiency causes copper levels to rise, making B_3 another potential antidote to copper.***
>
> ***As the animals became*** **[vitamin]** ***C deficient, the copper levels in the blood serum rose steadily until a level 2.5 times higher than normal was reached at death.*** *This may, in part, explain why the early treatment of mental illness with* ***large doses of vitamins B_3 and C often helped patients*** (pp. 18-25).

Copper: Your Best Friend, or Worst Enemy?

It all depends upon your level, (more is not always better). Some benefits of copper at proper levels are:

> **[Copper]** ***helps oxidize glucose and release energy.*** *Helps the body absorb iron.* ***Aids the thyroid gland in balancing and secreting hormones. Carries oxygen in the blood stream.*** *Supplies the body's tissues with oxygen.* ***Increases the body's energy levels. Aids in nerve and brain function.*** *Needed for the functioning of the amino acid, tyrosine. Essential for making red blood cells. Helps tyrosine work as a pigment factor.* ***Helps supply oxygen to the brain.*** *Enzyme component. Necessary for the synthesis of the hormone adrenaline. Associated with intestinal enzyme activity.* ***Acts as a brain stimulant.*** *Copper antagonizes*

manganese ions. ***Copper level in the body parallels estrogen levels. Copper is a natural yeast fighter. Copper improves epinephrine, norepinephrine and dopamine.*** *Low copper causes the cells to suffocate and lack oxygen* (http://www.healthvitaminsguide.com/minerals/copper.htm).

Sounds rather impressive, doesn't it? But what about elevated copper? You will soon find that's a whole different story. Copper is defiantly a two-edged sword, and as you will discover, a proper balance is absolutely critical in order to avoid complications. Following are some major concerns associated with elevated copper:

> ***High intake of copper may lead to*** *headaches,* ***Hypoglycemia,*** *Increased heart rate, and nausea.* ***Copper deposits in the brain and liver, Damage to the kidneys,*** *Inhibit urine production, causes anemia, Causes hair loss in women.*
>
> ***High copper interferes with zinc,*** *which is needed to manufacture digestive enzymes. Many high copper people dislike protein and are drawn to high-carbohydrate diets because they have difficulty digesting protein foods.*
>
> ***Excessive copper in children is associated with hyperactive behavior, learning disorders such as dyslexia, ADD and infections such as ear.***
>
> ***Psychological symptoms of high copper leads to autism type symptoms such as depression, Hallucinations, Hyperactivity, Insomnia, Paranoia, Personality changes, Psychosis, Schizophrenic type symptoms, Over stimulation, Disperception of the senses, time, body, self and others. Produces Hypomanic states*** (http://www.healthvitaminsguide.com/minerals/copper.htm).

As you can easily see, several of the side effects associated with elevated copper can not only contribute to schizophrenia, but also **the majority of symptoms noted above are actually those that many children are being placed on antidepressants and antipsychotic medications for**. The question is, **could they just be suffering from elevated copper?** It's just one possibility that is seldom considered.

Dr. Pfeiffer validated the fact that ***"Women taking contraceptive pills uniformly have raised copper levels"*** (*Nutrition and Mental Illness*, 1987, p. 25). He stresses the problem related to elevated copper and agrees that ***"High levels of copper can cause mental illness, often characterized by extreme fears, paranoia, and hallucinations."***

In fact, as far back as 1941, studies by Dr. Heilmeyer and colleagues reported findings of ***"elevated copper levels in twenty-three of thirty-seven schizophrenics"***

Bromine Intoxication

Bromine is a liquid heavy metal, and is often used as a dough conditioner in baked goods, as well as a clouding agent in many popular drinks. **Toxicity of bromine has been reported from ingestion of some carbonated drinks (i.e. Mountain Dew™, AMP™ Energy Drink, some Gatorade™ products), which contain brominated vegetable oils** (*Clinical Toxicology*, 1997, pp. 315-320). Bromine is also used in dyes, pesticides, as an antibacterial agent for pools and hot tubs, as fumigant for agriculture, and is still used today in many prescription medications (i.e. asthma treatment).

In his book, *Iodine: Why You Need – Why You Can't Live Without It,* (2004), Dr. David Brownstein, M.D. notes the following:

> ***Bromine intoxication*** *(i.e. bromism) has been shown to cause delirium, psychomotor retardation,* ***schizophrenia,*** *and hallucination.* ***Subjects who ingest enough bromide feel dull and apathetic and have difficulty concentrating. Bromide can also cause severe depression, headache, and irritability*** (p. 78).

Mental Illness – Or Just Physical Illness?
Improperly Diagnosed and Placed On Potentially Dangerous Drugs For Years

Kenneth Thomas, a Registered Nurse with 29 years of on-the-job experience in a wide variety of medical settings, has observed the following misdiagnoses, which he shares in an online documentary titled ***"TeenScreen Calls Physical Illness A Mental Disorder"*** (http://www.sierratimes.com/06/02/13/24_54_74_7_84499.htm), with a portion as follows:

> *In my work, I have seen first hand the finding of* ***heart valve prolapse****, which had gone undetected for years in some women.* ***This condition causes the sensation of rapid heartbeat, fluttering in the chest, sweating and anxiety. These are the symptoms of "panic attacks" and many of these women had been treated with anti-anxiety drugs. These are cases of actual undetected physical illness being passed off as "mental illness"*** *for months or years, only to eventually find that there is a REAL cause and it can be treated and resolved.* ***Half the battle today is the false advertising of psych drugs to treat chemical imbalances in the brain. A theory only with no clinical evidence, patients are put on mood-altering drugs at the whim of a psychiatrist or medical practitioner.***
>
> ***A friend of mine, also a nurse, was sent home recently from work because she was "acting erratically" and didn't seem to know where she was. After thorough medical testing, she found out that she has hypoglycemia. She had been suffering with that undetected condition on and off for 15 years. She had been through the whole regimen of expensive anti-anxiety medications in attempts to treat it****. After the actual cause of her symptoms were located, she changed her eating habits, the symptoms did not return and no drugs were needed to handle this condition.*
>
> ***Those are my observations of so-called "mental illnesses".*** *Many, if not all, can be found to have physical causes and can be handled in ways not requiring glossing over with dangerous mood and mind-altering drugs.* ***Our population, especially the elderly and the children, deserve better treatment.***

Although we do address solutions for the often-misdiagnosed hypoglycemia in this book, we don't address the heart valve prolapse that can lead to the "panic attacks" that Ken mentioned. That condition, along with cardiomyopathy and congestive heart failure, as well as the causes and natural solutions, is covered in considerable detail in my book *A Drug-Free Approach To Healthcare*, now available in a *Revised Edition* (2007).

A Little Off The Subject, But Extremely Important

By avoiding medications that damage the heart, and using a special form of vitamins (containing vitamin B_4), along with amino acids and CoQ10, the heart and the mitral valve prolapse can be restored back to normal! Both the heart and liver have a very restorative capability, (seldom does anyone need a transplant of either).

The statin (cholesterol lowering) drugs are one of the worst for destroying muscle (especially the heart). They can lead to kidney failure as well. Don't ever allow a doctor to convince you to take them! All you have to do is read "Al's Story" in my first book, *A Drug-Free Approach To Healthcare* (now available in a "Revised Edition" 2007), which is an example of an ex-body-builder and professor, who was losing his memory, and a ton of muscle that he spent decades building. Just a high dose of cholesterol medication, combined with a beta-blocker for hypertension, along with five hours a week of body building, destroyed his muscle and damaged his heart. And worst of all, he never really needed either one! I realize this is getting a little off the subject, but it's a critical issue that many in the nation are also unnecessarily dealing with. Elevated cholesterol never has been the risk it is made out to be, although if it's excessively elevated, in my other book I do provide several natural drug-free options for lowering it. In case you forgot, we were discussing causes of schizophrenia, so we'll now continue our discussion.

Possibly Predisposed During Pregnancy

The Medical College of Georgia recently announced that according to research performed at the University of Barcelona in Spain, and the University of Maryland, there is ***"mounting evidence that developmental problems, resulting from significant maternal stress in the second or early third trimester of pregnancy, may cause schizophrenia and related problems"*** (http://www.mcg.edu/news/2006NewsRel/Kirkpatrick082106.html).

Further research by Professor Marelyn Wintour of Monash University in Melbourne, found that ***"Vitamin D deficiency during pregnancy for example has been suggested to correlate with the later development of schizophrenia"*** (http://www.lafamily.com/display_article.php?id=1089).

Drug-Induced Schizophrenia - Often Just A Side Effect Of Drugs Such As Ritalin™ And Prozac™

Studies have shown that amphetamines such as Ritalin™ can generate a schizophrenic-like psychosis. Retired medical director, Dr. Heinrich Kremer, of Barcelona Spain, in his on-line article titled *"Ritalin – Target Brain"*, explains that ***"Patients have shown within a short time period, heavy psychotic reactions when given small amphetamine doses, after the paranoid and non-paranoid schizophrenic symptoms had subsided"*** (http://www.shirleys-wellness-cafe.com/ritalin.htm).

As reported in *USA Today*, (March 22, 2006), Rosemary Johann-Liang of the FDA's Office of Drug Safety stated: ***"We read case upon case of these children who do experience these hallucinations."*** And on March 14, 2006, a review posted on **the FDA website, listed nearly 1,000 reports of "psychosis" or mania possibly linked to ADHD drugs commonly prescribed to treat ADHD, which included Adderall™, Concerta™, Ritalin™, and Strattera™** (http://www.scoop.co.nz/stories/HL0607/S00162.htm). "Psychosis" was defined by the FDA as a mental disorder characterized by **the inability to distinguish real and imaginary events.**

As stated in an FDA report titled *"Adverse Events Associated with Drug Treatment of ADHD: Review of Postmarketing Safety Data,"* by Kate Gelperin and Kate Phelan, presented at the March 22, 2006 Pediatric Advisory Committee meeting, *"The most important finding of this review is that* ***signs and symptoms of psychosis or mania, particularly hallucinations, can occur in some patients with no identifiable risk factors, at usual doses of any of the drugs currently used to treat ADHD."*** The report went on to point out that ***"A substantial proportion of the cases occurred in children age ten years or less, a population in which hallucinations are not common"*** (http://www.scoop.co.nz/stories/print.html?path=HL0703/S00145.htm).

The following article was posted at http://www.idaho-observer.com/, by the Alliance for Human Research Protection, as follows:

> *The* ***astounding evidence*** *provided for the first time to an FDA Advisory Committee underscores the fact that* ***ADHD is both a gateway to prescribed psychoactive drugs, but also a gateway for major mental illness induced by those very drugs.***
>
> *The evidence also appears to support our observation that* ***the underlying cause that has led a U.S. diagnostic aberration "the Bipolar Child" – (not witnessed anywhere else in the world) is an effect of the drugs millions of children are being prescribed recklessly. Amphetamines and psychostimulants, SSRI antidepressants, and the most toxic of all the psychoactive drugs, antipsychotics, all may induce mania, psychosis, hostility, aggression, suicidal and homicidal behavior.***

And **not only are ADHD medications the problem, but as noted in both the prior article, as well as the following article, the SSRI antidepressants can also produce the very same conditions,** as pointed out by investigative reporter Evelyn Pringle:

> ***The symptoms of SSRI toxicity can also be mistaken for the progression of the underlying mental state,*** *"leading to use of more of the same and other offending SSRI drugs rather than to withdrawal of the causative SSRI agent,"* [Dr. Donald Marks, M.D., Ph.D.] *warns.*
>
> *An article from the Journal of Clinical Psychiatry researched at Yale University stated that 11% of all psychiatric hospital admissions were from antidepressant-induced mania and psychosis. It also noted another area of research showing that* ***Prozac and other SSRIs can simulate the effects of LSD.***

> *"In other words," Rosie* [Carr Meysenburg] *said, "this is saying* ***for some people, taking an SSRI is the same as taking LSD."***
> *According to Rosie, "About two million people enter a psychiatric hospital every year, 11% then is* ***over 200,000 people a year who have an antidepressant-induced psychosis and who are hospitalized****," she reported.*
>
> *"Not all are hospitalized," Rosie warns,* ***"Some of them have either committed suicide, a homicide, or a murder/suicide."***
> (http://www.sierratimes.com/05/08/13/24_164_252_187_48525.htm)

As noted by expert and author of *Talking Back To Ritalin* (1988) Dr. Peter Breggin, M.D., (http://www.lawyersandsettlements.com/articles/pharma_lawsuits.html), ***"as the child's emotional control breaks down due to medication effects, mood stabilizers may be added."*** And Dr. Breggin points out that **this is *"an all too common situation with children who are recruited by the mental health industry."*** He further warns that ***"Eventually, these children end up on four or five psychiatric drugs at once and a diagnosis of bipolar disorder by the age of eight or ten."***

One concerning study, reported in the June 2006 issue of the *Archives of General Psychiatry*, found that ***"there were about 201,000 office-based visits for youths aged 20 and younger that involved antipsychotic treatment in 1993. That number rose to 1,224,000 in 2002."*** That's a tremendous increase! **The obvious result of more kids being placed on drugs that are actually contributing to psychosis.**

And, according to an analysis by Medco Health Solutions, Inc., while **the number of children younger than age 10 taking ADHD medications increased almost 65 percent from 2000 to 2005, more than 6 percent of these young children on ADHD medications, were also taking an antipsychotic drug** (http://www.webmd.com/content/Article/112/110271.htm).

The Importance of Essential Fatty Acids (EFAs)

Malcolm Peet and colleagues announced, at the National Institutes of Health (NIH) Workshop on Omega-3 Essential Fatty Acids and Psychaitric Disorders, held in Bethesda, MD, September 1998, announced that ***"chronic schizophrenics have reduced levels of essential fatty acids in red cell membranes,"*** and went on to note that ***"Omega-3 supplements significantly reduced their symptoms."*** And as stated in the December 1998 issue of *Psychiatric Times*, from that same workshop, Jerry Cott, Ph.D., of the NIH, wrote in agreement: ***"There is evidence that deficiency of long-chain, omega-3 polyunsaturates may contribute to symptoms of schizophrenia,"*** and then goes on to point out that ***"Adequate long-chain polyunsaturated fatty acid, particularly Docosahexaenoic acid* [DHA]*, may reduce the development of depression and schizophrenia"*** (Vol. XI, Issue 12).

Cow's Milk and Schizophrenia – The Surprising Connection

Interestingly, on her audiotape *Help! I Can't Get Off My Antidepressants!* (1999), Dr. Ann Blake Tracy discusses the fact that some psychotropic medications, when combined with milk, actually convert to something called casomorphine, in the brain. And, she states that research preformed by Dr. Robert J. Cade, M.D. and his colleagues at the University of Florida, discovered **that *"80% of those diagnosed with either schizophrenia or autism found their condition totally resolved once milk was eliminated from their diet!"*** To me, it's amazing that something so simple could resolve a condition that serious!

Dr. Cade's research has also identified **a milk protein, casomorphine, as the probable cause of attention deficit disorder (ADD),** (*Autism*, 1999, p. 3). It has been documented that casein breaks down in the stomach to produce a peptide casomorphine, and eighty percent of cow's milk protein is casein! As you likely discovered earlier in Jeffrey's Story, just the elimination of milk and sugar from his diet resolved both his "ADHD" and nightly bed wetting, (which was also due to a milk allergy). Most importantly, his mom was able to get him off the Zoloft™ his doctor had placed him on (at age six!). Incidentally, that was after the highest allowable dose of Ritalin™, (which he was placed on at age four), proved ineffective, (as did the Zoloft™)! These drugs can be "extremely" dangerous, (especially with children), and most importantly, "totally unnecessary"!

Following is just one example of the potential side effects associated with ADHD medication, which clearly creates what I refer to as the domino effect. Marilyn Elias reported the following story, May 20, 2006, in *USA TODAY* (http://www.usatoday.com/news/health/2006-05-02-antipsychotic-side-effects_x.htm):

> ***Erin Evans is one parent who wishes she had never heard of anti-psychotics.***
>
> *Her son, Rex, 13, had trouble focusing in the classroom and **was diagnosed with attention-deficit disorder at age 6. He started on an ADHD medication** and began hallucinating about worms and bugs in his food.*
>
> ***Soon he was also on Prozac for anxiety**, but the nervousness and paranoia persisted.*
>
> ***At age 8, Rex was given Risperdal** by a child psychiatrist. He said the boy **probably had obsessive-compulsive disorder**, too, Evans says.*
>
> ***"(He) didn't tell us it had never been approved for children or warn us about any side effects," she says.***
>
> *For the first few weeks, Risperdal helped a little; Rex became less anxious and hyper. "But then it wore right off, soon **the doctor kept increasing the dose," she says.***
>
> ***After one month on Risperdal, Rex started having tremors: within a few months, his hands shook so severely that he could barely write at school, "and I'd have to guide the cup of milk to his mouth in the morning," Evans says.***
>
> *But the psychiatrist said the tremors weren't so bad, Evans says, and urged the family to continue the drug.*

*Then, about a year after Rex started Risperdal, the Evanses found out that **he might have schizoaffective disorder, a psychotic illness that children rarely get**. **A doctor's report said Rex probably would need to be institutionalized.***

*The parents started to learn more about Risperdal and, for the first time, they realized that Rex's symptoms could be side effects, so they started to wean him off the drug. **In a few weeks they noticed his jaw was scrunching up and his facial expressions were becoming distorted.** By then, Evans says, **they had read up on tardive dyskinesia (TD), a neurological disorder that can be caused by anti-psychotics.***

*Rex became less anxious, but the TD worsened. **"He had a horrible, ugly look on his face all the time,"** Evans says. Friends no longer came to play. **Rex went from winning an award for best reader in the third grade to claiming he couldn't remember how to spell his own name in fourth grade.***

*Then in fifth grade, Rex slowly began to improve. A medical exam showed **spasms in the thorax**, perhaps linked to the upper body spasms, **restricting the flow of oxygen to his brain.***

***He began oxygen therapy,** and he quickly became more responsive to others and did better at school, Evans says. At the end of elementary school, Rex had episodes only a few times a week.*

*But junior high has brought more stress and bullying, and the episodes have become more frequent. **"His movement-disorder specialist said he expected Rex to have this for the rest of his life,"** Evans says.*

*Now she is bitter. **"I trusted the doctors, I trusted the FDA...and I feel betrayed by both," she says.***

The Food and Drug Administration "does not regulate the practice of medicine," says Thomas Laughren, head of the division of psychiatry products. He adds that he's concerned about the use of such drugs in kids without systematic safety data.

***Nobody knows how many children on atypicals get TD**, says Ramy Mahmoud of Janssen LP, **maker of Risperdal**, but it's rare in adults. **"Our drug isn't indicated for children," he says. "It's a strong drug.** It has risks and benefits. Doctors and patients together have to weigh the benefits, at the start and on a continuing basis, along with the harm and suffering."*

One thing that immediately caught my attention was when Rex's mother mentioned that due to his tremors she had to guide the cup of "milk" to his mouth each morning. Then she mentioned that shortly thereafter, he had been diagnosed as having a Schizoaffective Disorder, (basically schizophrenia). Unfortunately, she didn't know about the potential connection, (the milk protein casomorphine that Dr. Cade discovered could very well be responsible for his condition).

In case you didn't notice, **the "Risperdal" this article was referring to, was just one of the drugs on the extensive list approved for use by children who are found to be mentally ill, by the new Bush-appointed NFC totally unscientific screening process, (although not approved for children by the FDA)!** Not only that, but **even the maker of Risperdal stressed that it's a "strong drug", and "not indicated for children"!** The obvious question is, **if they were aware of that serious concern, why in the world did they decide to promote it for children's use?** Apparently the income potential basically outweighed the potential for settling the lawsuits, (the only criteria that most companies seem to consider).

Drugs being prescribed for children's use are supposed to be clinically tested on children and, if proven safe and effective, should then receive FDA approval for children's use first. In the case of the 16 drugs promoted under TeenScreen, only the companies producing and marketing those drugs, (and not the FDA), made that determination! The obvious question is, **what authority does the FDA really have, and why would they just stand by and allow any drug manufacturer to totally ignore their normal drug approval process?** Especially when it involves our young children who are at the greatest risk, by far, for reactions to dangerous mind-altering drugs.

If the FDA is unwilling to assume that responsibility, and instead stand by and totally ignore an issue that serious, then our legislators should step in and see that it's addressed. They should propose legislation to assure that the FDA assumes their responsibility as mandated, and **no longer allow drug companies to use our children as guinea pigs, to test their dangerous drugs, (in a totally uncontrolled environment)!** This practice is in my opinion totally inexcusable, and absolutely must be stopped! Perhaps an entire overhaul of the FDA s in order. In my opinion, regulation of our food should be separated from drugs. And someone like Dr. David Graham, who has ethics, should head the FDA, and any employees with ties to a pharmaceutical company should be replaced.

Atypical Antipsychotics – Modern Medicine's Solution For Schizophrenia, and Sometimes Even Bipolar Disorder (Adding To The Domino Effect)

The first atypical antipsychotic medication was discovered in the 1950s, and introduced in clinical practice in the 1970s. Today's atypical antipsychotics (also known as second generation antipsychotics) are a class of prescription medications used to treat psychiatric conditions. All atypical antipsychotics are FDA approved for use in the treatment of schizophrenia, and some are also approved for treating acute mania, bipolar disorder, and psychotic agitation.

You may recall reading, at the beginning of this book, about how **the Bush-appointed New Freedom Commission on Mental Health (NFC) has a "preferred drug program"** in place. The program identifies drugs that can be used on children found to be mentally ill, **(although not approved by the FDA for children). This list just happens to include the atypical antipsychotics Clozaril™, Risperdal™, Zyprexa™, Seroquel™, Abilify™ and Geodon™.**

Although **none of these atypical antipsychotics are FDA approved for children,** doctors can (and quite often do) prescribe them to kids "off label". In fact, according to a new analysis of a federal survey by Vanderbilt Medical School researchers, ***"Prescribing atypical antipsychotics for aggressive children is leading the field in a growing pediatric business"*** (http://www.usatoday.com/news/health/2006-05-01-adult-antipsychotics-kids_x.htm).

This is obvious when you consider that Dr. Timothy Scott, author of *America Fooled: The Truth about Antidepressants, Antipsychotics and* **How We've Been Deceived,** reports ***"a 2005 study found there are approximately 30,000 children under 5 on these drugs"*** (http://www.sierratimes.com/07/02/27/75_7_243_126_94769.htm).

As usual, it all revolves around the money, as pointed out in the following article in the *New York Times* (May 10, 2007):

> *The sudden popularity of pediatric bipolar diagnosis has coincided with a shift from antidepressants like Prozac to* **far more expensive atypicals.** *In 2000, Minnesota spent more than $521,000 buying antipsychotic drugs, most of it on atypicals, for children on Medicaid.* ***In 2005, the cost was more than $7.1 million, a 14-fold increase.***
>
> ***The drugs, which can cost $1,000 to $8,000 for a year's supply, are huge sellers worldwide. In 2006, Zyprexa, made by Eli Lilly, had $4.36 billion in sales, Risperdal $4.18 billion and Seroquel, made by AstraZeneca, $3.42 billion.***

Notice, once again, the most costly drugs, (Zyprexa™, Risperdal™, and Seroquel™), which are all on the "preferred drug program" list, are those that are the most highly promoted!

Antipsychotics Are Being Written For All Kinds Of (Off-Label) Reasons

The following statistics were reported in the *Ambulatory Pediatric Association* (2006 March/April, Vol. 6):

> *In summary, analyses of NAMCS and NHAMCS data demonstrated* ***a nearly fivefold increase in antipsychotic prescribing for 2 – 18-year-old US children between 1995 and 2002. Over 50% of the antipsychotic prescriptions were for a diagnosis for which antipsychotics have not been studied in children. There may be little recognized benefits to these medications in many of the children receiving them, and potential risks do exist.***

Dr. Amita Dasmanapatra, senior director of medical affairs at Medco, worries that *"The sharp increase is noteworthy because the* ***powerful drugs are for individuals with serious psychosis such as schizophrenia*** *so* ***there is some concern the medicines may not always be prescribed appropriately,"*** and goes on to suggest that ***"it is possible that some doctors are prescribing the drugs for children with behavioral problems, which would be better controlled by other means"*** (http://www.msnbc.msn.com/id/12616864/).

Apparently, that is exactly what is happening. A review of Texas prescription records for the months of July and August 2004 found that, regarding **nearly 98% of the teens reviewed,** ***"the antipsychotics were prescribed off-label and in more than half the cases, the dosage***

appeared to be inappropriately high" (http://www.sierratiems.com/07/01/20/Pringle.htm). The study also stated that **almost half of the children did not appear to even have a valid diagnosis warranting the use of the drugs in the first place!**

"Off-label prescribing" of medication (especially to children, and especially these dangerous atypical antipsychotics), is a serious concern, and William Cooper, M.D., M.P.H., associate professor of Pediatrics in the Child and Adolescent Health Research unit at the Monroe Carell Jr. Children's Hospital at Vanderbilt agrees, stating that ***"there is limited information on the effectiveness of antipsychotic medications for behavioral and affective disorders, the conditions for which over half of the prescriptions were written"*** (http://www.mc.vanderbilt.edu/reporter/index.html?ID=4601).

Dr. Cooper goes on to warn: ***"These are really powerful medications and it's important that providers have a handle on both the potential benefits and potential risks. They haven't been studied in children yet and we don't know if they work and we don't know what the potential risks are."*** These are two serious concerns that obviously should be addressed! I believe you will agree, once you read the following excerpt from an article written for *USA Today*, (May 2, 2006), by Marilyn Elias:

> ***John March, chief of child and adolescent psychiatry at Duke University*** *School of Medicine says* ***prescribing them*** **[atypical antipsychotics]** ***for behavioral problems alone may be a mistake. "We have no evidence about the safety of these agents or their effectiveness in controlling aggression," he says. "Why are we doing this?"***
>
> ***A USA TODAY study of FDA data collected from 2000 to 2004 shows at least 45 deaths of children in which an atypical antipsychotic was listed in the FDA database as the "primary suspect." There also were 1,328 reports of bad side effects, some of them life-threatening.***
>
> [As noted by child psychiatrist Joseph Penn of Bradley Hospital and Brown University School of Medicine], ***"doctors often face time pressures that prevent them from finding out what's going on in kids' lives, knowledge that might suggest alternative treatments.*** *For example,* ***abuse of drugs such as methamphetamine, OxyContin and cocaine is fairly common among teens, he says. Kids begin acting strangely, hearing voices, becoming paranoid. The symptoms can mimic psychosis or behavioral disorders, and doctors can end up giving these children unneeded antipsychotic drugs",*** *he says* (http://usatoday.com/news/health/2006-05-01-atypical-drugs_x.htm).

If "at least 45 deaths in children" and "1,328 reports of bad side effects, some of them life-threatening" are associated with these drugs, why in the world are they still considered as "preferred" drugs, even for young kids under the age of 5? To the pharmaceutical industry, these unfortunate children are just millions of potential profit centers. They are also very much aware that one drug eventually leads to more drugs. They are basically looking for a way to dramatically broaden their potential market (by starting much sooner).

The following example is just one of the thousands of stories (many untold), regarding the inexcusable and totally unnecessary drugging of our innocent children, which clearly shows how the "domino effect" can quickly get out of control:

A Grandmother's Story - By Gloria Wright

We raised our grandson, Noah, the first 5 years of his life -- he was a happy, energetic, "normal" child who was a delight to be around. He was removed from our home by his mother (our daughter) at age 5 and was quickly entered into the world of legalized drugs by his mom through a willing doctor who was a stranger to him -- his own pediatrician having refused to put a normal child on amphetamines or psychotropic drugs. ***The gate of entry for Noah was via Ritalin, or methylphenidate, which led to his being placed on 16 more drugs, including psychotropic drugs.***

Noah's life was transformed from one of happiness and good health before his drugging, to one of severe depression, anxiety, diabetes, high blood pressure, severe migraines, severe hostility, homicidal tendencies, aggression, suicidality, etc., etc., etc. His history now includes involuntary commitment to 7 mental hospitals, *placement in 12 foster homes, and literally dozens of* ***so-called mental health "professionals"*** *pulling and tearing at his life & his psyche. At each turn, at each institution, while in the hands and/or care of these "professionals" Noah was taken deeper and deeper into the world of a severely mentally ill youngster, for he was being legally drug abused to the full extent of 1000 mgs per day (!) of psychotropic/antidepressant/SSRI drugs. He was only 14 years old!*

When we gained custody of Noah, after a 10 1/2 year court battle, he was in such poor condition mentally/physically and many of our friends were upset to look at him. ***His face was badly swollen, he drooled, his head hung down with his chin on his chest, he could not look directly at anyone or anything and his eyes frequently rolled back in his head, and he walked with a slow, shuffling gait. We learned via testing that he was on an early second grade level in his learning. He was 14 years old!***

During the 18 months we have had custody of Noah, we have had him in therapy with a wonderful psychiatrist, and psychologist and a neuro-psychologist.

It was during the second visit with the psychiatrist that he remarked our grandson was not ADD/ADHD, nor was he borderline personality, bipolar, manic, etc., etc. and that he should not be on any of the drugs! Drugs he had been LEGALLY ABUSED WITH for years! *He began removing him from the drugs -- a long and painful procedure for Noah and for us.*

> *Noah, after 6 months of detox/withdrawal, is now totally drug free and making progress toward a more normal life. He is looked upon by friends and neighbors as a miracle -- in fact, we are sure GOD has done just that in him -- a miracle!*
>
> *Prior to coming to live with us, Noah experienced anger, rage, violence, attempted homicide, and 2 suicide attempts that we are aware of, to mention just a few horrors.* ***Every time Noah was in trauma he was on a severe drug not approved for use on children.*** *What was the response from the mental health (psychiatrists) "professionals" or the medical "professionals"? Rather than removing him from the abusive drugs causing the trauma (had they bothered noting the NATIONAL INSTITUTES OF HEALTH or label warnings for dangerous side effects) they treated the behavior/symptom with an additional new psychotropic drug or greatly upped the dosage of the drug he was on -- WITH DRUGS NOT APPROVED FOR USE ON CHILDREN! Thus* ***Noah was sucked into the world of mental illness CAUSED BY THE PRESCRIBED DRUGS!!!*** *No child should loose their joy, their freedom, and the wonder of making marvelous memories of a happy childhood!*
>
> ***It is a miracle Noah is alive and able to function.*** *We are so thankful we were able to rescue him from the mental hospital where he had been placed and drugged into a stupor!* (http://www.ablechild.org/gloria%20wright.htm)

In my opinion, any doctor who would thoughtlessly subject a child to that many highly dangerous psychotropic drugs should have his or her license to practice revoked. Such a doctor can be even more dangerous than a criminal with a loaded gun! They can continue to "**legally destroy many children's lives"**, and never be held accountable for what is obviously malpractice, and outright dangerous.

Antipsychotics Are All Too Often Readily Paid For By Insurance

As pointed out in the *USA Today* article mentioned earlier, by Marilyn Elias, ***"Insurance coverage rules may encourage the soaring use of antipsychotics for children, as well. 'With some companies, the only thing they reimburse for is prescribing. There's little or no therapy,'*** *says Ronald Brown, editor of the Journal of Pediatric Psychology and a dean at Temple University"* (http://usatoday.com/news/health/2006-05-01-atypical-drugs_x.htm).

Investigative reporter Evelyn Pringle agrees, and **although the new atypical antipsychotics are NOT approved for children, doctors continue to prescribe these drugs off-label for unapproved uses, (especially when payment via insurance is guaranteed)**, as she explains:

> *The researchers analyzed data on children with an average age of 13, who were involved in annual national health surveys involving prescriptions issued during 119,752 doctor visits, and determined that* ***over half of the prescriptions were written for attention deficit or other non-psychotic conditions.***

*Even more disturbing finding was recently reported in a study led by Oregon Health & science University professor, David Pollack, that revealed that **246 preschool children under the age of 5, who were enrolled in the state-sponsored Medicaid program, were receiving antipsychotic or antidepressant medications.***

The review of Medicaid records, reported in the April 2006, Oregon Health News, found that 41% of the preschoolers were prescribed psychiatric drugs for ADD.

Experts say the prospect of children under 5, receiving psychiatric drugs intended for adults is alarming. Also alarming was the finding that about 50% of the prescriptions were written by primary care providers and not psychiatrists (http://www.lawyersandsettlements.com/articles/antipsychotics.html).

Apparently **both state-sponsored and publicly funded programs are all too willing to pay for these medications. And worst of all, the atypical antipsychotics are NOT even FDA-approved for use in children,** although doctors are free to prescribe the drugs as they see fit, (something most people are not aware of). And it's not just children – insurance companies are more than willing to make it a "family affair". Investigative reporter Evelyn Pringle tells of a frightening scenario, as follows:

The recent overdose death of 4-year-old, Rebecca Riley, in Massachusetts, demonstrates the dire need to educate the public about the practice of prescribing drugs for unapproved uses and the dangers of prescribing drugs like Zyprexa to children.

At 2-and-a-half-years-old, Rebecca was diagnosed with attention deficit disorder and bipolar disorder and was prescribed Zyprexa's atypical cousin, Seroquel, along with Clonidine, an adult high blood pressure drug, and Depakote, a drug approved to treat adults with epilepsy. None of these drugs were approved for children and they were prescribed in a combination that has never been tested even with adults.

***From age 2 on, Rebecca remained on this daily drug off-label concoction until she was found dead on the floor in her parents' home on December 13, 2006.** The autopsy report stated that **she died of the "combined effects" of the drugs** and that **her lungs and heart were damaged by "prolonged abuse of these prescription drugs**, rather than one incident."*

*The story behind Rebecca Riley's death, gives a clear picture of how blatant the off-label marketing scams have become. **After she died, investigators discovered that her 2 siblings, ages 6 and 11, were also fed the same 3 drug cocktail every day and that the parents were on psychiatric medications as well.***

> *Which means,* ***if not for the disruption by Rebecca's untimely death, this family represented five steady customers for the "mental health industry," with 100% of the costs for doctor's visits and prescriptions paid for by public health care programs.***
> (http://www.sierratimes.com/07/02/27/75_7_243_126_94769.htm)

The elderly are also at risk! A study reported in the June 13, 2005 issue of the *Archives of Internal Medicine* **reviewed antipsychotic use in nursing homes for approximately two and a half million Medicaid beneficiaries and *"found that over half (58.2%), received drugs that exceeded the maximum recommended dosage, received duplicate therapy, or had inappropriate conditions for the drugs to begin with."*** The study also revealed that that ***"more than 200,000 residents received antipsychotic therapy but had no appropriate indications for use"*** (http://www.sierratimes.com/07/01/20/Pringle.htm). This is obviously all about money when you consider that studies published in the October 2005 issue of the *Journal of the American Medical Association* (*JAMA*), reported that, **in trials of more than 5,000 elderly patients treated with atypical antipsychotics, *"patients had a 54% increased chance of dying within 3 months, compared to patients taking a placebo"!***

The Problem With Drug Testing Procedures (Or The Lack Thereof)

As we've repeatedly pointed out, these atypical antipsychotics have not only NOT been approved for use with children, but there is very little long-term research even done regarding the effects on children. Apparently, the FDA has asked five pharmaceutical companies to test these drugs on children with schizophrenia and bipolar disorder, which is what they are currently approved for in adults. Incidentally, all five companies are pharmaceutical companies that actually produce the drug!

According to a research review published in February 2006 ***"90% of drug-company-funded studies come up with findings that support the company's drug."*** This study, appearing in the February 2, 2006 issue of the *New England Journal of Medicine*, (http://www.ahrp.org/cms/content/view/70/29/), further reported the following findings:

> *An independent review by a team of German analysts published in the American Journal of Psychiatry confirms that corporate bias is ubiquitous in clinical trials.*
>
> ***The credibility of company sponsored tests of the so-called "atypical" antipsychotic drugs (neuroleptics)*** *including Johnson & Johnson subsidiary Janssen's Risperdal (risperidone), Lilly's Zyprexa (olanzapine), Novartis' Clozaril (clozapine), Pfizer's Geodon (ziprasidone) and Sanofi-Aventis' Solian (amisulpride)* ***is totally undermined by corporate bias at every step of the process--from design, subject selection, data analysis, and journal reports.***
>
> *Dr. Stephan Heres and colleagues (Technical University, Munich) found that* ***"Different trials comparing the same two drugs have had contradictory conclusions," the study notes. The reported results seem to be much like partisan politics—the drug favored depended upon who paid for the trial.***

Apparently the National Institute of Mental Health is also conducting pediatric studies regarding antipsychotics, but **the research is mainly funded and supervised by pharmaceutical companies,** (and you know that that means). David Graham of the FDA Office of Drug Safety agrees with previous findings, saying ***"Industry-funded trials are four to five times more likely than independent studies to show effectiveness for a drug"*** (http://www.usatoday.com/news/health/2006-05-01-adult-antipsychotics-kids_x.htm).

In a recent front-page story, ran in the *New York Times* (May 10, 2007), Steven Sharfstein, former president of the American Psychiatric Associations admitted that **psychiatrists have become too cozy with drug makers.** Following are other similar statements, made by other top psychiatrists:

- Daniel J. Carlat, an assistant clinical professor of psychiatry at Tufts University, told the Boston Globe (May 7, 2007), ***"Our [psychiatric] field as a whole is progressively being purchased lock, stock, and barrel by the drug companies:*** *this includes the diagnoses, the treatment guidelines, and the national meetings."*
- Steven E. Hyman, former director of the National Institute of Mental Health and provost of Harvard University, stated, *"There's an irony that psychiatrists ask patients to have insights into themselves, but we don't connect the wires in our own lives about how* ***money is affecting our profession and putting our patients at risk.****"*

According to figures from a *New York Times* analysis, **between 2000 and 2005, payments to Minnesota psychiatrists by pharmaceutical companies increased more than six fold, to $1.6 million**. Correspondingly, **antipsychotic prescriptions for children increased more than nine fold.**

Psychotropic drugs, including powerful atypical antipsychotics, are currently being prescribed to ten million children, although **the FDA has warned that the drugs actually cause mania, psychosis, suicidal thoughts and behaviors, homicidal ideation, heart attack, stroke and sudden death!**

The Rather Scary Results Of Clinical Trials

By using the Freedom of Information Act to gain access to FDA data on the drug trials for the atypicals, award-winning author Robert Whitaker reported in his book ***Mad In America***, the following findings, regarding **clinical trials for Zyprexa™, Risperdal™, Seroquel™, and Serdolect™,** as reported to the FDA:

1. ***One in every 145 patients died but the deaths were not mentioned in the scientific literature.***

2. ***The trials were structured to favor the atypicals*** *and most of the reports were discounted by the FDA as being biased.*

3. ***One in every thirty-five patients in Risperdal trials experienced a serious adverse event, defined by the FDA as life threatening or one that required hospitalization*** (http://www.lawyersandsettlements.com/articles/antipsychotics.html).

And then, regarding the specific **testing of Zyprexa™,** Whitaker found the following:

Based on the results of a six-week clinical trial sponsored by Eli Lilly, the FDA granted the company permission to manufacture and distribute Zyprexa on September 27, 1996. The trial involved 2,500 subjects, and two-thirds of them didn't even successfully complete the trial. Among those who stuck it out, 22 percent of the Zyprexa subjects suffered a "serious" adverse effect.

In addition, there were 20 deaths, including 12 suicides. Shockingly, these deaths went unreported in the scientific literature.

Information concerning these deaths was obtained from FDA documents through the Freedom of Information Act by science writer Robert Whitaker.

Bearing in mind ***these deaths****, which* ***occurred during very short trial periods****, the FDA's approval of three of the four atypicals cited* [Zyprexa, Risperdal, Seroquel, and Serdolect] *(Serdolect was unapproved) is appalling. It not only* ***condemns the agency's approval process*** *but also raises doubts about the agency's political independence* (http://www.thestreetspirit.org/August2005/zyprexa.htm).

It is unbelievable that a drug that potentially dangerous, is still being aggressively promoted and prescribed daily for children's use!

Another finding, reported in *The Lancet* (October 7, 2000;356:1219-1223), states that ***"People who take antipsychotic drugs, even those who are young and otherwise healthy, face an increased risk for potentially fatal blood clots."*** Research conducted at the Boston University School of Medicine in Lexington, Massachusetts, reported the following:

Researchers looked at nearly 30,000 patients on antipsychotic drugs over the course of 7 years.

Patients younger than 60 who had no risk factors for blood clots, such as heart disease or diabetes [were used].

They found that ***these patients were 7 times more likely to develop blood clots*** *known as venous thromboembolisms than drug-free study participants.*

Lead researcher Dr. Gwen L. Zornberg said in an interview with Reuters Health, that ***doctors have been noting for decades that antipsychotic drugs seem to trigger blood clots in some patients.***
She also notes that, ***despite accumulating evidence, blood clots are not listed as a potential side effect of antipsychotic drugs.***

Further information on other harmful side effects was reported by the Alliance For Human Research Protection, (http://www.ahrp.org/testimonypresentations/BestPharmaAct0803.php), regarding the "Best Pharmaceuticals for Children's Act of 2002", as follows:

> ***Among the reported severe adverse side effects experienced by the subjects during clinical trials of olanzapine* [Zyprexa™]*: cardiovascular complications (10% to 15%); acute weight gain (50%), an effect that signaled an increased risk for diabetes. Parkinson-like motor impairment (11.7%); and akathisia (mental and physical restless and agitation) (7.3%).***
>
> *It has been strongly suggested by senior psychiatrists at premier research institutions and in internal Eli Lilly documents that akathisia is the likely catalyst for suicidal and homicidal thoughts and acts. During* ***pre****-marketing clinical trials,* ***olanzapine*** [Zyprexa™] ***was linked to serious, in some cases life-threatening side effects requiring hospitalization in 22% of the adults in whom it was tested. According to FDA data, there were 22 deaths - 12 of which were suicides. The drop-out rate during 6-week clinical trials was 65%. In an extended (one year) trial, the drop out rate had been 83%.***
>
> ***Until the introduction of the atypical antipsychotic drugs, such as clozapine (Clozaril) and olanzapine (Zyprexa), diabetes was rare in children and adolescents. Since its approval, a review by officials of the Center for Drug Evaluation of FDA's MedWatch database reveals a causal association between Zyprexa and new onset diabetes that is ten times higher than in the general population.***
>
> ***How can anyone justify exposing healthy youngsters to a drug that has a ten-fold probability of causing diabetes?***

The real question is: Just how many children's lives must be sacrificed before this obvious deception, and unnecessary destruction of innocent lives, is finally terminated?

Other Tactics Used By Pharmaceutical Companies

According to an article in the *Register Guard*, (January 28, 2007), titled *"Reconsidering Psychiatric Drugs"*, by Susan Palmer, *"Zyprexa manufacturer Eli Lilly has already spent $1.4 billion to settle more than 20,000 claims by patients who say the drug made them sick."* So why are they still allowed to sell such a dangerous drug? Much in the same way they get away with selling all dangerous drugs. Following is just one example of the tactics Eli Lilly used with Zyprexa™:

> ***When Kentucky held public hearings to try to exclude Zyprexa from Medicaid's list of covered drugs, the most notorious Big Pharma backed front group in the US, the National Alliance for the Mentally Ill, bused in protesters for the hearings, placed full-page ads in newspapers, and sent faxes to state officials. However, a little known fact is that by funneling***

money through NAMI, Lilly paid for the buses, ads, and faxes, according to the December 18, 2003 New York Times.

Should the court continue to allow Lilly to hide the documents with the incriminating information, *it will not be surprising to many experts. For as pediatrician, Dr. Lawrence Diller, author of the book, "Should I Medicate My Child," stated in language relevant here, while testifying before an FDA advisory committee in September 2004, regarding* ***the conduct of companies concealing the adverse effects of drugs and promoting off-label prescribing:***

"The blame is clear: The money, power and influence of the pharmaceutical industry corrupt all. The pervasive control that the drug companies have over medial research, publications, professional organizations, doctors' practices, Congress, and yes, even agencies like the FDA, is the American equivalent of a drug cartel" (http://www.sierratimes.com/07/01/20/Pringle.htm).

I totally agree! The only difference is, it's very well disguised, and to date is totally legal. Not only that, but it has even been promoted by those sworn to protect us, (the FDA, and even our own elected officials in the federal government)! We spend billions of dollars, fighting the importation of illegal drugs by the drug cartel, while encouraging a far greater threat: the promotion of drugs known to be dangerous, to even our young children. This is a crime against humanity that we can no longer continue to ignore, especially now that we are aware of the devious and very aggressive perpetration of an obvious scam to deceive the public.

Nutritional Supplementation For Mental Health - The Importance of Nutrition

According to studies reported by the UK's Mental Health Foundation, ***"Scientific studies have clearly linked attention deficit disorder, depression, Alzheimer's disease and schizophrenia to junk food and the absence of essential fats, vitamins and minerals in industrialized diets"*** (http://www.newstarget.com/020268.html).

And in his book *Nutrition and Mental Illness*, (1987), the late Dr. Carl C. Pfeiffer, Ph.D., M.D. claimed that there are five main "biotypes" of schizophrenias, (and incidentally, **all responded to nutrition**). Dr. Pfeiffer provides some amazing insight, as follows:

1. ***Histapenia*** *– low blood histamine with excess copper: 50 percent of the schizophrenias.*
2. **Histadelia** *– high blood histamine with low copper: 20 percent of the schizophrenias.*
3. ***Pyroluria*** *– a familial double deficiency of zinc and vitamin B_6: 30 percent of the schizophrenias.* (NOTE: For more information on pyroluria, refer to the last chapter in this book under "Additional Technical Information".)
4. ***Cerebral allergy*** *– includes wheat-gluten allergy: 10 percent of the schizophrenias.*
5. ***Nutritional hypoglycemia:*** *20 percent of the schizophrenias.*

These percentages do no add up to exactly 100 percent because many patients have more than one disorder. In our outpatient clinic (The Princeton Brain Bio Center) we have treated over 5,000 patients labeled "schizophrenic." Of these, ***95 percent can be categorized into the five types just described. When the exact biotype guides the appropriate treatment, 90 percent of these patients will attain social rehabilitation*** (pp. 10-11).

Following are the benefits of several nutrients, proven beneficial in the treatment and/or prevention of schizophrenia and other psychotic conditions, as noted by several well-respected sources.

Vitamin C

- In her book *Natural Healing For Schizophrenia, 2nd Edition*, (1996/1998), Eva Edelman tells of the many benefits associated with vitamin C, as follows:

> ***The second highest concentration of vitamin C occurs in the brain.***
>
> ***Vitamin C supports formation of a number of neurotransmitters, including norepinephrine and serotonin. Depression, tension (anxiety), and paranoia have responded to treatment with vitamin C.*** *The vitamin may increase socialization and well-being, and* ***improve mood and general mental status in chronic schizophrenia.***
> ***Vitamin C may be a natural tranquilizer and antipsychotic agent.*** *Preliminary work by Tolbert suggests vitamin C occupies the same (dopamine) receptor sites as phenothiazines and that, gram for gram, it is as powerful as Haldol – without causing tardive dyskinesia or other such detrimental effects on the nervous system.*
>
> *Vitamin C and B have been used in treating drug-induced delirium and alcoholic psychosis. C has also been used to help counteract barbiturates, and amphetamines, and in treating addictions.*

- Following are the clinical experiences of Frederick R. Klenner, M.D., extracted from the booklet titled *Clinical Guide to the Use of Vitamin C* (1988), abbreviated, summarized and annotated by Lendon H. Smith, M.D.:

> *Six to 8 grams of C a day made the niacin work.* ***One schizophrenic took 1 gram every hour for 48 hours and was completely recovered for six months with no further treatment. These mega-doses halved the suicide rate. It has been demonstrated that schizophrenics burn up C ten times faster than the normal population.*** *Most people show some spill of C in the urine at 4 grams per day; schizophrenics have to take ten times this amount before it can be detected. Dr. Klenner noticed this spillage in patients severely affected with a virus only after two to three days of large doses of C and improvement had begun. (Could schizophrenia be due to a virus?)* (p. 36)

It might be worth mentioning that vitamin C, as well as every single one of the above B vitamins listed below, (which are very beneficial for both depression and schizophrenia), are included in the 16 nutrients depleted by the SSRI antidepressants.

The B Vitamins

➢ Eva Edelman also does an excellent job of explaining the many benefits of the B vitamins, (*Natural Healing For Schizophrenia, 2nd Edition*, 1996/1998), as follows:

> ***B3*** *supports the formation of the neurotransmitters, serotonin, histamine, and acetylcholine. It* ***is critical in treatment of the histamine-deficient biotype, histapenia (which may be involved in almost half of all cases of schizophrenia).***
>
> ***B6 has been used in the treatment of hyperactivity, epilepsy, depression, learning disabilities, nervousness and anxiety.*** *Along with magnesium, it is reported to be crucial in almost half of the cases of autism, agitation, insomnia, irritability, convulsions, (especially in children), depression, confusion, and brain wave abnormalities.*
>
> ***B12 is critical to nervous system metabolism. Deficiency symptoms include inability to concentrate, poor memory, confusion, fatigue, moodiness, agitation, incoordination, stuporous depression, mania, paranoia and psychosis.***
>
> ***Folic Acid supports formation of dopamine, histamine, and serotonin. Deficiency has been associated with fatigue, depression, <u>schizophrenia</u>, and Alzheimer's type dementia.***
>
> ***Riboflavin (vitamin B2) deficiency has been associated with*** *tremors, depression, fatigue, moodiness, irritability, compulsive eating,* ***hysteria, nerve damage and, in some cases, psychosis.***

➢ An article in the March 2006 issue of *Dr. Jonathan V. Wright's Nutrition & Healing* newsletter, points out that **it's been known for more than 70 years that *"A severe deficiency of niacin, a form of vitamin B_3, can lead to dementia in a relatively short period of time."***

➢ Researchers at the Centers for Disease Control and Prevention (CDCP) in Atlanta recently conducted a study, finding that ***"Even a slight deficiency* [of niacin] *over a much longer period could have the same devastating effects."*** The article goes on to point out:

> *Abram Hoffer, M.D. has demonstrated for more than 40 years that high doses of* ***niacinamide (another form of vitamin B3) can actually reverse many cases of schizophrenia if started soon enough after diagnosis*** *(Morris MC et al. "Dietary niacin and the risk of incident Alzheimer's disease and the cognitive decline." J Neurol Neurosurg Psychiatry 2004 Aug;p 75(8):1093-9).*

Dr. Hoffer just happens to have written a book on this very subject, titled *Vitamin B-3 and Schizophrenia: Discovery, Recovery, Controversy* (1998), which was reviewed by Dr. Andrew Saul, Ph.D., Assistant Editor of the peer-reviewed *Journal of Orthomolecular Medicine*, and posted on his personal website (http://www.doctoryourself.com/review_hoffer_B3.html). Following is a portion of Dr. Saul's review:

> *For half a century Dr. Hoffer has dissented. His central point has been this:* ***Illness, including mental illness, is not caused by drug deficiency. But much illness, especially mental illness, may be seen to be caused by a vitamin deficiency.***
>
> *I personally should have first become aware of a food-brain connection during those al-night, cookie-fired mah-jongg marathons I all-too-regularly indulged in while attending Australian National University. Though arguably somewhat less than psychotic, my mind was nevertheless pretty whacked out on sugar, junk food and adrenalin by 3 am.* ***My mood was destroyed; my mind agitated; unable to sleep, sit still, or smile. Of course, I never entertained even the thought of a nutrition connection. For we've all been carefully taught that drugs cure illness, not diet. And certainly not vitamin supplements!***
>
> *But the truth will out eventually. Three years later, I first saw niacin work on somebody else. He was a bona-fide, properly-diagnosed, utterly-incurable, State-hospitalized schizophrenic patient.*
>
> *The patient was a fellow whose parents were desperate enough to try anything, even nutrition. Perhaps this was because* ***their son was so unmanageably violent that he was kicked out of the asylum and sent to live with them.*** *On a good day, his Mom and Dad somehow got him to take 3,000 mg of niacin and 10,000 mg of vitamin C. Formally a hyperactive insomniac, he responded by sleeping for 18 hours the first night and becoming surprisingly normal within days. I'd seen him before, and I saw him after. I'd talked to his parents during the whole process.* ***It was an astounding improvement.***
>
> *Dr. Hoffer explains why this is so:*
>
> *1) As a rule, the more ill you are, the more niacin you can hold without flushing. In other words, if you need it, you physiologically soak up a lot of niacin. Where does it all go? Well, a good bit of it goes into making nicotinamide adenine dinucleotide, or NAD. NAD is just about the most important coenzyme in your body.*
>
> *2)* ***Niacin also works in your body as an antihistamine. Many persons showing psychotic behavior suffer from cerebral allergies.*** *They need more niacin in order to cope with eating inappropriate foods. They also need to stop eating those inappropriate foods, chief among which are the ones they may crave the most: junk food and sugar.*

3) ***There is a chemical found in quantity in the bodies of schizophrenic persons. It is an indole called adrenochrome. Adrenochrome (which is oxidized adrenalin) has an almost LSD-like effect on the body.*** *That might well explain their behavior.* ***Niacin serves to reduce the body's production of this toxic material.***

Dr. Hoffer has treated thousands and thousands of such patients for nearly half a century. At 83, he still is in actively practicing orthomolecular (megavitamin) psychiatry. He has seen medical fads come and go. What he sees now is what he's always seen: that very sick people get well on vitamin B-3.

Essential Fatty Acids (EFAs)

➤ In the December 1998 issue of *Psychiatric Times*, Jerry Cott, Ph.D., of the National Institute of Mental Health wrote ***"There is evidence that deficiency of long-chain, omega-3 polyunsaturates may contribute to symptoms of schizophrenia,"*** and then goes on to point out that *"Adequate long-chain polyunsaturated fatty acid, particularly Docosahexaenoic acid* [DHA], *may reduce the development of depression and schizophrenia"* (Vol. XI, Issue 12). Dr. Cott went on to comment on omega-3 therapy: ***"I don't know of any other preventive treatments for mental disorders. This is in a class by itself. It is extremely promising."*** As you are likely aware by now, there are many other supplements for treating various other mental disorders.

Some Final Thoughts on Schizophrenia

It's amazing that something so simple as eliminating milk from the diet, or adding one or more of the vitamins or minerals we just discussed, can resolve such a troubling condition. The disperceptions associated with schizophrenia can be very debilitating, as well as potentially dangerous. As you have just learned, quite often it is just a side effect of one or more medications. Most importantly, it can lead to disastrous results, such as the recent rash of school shootings that destroy the lives of innocent victims and families, (often for no apparent reason).

A prime example is Cho, the student at Virginia Tech who shot himself, along with 33 other students, for no apparent reason. The rage he expressed is, according to Dr. Ann Blake Tracy, an emotion some have expressed experiencing while on SSRI antidepressants. One example Dr. Tracy provided in her book *Prozac: Panacea or Pandora?*, was an individual who claimed it was as though someone else's brain was in their body. It's basically the potentially dangerous Jekyll-and-Hyde personality that these drugs can produce, where your mind is no longer your own. The obvious question is: who should be held responsible for their actions? And most importantly, should any drug, with that kind of mind-altering capability, be not only legal, but even promoted for young children's use? Considering their dangers, I see absolutely no justification for maintaining their legal status! How about you?

Although "I would never consider taking any drug", I would definitely prefer taking Vioxx™ (which was pulled, due to the increased risk for a stroke or heart attach), than any of the antidepressants or antipsychotics that millions of children are being placed on! They make Vioxx™ look like a walk in the park, and at least Vioxx™ would make the walk less painful, (although I can't think of "anything positive" to say about the antidepressants or antipsychotics).

CHAPTER EIGHTEEN

Conclusion

We Must Start A Movement To Stop The Madness In Medicine - Millions Of Lives Are At Risk, (But Especially Those Of Our Children)!

Although in this book I focus primarily on the many dangers associated with the "mind-altering drugs", that's not where the danger ends. All drugs pose a risk, yet there is one characteristic in particular that sets the mind-altering drugs apart from all the others. It's their ability to alter your brain, and thus your thoughts, and do so in an unnatural and unhealthy way, (sometimes permanently)! People have been known to do things that were totally out of character for them, things that they later admit they would never have considered doing, had they been in their "right mind". That's if they didn't take their life, (and thus live to tell of it)! Worst of all is when they take another's life, (an even greater tragedy)! It's as though you suddenly turn into someone else, that even you would never recognize. You are suddenly no longer in control of your actions, (what a scary thought)! Andrea Yates, a very caring mother who, without any provocations whatsoever, suddenly drowned her children, is a typical example. And we're not talking about just a few isolated cases, but tens of thousands of victims over the years. Some recognized the problem before it was too late, but unfortunately others didn't, thus many innocent lives have been needlessly sacrificed. Not only that, but as you are likely aware of by now, these same drugs also contribute to serious, life-threatening diseases, such as cancer and diabetes, (in both children, and adults).

The question is: If it wasn't for the side effects associated with all drugs, just how many of the drugs that most people are currently taking, would really be necessary, in order to suppress the primary symptom? Common conditions such as pain, depression, elevated blood pressure, or possibly blood sugar, are those that most people originally take medications for. Then we must also include the statins for lowering cholesterol (a non-disease), and drugs for acid reflux, (another non-disease). In my opinion, all drugs are seldom necessary.

"Confessions of an Rx Drug Pusher"

That's the title of a book written by a friend Gwen Olsen, which she shared with me. Both Gwen and her niece Megan eventually became victims of dangerous drugs. Unfortunately, Megan paid with her life, by committing suicide. She was apparently attractive and intelligent, but grew up in a very dysfunctional family. Megan had been placed on an extensive list of drugs, in dangerous combinations, by her doctor. After attempting to hang herself from the ceiling fan failed, she poured oil from a lamp, all over her body, and then lit herself on fire. She eventually realized what she had done and called 911, although it was too late. She had burns on 95% of her body, and died on the way to the hospital, (a terrible tragedy, and obviously not something that anyone in their "right mind" would ever consider doing). There are many other horror stories similar to Megan's.

For instance, in her audiotape, Dr. Ann Blake Tracy talked of an individual who shot his brother-in-law for no apparent reason while on antidepressants. He then called 911 (as Megan had), and kept him alive until the ambulance arrived. Luckily he survived. The 911 operator said he sounded more like a robot than a person. He then called his sister (his brother-in-law's wife), who also indicated that he sounded like a robot. His sister obviously knew how he normally sounded. His mind was obviously not his own.

Both Gwen and her niece Megan, (her sister's daughter), grew up in very dysfunctional families, which she describes in considerable detail in her book *Confessions of an Rx Drug Pusher: God's Call To Loving Arms* (2005). Following Megan's untimely death, Gwen did some serious soul-searching. She felt she could no longer pursue a career of marketing pharmaceutical drugs to doctors. Although very profitable, it was based totally on deception, and endangering lives, at least indirectly, by encouraging doctors to prescribe drugs and not disclosing their potential dangers.

Following is an extract of a story of another "ex" pharmaceutical rep, whose experience was very similar to Gwen's. Neither could, in good conscience, continue the deception that could indirectly place many at unnecessary risk of serious harm.

Prescription Drugs Under Fire Again

September 15, 2006

Kathleen Slattery-Moschkau spent ten years of her life selling drugs…legally, that is. She worked for one of America's corporate darlings – the pharmaceutical industry. Kathleen had it all – a big salary, a company car, a closet full of business suits, company perks, and ***a growing pit in her stomach.***

In this eye-opening interview with CRUSADOR editor Greg Ciola, Kathleen shares with the public the pill-pushing tactics of the pharmaceutical industry's leading companies and the reasons why we all need to be concerned about the drugs doctors are prescribing to patients.

"I'd say for the first three to five years, they basically told me what to say, and I said it. *They taught me how to say the big medical words."*

"I started to feel increasingly uncomfortable with what I was doing for a living. *Every day things were happening in the course of my career that in some cases were very humorous, and in some cases very shocking.* ***In the end, all of it was very scary when you think about the fact that people's lives were on the line based on information that I was giving these doctors."***

"Every time I was just sick enough to walk away, I'd get a big raise or a new company car. I found myself rationalizing or spinning that PR that they were giving me such as, ***'What would we do without the pharmaceutical industry,'*** *and,* ***'Oh, your role is so important in educating physicians.'*** *I found myself using that spin to rationalize why I was staying.* ***Then after ten years, I couldn't even look at myself in the mirror anymore. I was so uncomfortable that the information I was being given and then giving to physicians could potentially cause harm, I just had to walk away.*** *I didn't care if I had to flip burgers for a living."*

According to recent reports, ***"In 2004, spending for prescription drugs was $188.5 billion, almost five times as much as what was spent in 1990. Between 1995 and 2005, the number of drug reps in the US increased from 38,000 to 100,000"*** (http://medicine.plosjournals.org/perlserv/?request=get-document&doi=10.1371%2Fjournal.pmed.0040150#journal-pmed-0040150-t101).

With that many drug reps out there, my guess is that there has to be many other pharmaceutical reps, just like both Gwen and Kathleen, who do have a conscience. If so, it might be rather difficult for them to justify promoting drugs, known to be dangerous, to doctors for their patients, (especially young children), if they were better informed. It possibly might help ease their conscience if they didn't know, (obviously the company's objective).

If you just happen to know of such an individual, or someone who is considering such a career, you might share my book with them. They would obviously not be successful in selling drugs, once they know just how dangerous they are, as long as they share that critical information with the doctors they are promoting them to. If they are ethical, and truly have a conscience, they should consider looking for another career they can feel more comfortable with, (as Gwen and Kathleen did), even if it doesn't pay as much. **Money can't buy peace of mind.** It's not just coincidental that the majority of psychiatrist's patients just happen to be the wealthiest. The most important issue is, how they became wealthy. There is no crime in becoming wealthy, as long as you are honest in your dealings, and not knowingly placing others' lives at risk in the process.

Is Introspection and Serious Soul-Searching Possibly In Order?

If you're a relatively new pharmaceutical rep, out to make a million, or possibly a seasoned veteran, as Gwen Olsen "once was", you may need to seriously reconsider your priorities, (as Gwen eventually did). Even if you are a company exec, or possibly even the CEO of a very profitable pharmaceutical company, you must seriously consider if you can in good conscience, continue perpetrating the obvious deception. Can you go on placing millions of lives (especially innocent children) needlessly at risk, while pretending that the drug risks are somehow non-existent, while knowing full well how dangerous they truly are?

Sometimes, even doctors are victims. According to Gwen, doctors and pharmacists are some of the worst prescription drug abusers of all. And according to Dr. Joel Wallach, (the *Dead Doctors Don't Lie* guy), the average doctor lives for only 58 years! If doctors are the holders of all knowledge, they should live to be 90 or 100 years of age. Unfortunately for them, that privilege is reserved only for those who never heard of prescription drugs. Doctors are originally brainwashed in medical school, and then on an ongoing basis, by their pharmaceutical representatives. Not only that, but they have access to all those free samples, which often, to their own detriment, as well as their patients', many doctors totally believe in.

Would You Believe –
An Obvious Conspiracy To Deliberately Create Disease!

Gwen Olsen discovered a tactic one day that shows just how cunning and devious the industry she had been representing truly was, **(something she claims haunted her the remainder of her career).** It was regarding a non-steroidal anti-inflammatory drug (NSAID), for pain called Naprosyn™ (Naproxen). **The drug has a twelve-hour half-life. That basically means you would be required to take the drug, twice daily, in order to effectively relive the pain and basically maintain the drugs' effectiveness for 24 hours. Yet, the company's recommended dosage was *"one, three times daily"*, (which was obviously unnecessary).**

That prompted Gwen to raise her hand and ask the speaker (who was the product manager with Syntex, the maker of Naprosyn™), why they recommend the dosage of three daily, considering that twice daily should be adequate. Incidentally, this was a company-wide meeting, with nearly 1,000 reps throughout the country in attendance. **Gwen couldn't believe his response: *"Because we can sell more pills that way."* And he wasn't just joking!** Although he attempted to move on, Gwen persisted. She posed the obvious question that anyone familiar with NSAID drugs such as Naprosyn™ should ask: ***"Doesn't that unnecessarily increase the possibility of GI* [Gastrointestinal] *bleeding, and ulceration?"* To which the drug rep replied, *"Well, of course it does, but luckily for those patients, we have a new H2-blocker in the pipeline!"*** Gwen soon discovered that H2-blockers (h2-antagonists) were used to **treat stomach ulcers.** I guess that's what you'd call planning for the future, (obviously their future – not yours).

Ironically, Gwen herself had been a victim of the very same drug, due to samples she claims she had indiscriminately taken at one time for headaches and back pain. At the time, she wasn't aware of the risk. She claims she experienced a serious GI bleed from taking them, and later discovered, from research, that **there are 100,000 hospital admissions, and 16,000 deaths annually, attributed to NSAID use only.** And we're just talking about only one of many classes of drugs currently on the market, (some much more serious). **She indicated that the seriousness of those statistics was never brought to her attention by any of the companies she worked for that produced NSAIDs.**

Are Drug Companies Intentionally Creating The Typical Domino Effect? Is It Just Accidental, Or Possibly A Deliberate Marketing Tactic?

One can't help but wonder if the typical domino effect, which I often refer to, might very well be (at least at times) the result of a deliberate attempt to create an additional market they could in turn fill. As we learned, Gwen eventually discovered that is not just a possibility, but is instead a reality, as some companies deliberately recommend taking higher doses than necessary, and are doing so for that very reason.

Speaking of excessive dosages, if you consider for instance, the hundreds of potential side effects associated with Prozac™, and that it's even being prescribed for very young (and thus small) children, the potential for more serious side effects is considerably greater. As their livers are much smaller, and still in the developmental stage, more Prozac™ (and thus fluoride), which is known to be highly protein-binding, and thus very difficult for the liver to metabolize, will gain access to the child's brain, which is still developing as well. Drugs such as Prozac™ and Paxil™ pose an even greater threat for the very young (and old), who are the most vulnerable, (one reason that some experience a serious reaction shortly after being placed on an antidepressant, or antipsychotic drug). And worst of all, some children are being placed on multiple drugs, (a common practice today), which is even risky for an adult. And when a child reacts to the drugs, some doctors even add another drug, or increase the dosage, or possibly even worse, "suddenly" withdraw one or more drugs. That's a very dangerous practice, and when the most serious reactions often take place. The brain tends to over-react to any sudden change, (something many doctors fail to recognize). They thus place their patients at extreme risk, (especially when they're young children).

One tactic often employed by pharmaceutical companies is to hire a doctor, (it's a well-known fact that some doctors are for sale). They are paid to come to some pre-determined conclusion, such as a lower blood pressure level, or possibly lower cholesterol, for instance, is somehow advisable. It's then broadcast on the national news. The source for the announcement is often some organization such as the National Institutes of Health, (considered as a credible source), which just happens to have a surprising number of doctors, in key positions, with "two incomes" on their payroll! Their second job (some pharmaceutical company) normally pays considerably more than their NIH salary, which was discovered by research conducted by the *LA Times*. That greatly expands their potential market, allowing unsuspecting victims to unnecessarily be placed on more drugs, or have their dosage be increased by their doctor.

Just one such announcement, that cholesterol levels should be even lower, and that doubling their patients' dosage might be necessary, for instance, was all it took to prompt many doctors to do just that. These dangerous cholesterol medications not only contribute to a worsening of heart disease, but many other conditions as well. As Gwen eventually discovered, it's all about marketing and profit potential, (your health is their least concern). Although maybe I should qualify that statement, as your health actually is their concern. They know full well that, when you eat a healthy diet, and take your vitamins, (which doctors seldom recommend), you will be healthier. Thus, you wouldn't be going to your doctor nearly as often, (their primary drug pushers). That's the very reason that PhRMA, (who represents the pharmaceutical industry), continually attempts to convince you that many supplements, such as vitamins or herbs, are totally useless, or possibly even dangerous. Yet, you never once hear them warn you of how unsafe some dangerous drugs are, (even if they are known to be killing thousands), or that some were proven to greatly increase the risk for suicide. Not one single word of warning!

The pharmaceutical industry is in my opinion, even more dangerous than the drug cartels that produce and market illegal drugs (the same drugs once produced, and promoted, by the very same companies now producing legal drugs). The only reason many of the mind-altering drugs are still considered legal, and remain on the market, (and are even being promoted for young kids), is because the FDA somehow forgot who it was supposed to be protecting. Their compliance, and even total support, rather than oversight of the obviously corrupt pharmaceutical industry, has allowed dangerous drugs to not only be placed on, but also remain on, the market for years, even when the serious risks are well known. It's difficult any more to determine just who is really in charge of drug regulation. It's as though the companies are doing their own regulation, with their only criteria being the cost of litigation (lawsuits), versus the profit potential.

The reason I consider the legal drug pushers, (or the companies creating their drugs), as being even more dangerous, is obvious. It's totally legal, and the majority of adults in the nation are "unnecessarily" on one or more (often several) of their potentially dangerous drugs. And worst of all, our young children have now become their prime target. The class of drugs now being promoted for children consists of some of the most dangerous drugs on the market today, (mind-altering drugs that are very similar to the drugs now considered as illegal). And nothing could be more risky! Due to their crafty promotional campaigns, via their TV commercials, and deliberate cover-up of their known risks, many are totally unaware of their inherent dangers, (something that absolutely must change)! Every parent must be warned of the serious risks associated with the whole class of mind-altering drugs being aggressively promoted for their kids. If not, their children might very well be their next victims.

With that in mind, how can the FDA possibly justify allowing such dangerous drugs to remain on the market for decades? Even worse, they are now approving some even more dangerous antipsychotic medications. It's quite obvious they are not about to do anything about the obvious threat, unless they are somehow forced to do so, (our challenge). If we truly care, we can make a difference by making our voices heard! Tell your family and friends! Alert your senators and congressmen, (both state and federal)! Contact your local school administration, and put a stop to the "very aggressive" drug marketing campaign via the TeenScreen movement, (an all out effort to get as many of our children as possible on their very profitable, mind-altering, disease promoting drugs). Even some churches might consider getting involved, as they can have an influence on their congregation as well. You might also check with your local senior center. There are a lot of talented senior citizens just looking for a worthwhile cause. It gives them a reason for living, (one thing that helps keep them young and active).

Anyone who knows what these drugs can potentially do to our children should be concerned, although many adults are at risk as well. As stated by Gwen Olsen, the ex-pharmaceutical rep, ***"Be the difference that makes a difference",*** something she has set out to do herself. She has finally found peace of mind, since making that critical decision.

These drugs are not only destroying lives, both physically and mentally, but if the companies who produce and aggressively promote them are allowed to continue doing so, they will also totally destroy the very financial fabric of our nation. It's easy to see why our healthcare cost has been rapidly escalating, (several times the normal inflation rate)! If this corrupt industry is allowed to continue getting more and more children (and pregnant mothers) on their very profitable drugs, as they have been, (and fully intend to continue doing), we could soon begin experiencing an all-out epidemic of cancer, diabetes, and obesity, in our young children, (which is already being predicted). And although most are unaware of the underlying cause, now you know! We will also see a lowering of children's' IQs, and an increase in the rate of dementia and Alzheimer's disease, and at "a much earlier age" as well.

In my award-winning book, *A Drug-Free Approach To Healthcare* (now available in a "Revised Edition", 2007), I show the dangers associated with many other medications, and why they are seldom (if ever) necessary. If you recall, in Mary Lou's true story, she discovered that **she never really needed any of the nine medications she had been taking for years**, (including 2 antidepressants, and the dangerous lithium for **the bipolar disorder caused by Prozac™**). Most importantly, **she had been taking Prozac™ for a total of 16 years,** and **"in only 60 days she was totally drug free"!** There are many other similar stories; she is not somehow unique. **In my opinion, there are very few in the nation who couldn't quite easily accomplish the very same thing, if they so chose.** Our best defense is an offense, by saying ***"I no longer need your dangerous drugs",*** as Mary Lou and many others have done.

As I often stress, people's medications are by far the greatest contributor to their poor health, especially due to their well-known nutrient depletion, as well as their side effects that eventually leads to even more drugs just to suppress the side effects, (what I refer to as the typical domino effect associated with all drugs). The more drugs they are taking, the worse their health will become. Many have noted that when they were required to stop taking their medications prior to surgery, they discovered they felt much better after doing so. Maybe they should start paying more attention to what their body is attempting to tell them. Their bodies are obviously trying to tell them that those drugs are not really helping!

We should also consider that **"drugs are chemicals, created in a lab, by man, <u>for profit only</u>"**, (huge profits). God, on the other hand, created plants, and herbs, for our natural pharmacy. Plants contain many, (sometimes hundreds), of synergistic ingredients, and are far more complex than any drug that man could possibly create in any lab. Although drugs are normally far cheaper to mass-produce, they actually sell for "much more", (due to the obvious greed, as they are not really satisfied with a reasonable profit margin). There are also many concentrates, derived from natural sources that our body immediately recognizes as beneficial, versus the drugs that are recognized as the "toxins" they are, by our liver the detoxifier.

If you have even the least bit of apprehension about possibly withdrawing from your medications, just pray about your decision, and if necessary, find a natural practitioner that can help you in doing so. God created our bodies, which are organic, thus anything that can truly heal, or maintain our health, must be organic as well. **<u>Drugs just override and disrupt our normal processes</u>, such as maintaining "healthy", (<u>not "excessive"</u>), hormone levels in the brain.**

Another example is the **beta "<u>blockers</u>"**, or **ACE "<u>inhibitors</u>"**, (both blood pressure medications), which basically override natural processes that have important functions, such as providing adequate oxygen and nutrients where they are most needed, (especially the brain). If you noticed, they are designed to **<u>inhibit</u>, or <u>block</u>, normal functions,** which God created for an important purpose, (He obviously knew what He was doing)! I explain just how critical that can be, and how to eliminate the elevated blood pressure naturally, (if really necessary), in my book *A Drug-Free Approach To Healthcare*. I also explain how diabetes medications can actually worsen the condition, and often contribute to hypoglycemia (low blood sugar) as well. The symptoms of hypoglycemia are the exact same as those that mind-altering drugs are often prescribed for. Although, blood sugar can normally be easily stabilized with just a slight diet modification, and possibly a few supplements.

Diabetes medications also deplete the very nutrients necessary for producing "<u>quality insulin</u>", (no, <u>all insulin is not created equal</u>, and thus not as effective), although poor quality insulin is still effective in storing fat in fat cells, (obviously not our objective). By depleting nutrients necessary for producing insulin, diabetes medications actually contribute to insulin resistance. Insulin can't efficiently get glucose into the cells for energy when some of its parts are either missing, or in short supply.

The very worst combination, regarding your brain, is when the blood pressure medications, which can result in insufficient oxygen to the brain, are combined with one or more diabetes medications, which sometimes results in hypoglycemia, or low blood sugar, (a very bad combination). We then find that one more class of blood pressure medication in particular known as the calcium channel <u>blockers</u>, also pose a serious risk. According the Dr. Sherry Rogers, M.D., they were proven in brain scans to actually shrink the neurons in the brain, (as well as shrinking the brain itself), increasing the risk of acquiring dementia or Alzheimer's disease! Again, one more drug produced to <u>block</u> a critical function, and create a loss of neurons in the process. Other than Prozac™, with its high level of fluoride, and its ability to drastically increase the level of the "brain damaging" stress hormone cortisol (by 200%), these blood pressure medications, in my opinion, pose one of the greatest risks for developing Alzheimer's disease.

I might just add that the statin, or cholesterol lowering drugs (for a non-disease), also pose a serious risk, not only to the heart, kidneys, and liver, but also the brain, (where most of the cholesterol will be found). Many have discovered that once they stopped taking them, their muscles stopped hurting, their energy level returned, as did their memory! They are prescribed for a "non-disease", with absolutely no solid science to justify their use, (other than that, they are very profitable)! Never have they been able to show any connection whatsoever, between a person's cholesterol level, and their risk of experiencing a heart attack. Statistics don't lie, although some unscrupulous people sometimes do, (especially if there's enough money at stake). And unfortunately, even many doctors can be bought and paid for, (something that drug companies are very aware of, and all too often take full advantage of). Unfortunately, even some of our legislators have a price. Those are issues we should become aware of, and obstacles that must be overcome, (although when there is a will, there is always a way)! This is one of the most serious threats that we, as a nation, are facing today. Especially due to its broad (and continually widening) scope, via the aggressive campaign now targeting our kids, (from the cradle to the grave). A perfect long-term annuity, which just increases as each new drug is added.

A Very Effective Business Strategy – Proven To Be Effective: First Create A Demand For Drugs, And Them Provide Them

Eli Lilly has created several drugs, starting with the SSRI antidepressant Prozac™, and more recently the atypical antipsychotic Zyprexa™, which are very effective at "creating diabetes", (obviously not what they are promoted for). Diabetes is a well-known side effect associated with both drugs, and although Prozac™ is bad enough for creating diabetes, it appears that Zyprexa™ is even more effective in that regard.

Eli Lilly's second-largest income is derived from its diabetes care products, which actually grossed over $2.61 billion in 2004 (*Indianapolis Star*, January 27, 2005). Then, I understand that Eli Lilly is currently spending $325 million, building one of the largest factories ever devoted to making a single drug – **INSULIN!** They can see the writing on the wall, or should I say, they are the ones writing on the wall. A common saying is: If you want to be successful in any business venture, all you have to do is find a need and then fill it. And companies such as Eli Lily have actually found an even better business strategy. **They discovered how they could instead "create a need", and then fill it.** The very first step would be to get everyone possible on just one of their drugs initially, and then everything else would be automatic. The typical domino effect soon takes over.

They definitely came up with a winner to launch the demand for drugs when they created Prozac™ with its ability to create a serious nutritional deficiency, along with an "extensive list" of potential side effects. Only sick people go to doctors, and only doctors can prescribe medications. Then they went all out marketing Prozac™, initially targeting both doctors and their patients. Their promotional campaign made Prozac™ appear as a panacea that was perfectly safe, and a drug that nearly everyone could somehow benefit from. They then set out to broaden their market by encouraging doctors, via their drug representatives, to begin prescribing Prozac™ for off-label uses, (a practice that should be illegal). They are not even required to prove it's any more effective than a placebo for the conditions it is being prescribed for, although it definitely outdoes the placebo when it comes to side effects. That's obviously a far more cost-effective approach than creating several different drugs, (one for each condition), and then getting FDA approval for each one of the conditions that they encourage doctors to prescribe Prozac™ for.

Then there's the promotion of drugs, by the crafty commercials on TV, (that other countries don't allow – and for good reason), encourages people to request drugs that they often don't really need, although they are often prescribed by their doctor, due to the patient's request. If it wasn't working, the commercials would soon stop, (and they obviously haven't been stopping), and are instead continually increasing. You can't even watch the national news nowadays, without seeing one commercial after another, (and guess who is paying for them)! Not to worry, it's coming out of their research budget, (and just added to the cost of their drugs)! Unfortunately, many unsuspecting victims falsely assume that their survival somehow depends on their medications, although in my opinion, nothing could be further from the truth. They are instead the best possible way you can not only shorten your life, but also reduce your quality of life in the process. That doesn't sound much like a benefit to me, and just think of it – you are paying for it as well, (such a bargain)!

It's strictly a well thought out business plan, and their success hinges on total deception, by convincing you (via your doctor and their crafty TV commercials) that you can't possibly live without their drugs. If the general public only knew the whole truth, and nothing but the truth, their house of cards would soon begin to crumble. They would have to stop playing dominoes, and no longer create a lifetime of symptoms. And we could finally begin experiencing the quality of health that we all deserve, and should expect, (a goal that is in my opinion totally achievable). It's just a matter of exposing their tactics, and the many dangers associated with their drugs, and then spreading the word, (my goal, and hopefully yours).

For anyone promoting these drugs, the question remains: Is all that money really worth the damaged lives (both physically and mentally) to literally millions? This life is relatively short, compared to eternity. When your life is nearing its end, how will you feel about your contribution, and the legacy you will leave? Our children will respect us much more for our values, than how much money we might make (or even how much money we might leave them). We have only one opportunity in this life, to prove whom we choose to serve. Hopefully, your choice will be the right one. And don't forget, there is such a thing as repentance, (it's never too late). Pray about your decision if there is any doubt in your mind. Just listen to the spirit, and don't attempt to rationalize. I believe I know what your answer will be.

We must begin a movement, like none in our history; a movement even more aggressive than the pharmaceutical industry's. That means we definitely have our work cut out for us, but **"they absolutely must be stopped"! We need to "Just say no to <u>all drugs</u>", (legal or illegal)!** We must begin by taking back our healthcare system, and our health. For decades, our healthcare system has become totally corrupted by the pharmaceutical giants, with the aid of their tremendous financial resources. As their income continues to increase, our national debt will increase accordingly. The current trend is unsustainable. Due to their insatiable greed, the pharmaceutical giants will be responsible for their own demise. You mark my words, in the not-too-distant future, they will finally be exposed for what they are, and their deception unveiled, for all to see. We as a nation can no longer afford their disease-promoting drugs, sold to the unsuspecting public, for huge profits. They pose a far greater threat to us as a nation than the terrorists we're all so concerned about. Our most serious threat is within, and unfortunately still perfectly legal. Hopefully that will soon change.

CHAPTER NINETEEN

Additional Technical Information – In Simple Terms

This chapter is devoted primarily to discussing in more detail, exactly what I believe is happening, and in as simple terms as possible. It's basically for those (like me) who are curious and always analyzing the details, and attempting to truly understand why a particular drug or supplement might have an influence that a person might possibly experience. I likely tend to question, and at times analyze some things in more detail than the average researcher might. Thus rather than overwhelm some of my readers with the details, (and discourage them from reading the remainder of the book), I chose this approach. Thus they won't miss some valuable information that I cover. I'm basically attempting to isolate, yet include the more technical information, and provide it in this chapter.

As a research scientist, I tend to apply the very same approach to my medical research, as I did years ago, as a computer programmer/analyst developing software, (nothing is impossible). For example, I developed a complex, but extremely efficient operating system that two IBM engineers assigned to the project considered as impossible. It involved an innovative yet unproven approach that had never been attempted before. I designed, and programmed, the software myself, (and did so without any assistance from the IBM engineers). It not only worked, but was thousands of times faster than the traditional approach would have been! That was about 43 years ago, while working as a computer operations supervisor for Boeing, in Huntsville Alabama.

In order to speed up my progress, I basically research the research, constantly looking for new discoveries, uncovered by what I consider some of the most brilliant and dedicated scientists in the world. I then go a step further, and look for explanations, and possible connections. It's quite amazing how many new discoveries are constantly being made. Many doctors and scientists are spending years conducting clinical trials, a service which we all can benefit from. Although, rather than conduct studies as they do, I instead look at their results, which allows me to compile more valuable information faster, (my primary goal).

First I would like to say that in my opinion, **alternative healthcare is basically "light years ahead" of traditional medicine,** which has continually depended on drugs or surgery as the only solution for decades. During a recent survey conducted in 2001, less than 5% of the doctors interviewed were very knowledgeable about alternative therapies, (a major concern). Then as more natural therapies are being discovered on a daily basis, the gap will continue to widen. **We are also beginning to discover just how dangerous and unpredictable the many "FDA approved" drugs really are,** and how little safety our current drug approval process actually provides. I cover this issue in considerable detail in my book, *A Drug-Free Approach To Healthcare*, (now available in a new *Revised Edition, 2007*). I not only discuss the many dangers associated with these drugs, but also the serious nutrient depletion they are responsible for. Most importantly, I explain why **they are seldom (if ever) necessary**, and how easily then can normally be withdrawn from. In my opinion, **they are one of the greatest contributors to poor health in the nation.**

I believe you will find that at least some of the things you are about to learn are actually recent findings that were uncovered by other researchers, as well as some of my own. Thus, you will more than likely encounter some discoveries that even most natural practitioners are yet unaware of. Many don't have the time to devote to research that I do. **I believe that valuable discoveries are basically useless, unless they are shared (my goal), and then applied for the benefit of mankind, (your job).**

Understanding Iodine Receptors In The Brain and The Thyroid Connection

(Additional Technical Information Regarding Chapter 13 "Hypothyroidism")

The fact that iodine concentrates at the highest level in the area of the brain called the basal ganglia, where dopamine is produced, and the area associated with Parkinson's disease, might be a clue to one underlying cause of the uncontrollable Parkinson's-like symptoms that Dr. Glenmullen discusses in his book *Prozac Backlash*. First, he claims that **SSRI antidepressants such as Prozac™ and Paxil™, actually deplete dopamine by over 50%.** Although another potential contributor to the condition could very well be **the disruption of the iodine receptors in the brain, by the fluoride found in Prozac™**, (an issue that, at least to date, I have yet to see addressed).

The obvious question is, what might the function of all those iodine receptors in the brain possibly be? The only logical explanation would be modulating or regulating the action of thyroid hormones in the brain. The number of iodine molecules in the thyroid hormone at any one time, has a great deal of influence on its action, (or lack thereof). For example, the T_3 thyroid hormone is by far the most active form, with the T_4 thyroid being considerably less active, and then we have the T_2 (often referred to as R-T_3, or reverse T_3), which is basically inactive.

So any time there is a high-energy demand in the brain, it would likely utilize more of the active T_3 thyroid. The T_4 could then be useful in moderating the action of T_3, (possibly utilizing a combination of both T_3 and T_4). Then at night, when the brain is much less active, the T_4 would likely be more appropriate. Also, if there happened to be an excess amount of T_3, and a deficiency of T_4 at any one time, the extra molecules of iodine found in the brain could be utilized to convert some T_3 to T_4. And finally, if it was discovered that there was a deficiency of T_3, adding an iodine molecule to the T_2 (or RT_3), could then activate the inactive form, by converting it into T_3, the most active form. If you stop to think about it for a moment, it makes perfect sense.

When I first discovered that the liver sometimes removes an extra iodine molecule, producing the T_2, (or inactive R-T_3, referred to as a reversing hormone), at the time it didn't quite make sense. Although the logical explanation would be that the inactive T_2 (or R-T_3) is just a reserve that the body could draw from by activating it when necessary. That would help explain at least one function of the iodine receptors found throughout the brain.

Evaluating The Iodine / Fluoride Interaction

Then, along came the fluoride molecules found in Prozac™, (actually three molecules of fluoride for every molecule of Prozac™). Fluoride is well known for disrupting the iodine receptors, (not only in the thyroid gland, but also the brain). Yet, that's not the only concern associated with fluoride. Another is fluoride's well-known enzyme suppression, which leads to another problem. Either the addition, or removal, of an iodine molecule in the thyroid hormone, <u>involves enzyme action</u>. Not only that, but we can't forget another problem, the damage to receptors caused by the fluoride in Prozac™. That means that not just the thyroid hormone, but the activity of all hormones in the brain (including serotonin and dopamine) would be reduced accordingly, which could have tremendous implications. And then the effectiveness of the hormone feedback receptors in the hypothalamus would also be reduced, thus the hormone regulation would be less effective as well.

As we gradually assemble the pieces of the puzzle, we can better appreciate the tremendous potential for long-term reduction in normal healthy brain function caused by Prozac™. The overstimulation of elevated serotonin temporarily masks the underlying damage that is slowly taking place. The sooner we intervene, and eliminate the problem (Prozac™), the less potential there will be for serious brain damage, and eventual mental decline, basically leading to lower IQs in our children, as well as the increasing rate of dementia and Alzheimer's disease in adults. We'll now look at some research studies that show how fluoride (found in Prozac™) can easily disrupt this process.

> *1955 – Korrodi, Webmann, Galetti and Held also verify a* ***fluoride – iodine antagonism, presuming that the fluoride ion pushes out the iodine in the thyroid gland.***

> *1960 – Gordinoff and Minder describe the results of experiments with radioactive iodine (I131) which shows that* ***fluorides remove an iodine atom during the conversion process (T4 to T3).*** *Effects are dose-responsive, meaning* ***the higher the fluoride intake the lower the iodine measurements.***

> *1962 – Spira reports on the* ***fluorine-induced endocrine disturbances in mental illness.***

> *1963 – Gorlitzer von Mundy reports on the [then] current knowledge gained from experiements by Gordonoff with I131 as to* ***how the effects of the enzyme responsible for the T4 to T3 conversion were inhibited if a fluorine ion was absorbed before the conversion from T4 to T3 occurs.***

> *1972 – Willems et al. documents that* ***sodium fluoride blocks thyroid hormone.***

> *1991 – Lin Fa-Fu et al. report that a low iodine intake coupled with "high" (0.88ppm) fluoride intake exacerbates the central nervous lesions and the somatic developmental disturbance of iodine deficiency.* ***The authors considered the possibility that "excess" fluoride ion affected normal de-iodination. Fluorides caused increase of reverse T3 (rT3) and elevated TSH levels,*** *as well as increased I131 uptake (see: Bachinskii et al, 1985)* (http://www.bruha.com/pfpc/html/**thryroid**_history.html).

Another factor regarding fluoride that comes into play is, Dr. Cade's discovery that Prozac™ (and thus fluoride) accumulates at surprisingly high levels in the brain, (and can remain there for years)! Thus, one would suspect the likelihood that the brain's metabolism could very well be compromised for years, as well. Does taking Prozac™ appear to you to be a risk worth taking, especially due to its very poor performance record? Then we can't forget Prozac's success in effective nutrient depletion, as well as its outstanding record for creating side effects!

Understanding Pyroluria – An Unsuspecting Possible Cause of ADHD, Bipolar Disorder, and Schizophrenia

(Additional Technical Information That Could Be Applied To Chapter 6 "ADHD", Chapter 16 "The Bipolar Disorder", and Chapter 17 "Schizophrenia")

Pyroluria is a stress-induced mental disorder, that was first connected with psychosis (or a "manic" phase), way back in 1958, and is just one more way Prozac™ can contribute to the bipolar disorder (as it produces the stress hormone). And keep in mind that pregnant women are being placed on Prozac™, as well as being aggressively marketed for children's use under the new TeenScreen, (an obvious drug promotion program).

According to Dr. Carl C. Pfeiffer, Ph.D., M.D., **hyperactivity, compulsiveness, teenage depression, or delinquency,** as well as allergic symptoms, as are all typical with Pyroluria. And then, if you were to see a doctor and complain of "hyperactivity" and then "depression", you would likely be diagnosed with bipolar disorder.

In her book *Depression –Free, Naturally*, (2001), Dr. Joan Mathews Larson, Ph.D. warns that, if you have pyroluria *"you can relapse into an episode of illness when you are severely stressed – from a car accident, the breakup of a marriage, the loss of a loved one, or any major anxiety-creating event"*, and claims that she has seen ***"lab levels of kryptopyrroles double because of such unavoidable stress"*** (p. 155). Incidentally, an elevated level of kryptopyrroles is diagnosed as the condition known as pyroluria.

And if we consider that just one 30 mg dose of Prozac™ increases the "stress hormone cortisol" by 200%, you can easily see how Prozac™ contributes to both the bipolar disorder and pyroluria! While on these drugs, it's as though you are stressed all day, every single day. In fact, even "dehydration is considered as a stress" to the body. Thus, the environmental toxin fluoride, found in Prozac™, is also considered as a stress to the body as well.

It was also found that fully one-third of all psychiatric patients with a diagnosis **"other than schizophrenia"** actually have Pyroluria, (which contributes to a deficiency of both vitamin B_6 and zinc, causing elevated copper). According to Dr. Pfeiffer, the majority of his pyroluric patients responded well to B_6 and zinc, which he refers to as "the missing link". He discovered that many mental ill people are deficient in both B_6 and zinc. Incidentally, both are depleted by Prozac™.

Dr. Pfeiffer also found that pyrolurics (those suffering with Pyroluria) do not metabolize drugs efficiently, and are thus more inclined to experience a drug overdose than others normally would. That is especially a concern with those taking SSRI antidepressants such as Prozac™, Paxil™, and Zoloft™, as they are known to be highly protein binding, and thus very difficult for the liver to metabolize. This would basically compound the problem of the inefficient metabolism of drugs, greatly increasing the risk of drug overdose. Then if a person was also experiencing stress as well, it could easily result in an overdose of the antidepressant itself, and help explain the more serious reactions that some suddenly experience. Your liver is fully aware that these drugs are toxins, and the very same P450 enzyme in the liver that metabolizes and removes alcohol, is attempting to remove the SSRI antidepressants as well.

The Bipolar Disorder and Lithium Carbonate Therapy Hyperparathyroidism – A Possible Dangerous Side Effect

(Additional Technical Information Regarding Chapter 16 "Bipolar Disorder")

Hyperparathyroidism is the overactivity of the parathyroid glands, stimulated by lithium carbonate, and normally treated by surgery, resulting in the removal of all, or part of the parathyroid glands. The question is: If part is removed, then what par, (or how much), of the glands should be removed?

According to a fairly extensive report on lithium, (obtained at http://www.healthyplace.com/medications/lithium.htm), not only is **"hypothyroidism"** and neurogenic **"Diabetes Insipidus"** mentioned as possible conditions caused by taking lithium carbonate, but in addition, **"hyperparathyroidism"** is also included as **one of just three conditions that apparently can persist even after the discontinuation of the lithium therapy.**

This raises some important questions. Do these conditions ever become resolved after lithium therapy is discontinued, or do they become permanent? And if not, how long can they persist, and what is the approximate time frame for resolution? Obviously some important issues.

How Does Lithium Create So Much Chaos In Both The Body & Brain? Answer: By Depleting The Following Important Nutrients

1. Inositol. In the second edition of the *Drug-Induced Nutrient Depletion Handbook* (2001/2001), written by Ross Pelton, R.Ph.D., C.C.N., and three other registered pharmacists, we find that *"although depletion has been noted, routine **replacement of inositol is not recommended** due to a possible relationship to lithium's therapeutic effect"* (p. 167). Apparently, "lithium's therapeutic effect" is something they chose not to discuss, so I'm not sure what the concern might be, or why inositol replacement is not recommended.

Dr. James Balch observes that one important function for which inositol is known for, is assisting in the prevention of several cardiovascular problems, particularly helping remove fats from the liver. He also lists **irritability and mood swings** as two potential problems **related to inositol deficiency**. Once again, it appears that **lithium might be contributing to the very problem it is being prescribed for.** Interestingly, Dr. Balch also notes that *"Research has also shown that **high doses of inositol may help in the treatment of depression, obsessive-compulsive disorder, and anxiety disorders, without the side effects of prescription medications"*** (*Prescription for Nutritional Healing, 3rd edition,* 2000, p. 19). Thus, it's obvious that **the depletion of inositol is a real concern.**

2. Sodium. In the *Drug-Induced Nutrient Depletion Handbook* (2001/2001), although inositol was the only nutrient listed under "Nutrients Depleted", we find that's not really true, as in that very same handbook, in a study titled "Lithium and Sodium Depletion", it was discovered that the administration of lithium carbonate resulted in ***"renal sodium wasting."*** So, although sodium was not listed under "Nutrients Depleted", we find that it actually is depleted as well.

Not only are sodium and potassium necessary for transporting nutrients into the cell, as well as removing toxins from the cell, but an adequate level of sodium is also necessary for maintaining sufficient water levels in the body, (an area in which lithium definitely falls short). And one important function of sodium (salt) is attracting water. If this doesn't happen, **dehydration then follows, resulting histadelia (elevated histamine).**

The rise in blood sugar, one of the severe side effects associated with lithium carbonate, is actually exacerbated by a sodium deficiency. Then, Dr. Batmanghelidj, M.D. states that ***"a deficiency of salt makes it impossible for the body to regulate blood sugar levels,"*** which is at least one reason for the elevated blood sugar associated with lithium. Then, if you are also taking Prozac™, as Mary Lou was, the elevated stress hormone cortisol (caused by Prozac™) contributes to elevated blood sugar as well. **An excessive rise in blood sugar stimulates insulin secretion, often resulting in hypoglycemia, which, like hypothyroidism, also promotes both depression, and mood swings,** which are again the very same symptoms lithium is normally prescribed for.

3. Choline. From another source, we discover that inositol and sodium (salt) are not the only nutrients depleted by lithium, as Eva Edelman suggests otherwise, noting that ***"choline can be depleted in histadelia*** **[elevated histamine]."** Choline plays an important part, as it is the precursor of acetylcholine, a calming neurotransmitter, and one deficiency that lithium indirectly contributes to.

Both choline and inositol have many important functions, including efficient neurotransmitter function, relieving anxiety and depression, and also promoting sleep. Edelman points out that **choline and inositol actually play a role in the absorption of the important minerals calcium, magnesium, manganese, and zinc,** and goes on to explain that:

> ***Choline and inositol nourish and strengthen nerves and brain.*** *They have been used* ***to help relieve anxiety and depression, and promote sleep. Choline is the precursor of acetylcholine, a neurotransmitter essential to memory, nerve/muscle communication, and parasympathetic activity.*** *Choline also helps maintain the myelin sheath which surrounds certain nerve axons. DMAE* [**Di**methyl**a**mino**e**thanol], *a potent form of choline, is reported to sometimes* ***benefit behavior disorders, and frequently be effective in hyperactivity.***
>
> ***Choline can be depleted in histadelia,*** *and* ***supplementation may improve mood.*** *In certain cases,* ***choline may be helpful*** *(once biotype imbalances are reduced)* ***in moderating the racing thoughts and hypomania*** *which can occur in paranoid schizophrenia.* ***Inositol is reported to have a mild sedative action and be useful in promoting sleep and reducing anxiety*** (*Natural Healing for Schizophrenia*, 1996/1998, p. 31).

So as we can see, **anything such as lithium carbonate that can lead to the depletion of choline, could actually contribute to hypomania – again, what lithium is normally prescribed to prevent.**

4. Calcium. As you are about to learn, there is also the potential for calcium depletion, and only by researching multiple sources, looking for answers, and evaluating the interrelation between different nutrients, (which I have done here for you), can we fully recognize the tremendous influence that a drug such as lithium carbonate can have on the body and brain.

For example, as we previously discussed, **lithium carbonate can cause hyperparathyroidism,** (and is just one condition that can actually persist even after lithium therapy is discontinued). If we dig a little deeper, we find that **the "parathormone" hormone is produced by the parathyroid glands, and is responsible for the distribution of calcium and phosphate in the body. Thus, hyperparathyroidism would be the overactivity of the parathyroid, (and overproduction of the parathormone hormone).**

Then we find in the *Bantam Medical Dictionary, 3rd edition* (1981/2000), that ***"a high level of the* [parathormone] *hormone causes transfer of calcium from the bones to the blood"*** (p. 240). The first, and most obvious conclusion is: **The onset of calcium depletion of the bones would lead to osteoporosis.**

Another concern, stressed by Dr. James Balch (*Prescription for Nutritional Healing, 3rd edition,* 2000) is that ***"a proper balance of magnesium, calcium, and phosphorus should be maintained at all times"*** (p. 31). He then explains that ***"Excessive amounts of phosphorus interferes with calcium uptake."*** This brings to light the importance of vitamin K supplementation, as it would likely reduce some of the problems associated with elevated levels of calcium in the bloodstream, due to an overactive parathyroid hormone, potentially resulting from lithium therapy.

An adequate level of vitamin K is also important for maintaining the integrity, and permeability, of the critical blood-brain barrier). Its function, whether preventing unwanted toxins, or just the opposite, by allowing the many nutrients necessary for healthy brain function to penetrate, is extremely important.

It has been proven that **vitamin K deficiency increases with age,** and according to Dr. Richard Wood, Ph.D., a researcher at Tufts University in Boston, ***"Poor vitamin K status has been found to triple the risk of severe vascular calcification"*** (*Life Extension* magazine, February 2003, p. 86). Thus, **a deficiency of vitamin K, combined with an excessive level of calcium in the blood, could be a serious combination,** and as Dr. Wood points out, especially in light of **vitamin K's ability to *"reduce neuronal damage*** *by protecting the vascular system, guarding against inflammation and* ***blocking excess calcium into brain cells."*** Dr. Wood notes that ***"Vitamin K is also involved in regulating important brain enzymes and growth factors."***

Not only does the lithium carbonate create several deficiencies, (some obvious and others not so obvious, at least initially), but as we can see, we also have another concern. The high level of calcium in the bloodstream, caused by lithium, can be potentially serious unless an adequate level of vitamin K is also present. Thus, it's also creating an increased demand for vitamin K, which many are already deficient in.

Then, anything that can compromise the integrity of the blood-brain barrier is a major concern, as would the influx of excess calcium into the brain cells be.

We're not only increasing the risk for serious brain damage, but also osteoporosis and vascular calcification. Then as we are about to discuss, we're also facing another problem, due to the mineral imbalance caused by the excessive calcium in the bloodstream. I might add that many, placed on lithium carbonate, are left on Prozac™ as well, (which incidentally was true in Mary Lou's case). And we can't forget that **Prozac™ depletes a total of "sixteen nutrients", including the critical minerals magnesium and zinc, discussed next,** (although their deficiency can also result from an elevated level of calcium in the blood stream).

5. Magnesium. You are about to learn another factor resulting from elevated calcium in the blood, which might be of even greater concern. According to Dr. Balch, ***"excessive calcium levels would interfere with the absorption of the two critical minerals: magnesium and zinc"*** (*Prescription for Nutritional Healing, 3rd edition,* 2000, pp. 25-26). Many potential problems could easily result from a deficiency of either one or both of these two very important minerals.

According to Edelman **magnesium is:**

> ***Calming to the nervous system.*** *In a study of 165 boys,* ***those with schizophrenia, depression, autism or sleep disturbances had low levels of magnesium.*** *In other studies,* ***psychiatric patients who tried to commit suicide were also found to have depressed levels****. Magnesium affects cell membrane permeability, helps maintain cellular electrical potential, and supports formation of tyrosine.* ***A deficiency may produce*** *apathy,* ***agitation, irritability, personality changes****, disorientation, bizarre movements,* ***sleep disturbances, depression*** *and, in some cases, hallucinations* (*Natural Healing for Schizophrenia,* 1996/1998), p. 35).

Also, according to Dr. Balch (*Prescription for Nutritional Healing, 3rd edition,* 2000), **magnesium aids in *"maintaining the body's proper pH balance and normal body temperature,"*** and he adds that *"some possible manifestations of magnesium deficiency include poor digestion, rapid heartbeat,* ***chronic fatigue****,* ***seizures****, and* ***tantrums; often a magnesium deficiency can be synonymous with diabetes****.* ***Magnesium deficiencies are at the root of many cardiovascular problems****"* (p. 30).

Dr. Balch also stresses that ***"a low magnesium level makes nearly every disease worse."*** Thus, as we can easily see, a magnesium deficiency definitely has widespread implications.

6. Zinc. As with magnesium, an elevated blood level of calcium also interferes with the absorption of zinc, thus elevated copper levels. Eva Edelman stresses the many benefits of zinc, as follows:

> ***Zinc is abundant in the brain hippocampus and may function as a neurotransmitter. It is needed in neuron development neurotransmitter synthesis, and copper chelation. Zinc also enhances resistance to stress; and helps maintain intellectual function, memory, and level moods. Deficiency can lead to*** *headaches, lethargy, amnesia, other* ***memory impairment, irritability, behavior disorders,*** *and* ***paranoia. Zinc is used in treating histamine imbalances, pyroluria, and blood sugar disorders*** (*Natural Healing for Schizophrenia,* 1996/1998, p. 34).

Another important function of zinc is counter-acting some important excitotoxins. According to neurologists John Olney and Russell Blaylock, **when certain chemicals exceed critical levels, they can overexcite brain neurons, causing nerve cell death** (*Natural Healing for Schizophrenia,* Edelman, 1996/1998, p. 145).

Some other uses for zinc are blood pressure moderation, protein and **fatty acid synthesis, insulin storage, thyroid functioning,** and thiamin, phosphorus and **protein**

metabolism. You might notice that **a zinc deficiency actually contributes to many of the same conditions that lithium is responsible for creating, (i.e. behavior disorders, histamine imbalances, Pyroluria, and blood sugar disorders).** This might possibly be due to the fact that **a zinc deficiency naturally produces elevated copper levels,** which **cause pyroluria, depression, obsession, compulsiveness, and contributes to the bipolar disorder!**

Considering that according to Eva Edelman, ***"It is unknown whether lithium is needed or contraindicated for humans, much less, what daily intake should be,"*** and that ***"Rosenblatt believes lithium may act as a substitute for sodium,"*** and that ***"Snyder warns that lithium might disrupt critical sodium balances"*** (p. 155), one can't help but question the reasoning behind the conclusion that inorganic lithium therapy should even be considered, especially in light of the serious side effects associated with its use. As usual, there are much better options available.

Additional Information Regarding The Connection Between Elevated Homocysteine and Depression

(Additional Technical Information Regarding Chapter 15 "Depression")

Let's first take a look at the part Prozac™ plays, and exactly how it contributes to elevated homocysteine. Quite simply, the primary problem is the nutrient depletion that Prozac™ is so proficient at. Of the sixteen nutrients Prozac™ depletes, three in particular (folic acid, vitamin B_6, and vitamin B_{12}), in adequate supply will prevent elevated homocysteine. Through a process called methylation, these three B vitamins convert homocysteine into one of two beneficial amino acids (methionine, or cysteine). Then, through additional methylation, (also requiring enzyme action), the body can convert the amino acid methionine, along with the energy molecule ATP, into SAMe, which incidentally does an excellent job of "preventing depression"! This is just one more example of how Prozac™ can actually contribute to depression, (which we discussed earlier in the chapter on Depression). I'll just mention here that SAMe is available as a natural supplement (it's not a drug), and in my opinion, and that of other doctors, SAMe is totally side effect-free, and "much more effective" than any antidepressant on the market.

If you're getting a sufficient supply of B vitamins (not available in some cheap Once-A-Day vitamin-mineral pill), and not taking medications that are responsible for depleting them, your body should eventually be able to create its own SAMe. The greatest contributors to depression appear to be a nutritional deficiency, or a low thyroid condition, (especially common with women). Doctor Kilmer McKulley, M.D. discovered, more than 30 years ago, that elevated homocysteine (rather than cholesterol) was the major contributor to cardiovascular disease. When he decided to publish his findings, he soon lost his funding, and his job. So what prompted his demise, you might ask? There's a lot of money in cholesterol lowering drugs, called statins, (which in my opinion no one really needs), yet elevated homocysteine can only be controlled by vitamins, something pharmaceutical companies are fully aware of, but would rather you remain in the dark about, (and an area they made sure your doctor wasn't trained in). Incidentally, one common cause of excessively elevated cholesterol is again "a low thyroid condition", which as we just learned, Prozac™ contributes to. Interestingly, in one study conducted in 2001 on 2,000 individuals, it was discovered that ***"About two-thirds of those diagnosed with hypothyroidism* [low thyroid] *had cholesterol levels nearly 4 times higher than normal"*** (*Life Extension Foundation's Disease Prevention and Treatment, expanded fourth edition,* 1997/2003, p. 414). It's difficult to avoid discussing the thyroid, as it's so intricately involved in so many different processes in the body, and there are so many things that can influence the thyroid, (either directly or indirectly).

Although we learned that homocysteine is a major contributor to cardiovascular disease decades ago, thanks to Dr. McKulley, we now have some more recent findings that identify some other conditions that are associated with elevated homocysteine. I might add that, although our body is continually producing homocysteine, it only becomes elevated when there's a deficiency of the vitamins necessary for converting it via methylation, to the beneficial amino acids.

Researchers also determined that **about 90% of those in the U.S. who were hypothyroid (low thyroid), had either elevated homocysteine or cholesterol,** contrary to 31% who had normal thyroid. As I mentioned earlier, it's quite amazing how many things are influenced by proper thyroid function. Although we're supposed to be back on the subject of homocysteine, it appears that we're also back on the subject of the thyroid! One possible explanation is the methylation process involved in converting homocysteine into one of the two beneficial amino acids, methionine, or cysteine, requires enzyme action. Then, Dr. E. Denis Wilson, M.D. discovered that with a lower body temperature (hypothyroid condition) the action of all enzymes is greatly reduced, and there are about 3,000 enzymes in the body that are influenced. Then the fluoride in Prozac™ actually adds to the problem, as it's known to reduce the action of enzymes as well. Aren't drugs fascinating? You can now begin to better understand why so few adults in the nation actually experience optimum health.

While the primary focus of homocysteine's influence has been on its contribution to cardiovascular disease by thickening and thus stiffening the vascular wall (arteries and capillaries), and increasing the incidence of blood clot formation, there is much more to the story. For example, it was discovered that ***"individuals suffering with Alzheimer's disease, depression,*** *eye problems,* ***liver damage, Crohn's disease, ulcerative colitis, irritable bowel disease,*** *pernicious anemia, and Parkinson's disease* ***often present with elevated homocysteine levels"*** (*Life Extension Foundation's Disease Prevention and Treatment, expanded fourth edition,* 1997/2003, p. 421). **Yet elevated homocysteine is something most doctors have continued to ignore, even decades after its discovery by Dr. McKulley!** Then if you consider that such a broad range of conditions appear to be related to elevated homocysteine regarding adults, **could you possibly imagine the potential for damage to the developing fetus?** Let's just focus on some of the more important ones for a moment.

We'll begin with those that might normally be considered as the least likely to be associated with depression, (although you'll find that's not actually true). They just happen to be the intestinal disorders (**Crohn's disease, ulcerative colitis, and irritable bowel disease**). What's the connection, you might ask? Would you believe that **at least 90% of the serotonin that Prozac™ is targeting, (but can't actually produce), just happens to be produced in the intestinal tract? Any unhealthy intestinal condition will reduce the efficiency of serotonin production.** So it's obviously important to maintain a healthy intestinal tract, and avoid elevated homocysteine.

Then we come to another unlikely suspect, pernicious anemia. Two major contributors are a vitamin B_{12} deficiency, (if you recall, one vitamin that Prozac depletes), and the other is a low thyroid, which both Prozac™ and elevated homocysteine contribute to. Not only does a low thyroid condition (and thus lower body temperature) reduce the efficiency of the 3,000 enzyme actions in the body, but there's another concern. **When the body temperature is lower, (a hypothyroid condition), the bones are colder as well, which reduces their efficiency regarding their production of red blood cells, contributing to anemia.** Looks like we're back to the thyroid again. As you can see, it plays a vital role regarding our overall health, (both physical and mental), or lack thereof.

Anemia not only contributes to fatigue, but also cancer. **The more anemic you are, the less efficient the oxygen delivery to the cells.** Then, anything that can damage the liver is a major concern, (especially when taking antidepressants). Other than the brain, the heart and the liver are two of the three most important organs in the body. You can't possibly be healthy if your liver is in any way compromised, due to the many critical functions it's responsible for. And regarding the brain, according to author Eva Edelman, in her book *Natural Healing for Schizophrenia*, **homocysteine damages the neurons in the brain**. **Then, it's found that most people with Alzheimer's disease not only have elevated homocysteine, but also low levels of vitamin B_{12} and folic acid. As we learned, Prozac™ actually contributes to elevated homocysteine, as well as a deficiency in both vitamins! And Prozac™ contributes to Alzheimer's disease, as well as diabetes and cancer, (a rather risky drug, to say the least)!**

Now we'll see how elevated homocysteine contributes to another condition on our list, "depression," which it all started with.

Scientists claim that ***"a clear association exists between elevated homocysteine and major depression"*** (*Life Extension Foundation's Disease Prevention and Treatment, expanded fourth edition,* 1997/2003, p. 626). They also note that **those with a folic acid deficiency had decreased synthesis of both "serotonin and dopamine," which obviously would contribute to major depression. They also indicate that either a folic acid or B_{12} deficiency can cause severe depression** (*Life Extension Foundation's Disease Prevention and Treatment, expanded fourth edition,* 1997/2003, p. 635). And of course, a deficiency of either would contribute to elevated homocysteine, and again, Prozac™ is a contributor to all three. Then as we just learned, all three could contribute to Alzheimer's disease as well. **It's a rather vicious cycle that begins and ends with Prozac™.**

It's quite amazing when you consider how many different problems are related to elevated homocysteine, yet many doctors seem to be totally oblivious to the fact. Thus their patients often are, as well, (at least you now know). Although I have been fully aware of the concern of elevated homocysteine for decades, even I was surprised at how extensive the damage to both the body and brain that homocysteine can potentially create, as many of the findings are more recent. And due to the damage to the arteries feeding the brain, (especially the carotid arteries), that could also contribute to Alzheimer's disease, due to the reduced circulation supplying nutrients and oxygen to the brain. And don't forget, the thyroid plays an important part in the metabolism of not only the entire body, but also the brain. It plays a major role in the energy process and the efficiency of all enzyme actions. Thus, efficient thyroid function (optimum metabolism) is critical to optimum heath and brain function.

INDEX

A

B

C

D

E

F

G

H

L

M

N

O

P

Q

R

S

T

V

W

X

Y

Z

Alternative Healthcare Professionals

- **Alternative Medicine Connection Directory of Practitioners**
  MedSearch claims to be *"The World's most complete directory of holistic practitioners, currently hosting well over 10,000 records and expanding every day."*
  For a practitioner nearest you, see their Website:
  http://www.arxc.com/medsearch.htm

- **American Board of Holistic Medicine**
  For a roster of board certified physicians, see their Website:
  http://holisticboard.org/roster.html

- **American College for Advancement in Medicine (ACAM)**
  For a list of natural practitioners in your area call:
  (888) 439-6891
  http://www.acam.org

- **American Holistic Health Association (AHHA)**
  Searchable database of over 270 AHHA Practitioners Members who work in partnership with their patients, and encourage a holistic approach to wellness.
  For a healthcare practitioner nearest you, see their Website:
  http://ahha.org/ahhasearch.asp

- **American Holistic Health Association (AHHA) Healing Centers in North America**
  For a list multidisciplinary health care centers, affiliated with the AHHA, that are integrating alternative therapies and conventional medicine or exclusively offering alternative therapies, see their Website:
  http://ahha.org/ahhainstit.htm

- **International Guide to the World of Alternative Mental Health**
  To find an alternative mental health practitioner nearest you, see their Website:
  http://www.alternativementalhealth.com/directory/search.asp

- **Dr. Jonathan Wright / Tahoma Clinic**
  801 SW 16th
  Renton, WA 98055
  (425) 264-0059
  http://www.tahoma-clinic.com/

- **Dr. Julian Whitaker / Whitaker Wellness Center**
  4321 Birch Street
  Newport Beach, CA 92660
  (800) 488-1500
  http://www.whitakerwellness.com/